Nutrition in Action

Nutrition in Action

ETHEL AUSTIN MARTIN

HOLT, RINEHART AND WINSTON

New York — Chicago — San Francisco — Toronto — London

Library of Congress Catalog Card Number: 63-11912

25476-0113

Printed in the United States of America

PREFACE

Nutrition in Action is planned primarily as a text for the growing number of university courses in nutrition and health that are offered for majors in such areas as elementary education, nursing, health and physical education, and social service. It has two main objectives:

> To provide a background in nutrition subject matter for students who may not have specific science requirements.
>
> To interpret nutrition to such students in terms of their own well-being, and, in a more general way, the nutritional welfare of those they may serve.

Such a course does not seek to turn out "experts" in the field of nutrition. It does try to give a down-to-earth, functional knowledge of the subject, and some appreciation of the student's eventual niche in nutrition education. Emphasis in the text is placed on the nutritional needs of the average normal adult, as representative of the student or young person in professional life. This is done in the belief that once he, himself, is "sold" on the importance of nutrition, he is ready to make nutrition important to others.

The text is planned for use in a variety of classroom situations where greater or lesser emphasis is placed on nutrition. Its use can be extended as the time, the interests, and the backgrounds of the students permit. Broadened use has been provided for by documenting main topics in each chapter with selected references and by listing additional readings of a more general character. Both references and readings furnish further bibliographical material on the subjects discussed.

Brevity in the text has been necessary because of the limited time usually devoted to courses for which it is intended. The aim has been to be brief without being superficial, and to simplify explanations without implying that nutrition itself is a simple science. If students are to develop a real interest in the subject and gain some confidence in its application, they must do more than "skim the surface." They must know the basic principles of nutrition and be given the tools necessary to discover for themselves how these principles "work."

In an effort to condense the text and make it more readable, the names and titles of scientists whose research is reported and the institutions they represent have been omitted in most cases. This information is provided in the books, articles, and pamphlets cited in the text and listed at the end of each chapter. Scientific terms have been used for the most part without accompanying explanation. Where unfamiliar terms are not defined in modern collegiate dictionaries, a brief, parenthetical explanation has been included at the point of use.

Nutrition in Action is considered under three main divisions: Section One, background understandings of food and food habits in relation to nutrition; Section Two, basic nutrition subject matter; Section Three, practical interpretation of nutrition information in terms of daily meals.

For those concerned with teaching children, a fourth section is provided as a separate volume under the title, *Nutrition Education in Action—A Guide for Teachers.* It introduces teachers and prospective teachers to some of the acceptable ways of implementing nutrition education in the elementary school program. This *Guide* is designed for use with the present text in courses for students of elementary education and for inservice teaching programs, such as workshops, refresher courses, extension lectures, home-study series, and small study groups. The text and *Guide* offer suitable reference material for curriculum supervisors, home economics teachers, health educators, school nurses, lunchroom supervisors, and all others who cooperate in the school health program.

Many persons served in many ways to make this project a reality. Some prodded me to attempt the task; others contributed ideas and counsel during its development. Only a few can be named. Mary Alice Banks, Mary Reeves, and Mary Alice Tarulli gave encouragement and aid from the beginning. Mary Rich, Marie Balsley, Margaret Dunham, and Fannie Lee Boyd read portions of the manuscript. Lydia J. Roberts and E. Neige Todhunter read the manuscripts for the text and *Guide* in their entirety. All left their individual imprints on the material. D. Laurel Bocobo supplied food guides from other nations. The National Dairy Council, through its staff and its library, graciously gave continuous assistance. Edward M. Martin provided at all times that indefinable ingredient called moral support, which is essential in any undertaking. To these and to the many others who gave generously of their time and talents, the author extends thanks.

CONTENTS

FIGURES AND TABLES

Figures

Figures

Figures

Tables

Tables

Tables

Nutrition in Action

SECTION ONE

Nutrition begins with food

Nutrition *does* begin with food, but it is *more* than food. It is the food itself plus all the things that happen to it from the time it is eaten until it actually nourishes the body. Nutrition is really a *process* in which food is digested and its nutrients are absorbed and finally distributed to the parts of the body where they are utilized in all metabolic activities. This process may be entirely successful, or it may be faulty in varying degrees at different points. The faults may consist of too little, too much, or the wrong kinds of food; or there may be functional failure in any of the steps through which food passes before it is ready for body use.

Food goes beyond its purely physical functions. It is said to be essential for "the spirit" as well as the body. Food is associated with every human emotion. For the individual it may symbolize joy or sorrow, comfort or fear, security or conflict. As these psychological factors operate, they may affect the amounts and kinds of foods one eats and how well the body utilizes food for its own nourishment.

The outcome of such physical and emotional processes—the product of them—is the individual himself. How well he is nourished depends on how well these physical and emotional factors function. His level of nourishment is referred to as his *nutritional status* or his *nutriture.* A person may be described, roughly, as being in *good* or *poor* nutritional status or nutriture. His nutritional status is an essential aspect of his total health, which implies not only freedom from disease, but physical, mental, and emotional fitness as well.

Food itself is the most important factor in the concept of nourishment. Therefore, the foods people eat and the ways they respond to different patterns of eating offer a logical point to start a study of nutrition.

CHAPTER 1

Your food habits and what they mean

The food habits of a nation determine in large measure the nutritional level and health of its people. Both kinds and amounts of food are involved. If people do not have enough to eat, they will obviously be hungry and poorly nourished. But abundance of food in itself does not guarantee that they will be *well* nourished. Even when the food supply is plentiful and varied, they may suffer from "hunger" of a different sort if they choose the wrong kinds of food or if they eat more food than they need.

Whether their food supplies are limited or abundant, people everywhere tend to develop patterns of eating. These patterns settle into fixed habits. Eventually, they may characterize national eating practices. Ultimately, the food habits of a country—good or poor—furnish presumptive evidence of the nutritional status of its population. Recognizing patterns of eating and appreciating their significance, therefore, provides a base line for approaching nutrition and the processes involved in nutrition education. And since the food habits of an individual tend to reflect those of his group, we propose to explore with you first some of the more obvious influences that may affect individual eating patterns, including your own.

» EATING PATTERNS

Everyone eats certain foods and refuses other foods for many different reasons. Often these reasons have little to do with the foods themselves. Favorite foods, for example, may be traced to childhood memories of happy family meals or special gatherings with relatives and friends. Perhaps your favorite fried chicken now was a Sunday dinner specialty when everyone was at home; you may associate chocolate cake with your birthday, when you received gifts; you may identify homemade bread with your memory of a warm kitchen filled with the aroma of baking bread on a winter afternoon; or you may enjoy sandwiches grilled on an outdoor fire because you connect them with the fun of picnics and the smell of a wood fire. Foods unavailable to you as a child may also affect your food habits. Do you have a special fondness for beef steak now because at one time the family could not afford it? Have you learned to eat so-called "status" foods, such as wild rice or artichokes, because your affluent friends do so? Probing along these lines can give you a new conception of your own food habits.

Rejected Foods

A pattern of eating reflects the foods refused as well as those accepted. As food habits are acquired, negative as well as positive influences are operating. They are usually the opposite of those mentioned above, i.e., unpleasant associations with family, friends, and events. You may reject stew now because it was always served on wash day, when your mother was cross and you felt neglected; you may avoid baked beans because you had them on the days your mother cleaned house, when your room was upset and your routine was disturbed; or you may leave alone any of the foods that made you sick because you ate too much of them.

Negative influences are also linked with the very character of foods themselves. For example, you may refuse liver because it was always "leathery"; orange juice because it was used to help cod-liver oil go down; or spinach because it was stringy and hard to eat. Ways of eating, based on experiences of a lifetime, help to make up food habit patterns. Their exploration makes a fascinating study.

► *As a means of focusing attention on your own food habits, keep a record of the foods you eat for a period of three days.*[1]

Choose days that are representative of your normal eating pattern. When the record is completed, classify the major items as follows: your favorite foods; those foods which you have learned to like and take some pleasure in eating; those which you merely tolerate; and finally, list some of the foods that do not appear on your meal record because you "never touch them." Make a serious effort to account for your attitude toward the foods in each category.

The analysis of any one food record will suggest some of the factors involved in forming food habits. A compilation from the class should bring forth many of the more apparent reasons why people eat or refuse to eat foods. Underlying factors in food-habit formation may not come to light in such a survey. True origins in some cases may lie far beyond the memory or knowledge of class members. A brief examination of some of the roots from which food habits develop will show how deep such roots may lie.

Deeper Meanings of Food

Food habits obviously do not spring full-blown. They are gradually developed from infancy through childhood by the types of experiences cited and by others—some favorable, some unfavorable. Eating habits, in effect, are merely the symbols of these influences and experiences. They are the outcome of multiple factors that operate singly and together.

Basic influences in food habit formation include the following:

Food Supply—the quantity and kind of food available to a population from all sources are the basic ingredient of eating patterns.

Economic Welfare of the People—the ability of individuals and families to afford the foods that are available controls the amounts and kinds to be eaten.

Family Eating Practices—family meal customs may be deeply rooted in racial, religious, and national practices, or in family beliefs and habits developed over generations.

Social Customs—attitudes and practices of peoples with respect to eating

---

[1] See Appendix A for the form and method of keeping your meal record. As this record is to be the basis for other class activities, suggestions for keeping the record should be followed carefully.

with friends, with social groups, or even with strangers may be based on ancient customs, or on racial or religious rites.

Emotional Climates—situations that generate pleasure, annoyance, or frustration with respect to foods may be responsible for favorable or unfavorable attitudes toward food and eating.

Sensory Reactions—individual variations in response to the taste of foods.

Educational Influences—knowledge of food values may provide the basis for judgment in selecting foods.

These basic influences form the background against which the food habits of the people of any country develop. They provide the framework for the culture in which eating practices of families and neighbors gradually become those of the individual. The individual absorbs these habits as his own, and through the ideas associated with them, he sees and interprets all his experiences with food and eating. Food habits are particularly static when cultures are old and tradition rules the way of life, when people live together in closely integrated units, and when food supplies have been limited for generations to a few staple items. Under such circumstances, people literally go hungry rather than fly in the face of tradition by eating foods not specifically prescribed by their pattern of eating.

To understand such deep convictions one must know their sources. The situation in one South African community serves as an example[1].[2] Health conditions in the tribe were poor. The tribal diet, which was grossly inadequate in several respects, contained only negligible amounts of milk. Milk was associated with a deep-seated custom that dictated that only members of the kin group of the head of a household could use milk produced by that man's herd. This restriction applied to all members of the household, but for women and the older girls the situation was more complicated. During her menses or when pregnant, a woman was thought to exert an evil influence on cattle and was not allowed to go near the herd or to use milk. When a girl married and went to her husband's family, she was further separated from the only milk supply for which she was eligible. The practical outcome was that women used no milk.

The origin of this custom had long since been forgotten. Not even the oldest members of the tribe could recall the basis for it. It undoubtedly stemmed from native religious beliefs centered around ancestors. Cattle were the link between man and his ancestors. Any possible evil influence in this relationship became a powerful taboo. Therefore, although the exact origin of the custom was lost, the custom itself remained intact. Professional advice that milk was needed by women for health reasons, particularly during pregnancy and lactation, fell on deaf ears. The habit, a relic of the past, remained unchanged.

The United States is generally regarded as a melting pot of races and cultures with no distinctive food habit pattern of its own. The variety and abundance of its food supply, the people of mixed racial origins who comprise the population, and its vast geographical area, would seem to support this view. But the very size of the country creates the conditions that give rise to subcultures and regional food habit patterns. Certain geographic regions, for example, have well-known, characteristic eating patterns: Boston baked beans, clam chowder, and pie for breakfast are food customs associated with New England; fried chicken,

[2] Numbers within brackets are keyed to the numbered references at the conclusion of each chapter.

turnip greens, and hot biscuits are part of the traditional meal pattern of the South. Racial, national, and religious groups have retained some of their food practices for generations. These groups include the Pennsylvania Dutch, the Seventh Day Adventists, and the orthodox Jews. Food customs of the types represented have many origins. They have come to be inseparably linked with the lives and living of those who practice them. And they are not easily changed!

Food Habit Origins in the United States

The most distinctive food patterns are those of persons who have recently migrated to this country. Often nationality groups colonize in certain areas and retain their native eating customs practically intact. The longer they stay in this country and the more outside influences creep in, the more is their original diet subject to change. They learn gradually to like and to use foods of their adopted country. This is to be expected. The remarkable fact is that they retain as much as they do of their native foods and eating customs. The history of food habits in this country is the story of how the hard core of such customs is handed down through generations [2]. Like the African food habits, their origins may be lost, but their foothold in the regions where they are practiced remains strong.

The so-called "historic core" of the "old German" diet in this country is characterized by such foods as heavy soups, sausages, boiled potatoes, rye bread, foods made from barley, and pickled pigs feet [2]. These foods are used now by people of all nationalities, but it is largely those of German descent who have retained them as a regular part of their eating pattern. This is true of families that have been in this country for several generations and have been exposed constantly to other foods and meal customs.

The tenacity with which *Italian-Americans* cling to their native diet is legendary [2]. They may add foods new to them, but the core of the diet always symbolizes the homeland. The day's meals listed here could be considered typical in many homes of second- and third-generation Italian families [3].

The Italian bread, the minestrone soup, and the pasta are clearly the Italian dishes in these meals. The fried peppers, the tossed greens, and the fruit at every meal are also suggestive of Italian influence. The Italian diet often follows a cycle of foods to be served on specified days. The traditional spaghetti and tomato sauce is generally eaten twice a week, usually on Thursdays and

Breakfast	Lunch	Dinner
Seasonable fruit	Minestrone soup with grated cheese	Pasta fogiali with grated cheese
Italian bread	Italian bread	Italian bread
Egg if desired (never cereal)	Fruit	Fried peppers or broccoli
Coffee with milk	Milk for preschool children	Tossed greens with tomato, oil and vinegar dressing
	Coffee for adults	(Veal steak, sometimes)
	Soft drink for school-age children and women	Seasonable fruit
		Milk for preschool children
		Coffee for adults
		Soft drink for school-age children and women

Sundays. Native Italian food habits, transplanted to this country, thus follow a carefully laid-out plan. In city centers where Italians settle, neighborhood stores stock the native foods; children of Italian parents learn to eat and enjoy them at home. The features of the native eating pattern are thereby perpetuated.

People from *Spanish-speaking* countries coming to this country also have well-defined and distinctive food habits that resist change. Mexican families, for example, who have been in the United States as long as 6 years, often continue to use tortillas as bread at each meal. Sample meals of a 3-year-old child in such a family are given below [3].

Children and adults eat essentially the same foods except for milk, which the children drink, until they enter school; then they change to coffee. Adults take no milk, but drink coffee at each meal. At lunch, other foods are often placed *in* the tortillas and eaten as sandwiches or "tacos." Food is fried in lard and little butter or margarine is used.

When Mexican families are housed together with little outside contact, they cling more closely to their native diet than would be suggested by the menus below. This has been demonstrated with children of Spanish-speaking migrant workers. These children travel with their parents and live with them in temporary colonies while they follow the crops. The rigidity of their food pattern was demonstrated in Colorado, where an attempt was made to adapt the school lunch to their needs. Their diet at home consisted largely of tortillas and frijoles, supplemented with candy and soft drinks. They often refused even to taste dishes in the school lunch that did not fall within their limited range of acceptable foods. They preferred to go hungry, rather than eat a lunch they did not like.

► *Obtain a typical day's menus of an individual or family that are quite different from your own menu. Try to identify religious, national, racial, or other influences in these menus.*

Food habit patterns in this country have been discussed here briefly to suggest that there are more different patterns than most people realize; that many of these patterns are deeply entrenched, with long histories of family, national, and racial practices; and that an awareness of habit backgrounds and the need for analyzing them in terms of possible educational approaches is the first step in habit improvement.

Cutting across all food habit patterns, regardless of origin or locale, are personal preferences for individual foods and food groups within the patterns. When likes and dislikes for certain foods are strong enough to influence meal selection, they may seriously distort the original eating pattern. Individual food preferences may therefore be an important factor in determining the nutritional adequacy of the diet.

Variations in Food Preferences

The food preferences of a considerable number of men and women, boys and girls, in this country have been obtained by interview, observation, questionnaire, and food

Breakfast	Lunch	Dinner	Between meals
Orange	Fried rice	Meat and bean stew	Crackers
Oatmeal with milk	Refried pinto beans	Fried potatoes	Milk (sometimes)
Fried egg	Milk	Milk	
Tortilla	Tortilla	Tortilla	

check list. They indicate attitudes toward main groupings of foods and toward specific foods—those widely accepted and those rather universally rejected. A few highlights of several of these studies are summarized here.

Vegetables—particularly cooked vegetables—are the most unpopular food group. Strong-juice vegetables, especially those green or yellow in color, are more disliked than others. "Greens," parsnips, cabbage, carrots, and rutabagas are frequently on the rejected lists. Unfamiliarity with a vegetable, rather than dislike for it, is often given as the reason for rejection.

The attitude of the majority of individuals toward most of the other food groups is, on the whole, favorable. Milk, meats, fruits, most cereals and breads, a few vegetables and almost all desserts usually rank high on the lists of liked foods. There are 2 chief drawbacks to the full use of these food groups. First, dislike of certain items *within* food groups, which limits selection. For example, beef and chicken are popular among meats, but organ meats are almost universally rejected; fish and lamb are rejected by many. Second, the use of nutritionally important foods in too small quantities. Most persons profess a favorable attitude toward citrus foods and milk, for example, but use them in less than recommended amounts.

Food Preferences by Age [4,5,6] In studies that permit comparisons of food preferences by age, a few findings stand out: Health aspects of food have greater appeal for middle-aged persons than they do for boys and girls; flavor of foods, on the other hand, appeals more to the young than to the older group. Strong taste is more acceptable to older children than to younger ones.

With respect to individual foods, milk is preferred and used more by the young than by the old. Children in upper grades showed less preference for milk than did those in lower grades; and nearly 60 percent of the latter took 2 cups of milk daily, but only 20 percent of the middle-aged adult group used that amount. The situation is reversed with eggs. Older people show a higher preference for them than do children.

Meats, with the exception of organ meats, lamb, and fish, are popular with both old and young. Preferences in the young run to frankfurters, luncheon meats, and bologna. At each age studied, vegetables as a group were declared to be the least preferred.

Food Preferences by Sex [4,5,6,7,8] There appears to be little sex difference in children's preferences for foods below about the tenth year. In older children sex differences become important. In one study, girls registered more dislikes for foods than did boys from the fifth grade through high school, except for the eighth grade, which brought the largest number of dislikes from both boys and girls. Women have more dislikes than men.

More boys than girls accept milk and dairy foods. More college men than women select milk in college dining halls. In older adult groups the ratio is similar; more men like and choose milk than do women.

There is also a sex difference in attitudes toward vegetables, although they are unpopular with both sexes. More boys will accept green and yellow vegetables than girls; strong-juice vegetables are more acceptable to boys than girls; and more boys than girls are "willing to eat" cooked cabbage and "greens." College women, on the other hand, rate vegetables higher than men do, and favor salads in particular. Homemakers list vegetables as the most disliked (by their families) of the food groups, but women personally favor the *use* of vegetables more than men do. It is likely that the positive effect of serving vegetables at the family table is offset, in terms of the children's acceptance of them, by the parents' own dislike for vegetables.

The negative attitude toward vegetables revealed in the studies reported here points to the need for children to learn early to know and like a wide variety of common vegetables. The attitudes of teachers and parents, particularly fathers, toward all foods, are major influences in creating children's preferences. Tasting lessons at school can help children to know favorably and to like many foods, including vegetables. But such programs must, in some way, reach parents as well as children if preferences are to be translated into food habits.

Despite general trends in food preferences, there are vast differencs in individual likes and dislikes within groups. The significance of such variations, as applied to the nutritional adequacy of diets, will take on meaning as your study of nutrition proceeds. In the meantime, it is of interest to speculate briefly on *why* individuals differ in their reactions to foods. Are there real bases, for example, for dislikes of certain foods—actual distaste for them? Studies in this field show that *taste* may be one of the many factors involved.

Food Preferences by Individual Taste Some individuals have a much sharper taste than others. In one series of taste tests, for example, one person found saccharine 2000 times as sweet as sugar; another found it only 32 times as sweet as sugar [9]. There are also variations in the sense of taste of the same individual from one time to another. A food may actually taste differently to a person today than it did yesterday. Recognition of variations in taste may therefore offer some insight into the differing food likes and dislikes of individuals and into the reasons some children and adults are more serious feeding problems than others.

Taste buds vary in their location and activity throughout life [10]. In early childhood they are present in the throat, tongue, and cheeks. At different points in the mouth area they register the different basic taste sensations of sweet, sour, salty, and bitter. A young child's taste buds are more numerous and sensitive than an adult's. It is therefore reasonable that a food too sour or too salty might permanently affect a child's attitude toward it. Taste buds disappear gradually until by the twelfth year, chiefly those in the tongue remain. (Fig. 1.1). In early and middle adult life there is little further change. In elderly persons the functioning of taste buds is drastically curtailed. These observations offer some explanation of the reactions to foods of persons at different points on the age scale.

Flavor is a broader term than taste. It is a complex sensation that involves various environmental factors, including aroma, texture, and temperature, as well as taste. A well-known investigator in this field suggests the complexity of the concept of flavor by saying that research on flavor "cuts across a wide spectrum of problems and methods, from psychophysics and psychophysiology to the psychology of personality and education," and adds humorously, "with advertising thrown in for good measure" [11]. Thus flavor, in a broad sense, is conceivably the basis for many likes and dislikes of foods.

» ENJOYMENT OF FOOD

Enjoyment of food has even wider implications for food habits than taste or flavor. It includes the atmosphere in which food is eaten and the companionship enjoyed with it. Eating is a social rite among all peoples. It is endowed with symbolism for friendliness, sociability, and rapport. Eating alone is usually a dreary experience. Lone eaters are apt to eat a limited variety of foods, to undereat or overeat, and to hurry through their meals without enjoying them.

People come to like what they are accustomed to eating under pleasant circumstances. Efforts to transform their patterns of eating should be made with caution lest they lose their pleasure in food. Eating attractive food in pleasing surroundings with congenial company is not only a satisfying social experience but also creates the most favorable conditions for physiological utilization of the food. Some of the ways in which enjoyment of foods can shape food habits have already been pointed out.

For those who have a good appetite for meals, there is added enjoyment. People say they are "hungry" at meal time. But hunger and appetite are not identical, and the difference between them is important in understanding food habits [12]. Hunger indicates the actual need for food—we suffer from "hunger pangs"—and appetite pertains to the desire to eat. Appetite often functions long after hunger is satisfied. The habit of overeating may arise from an uncontrolled appetite.

Contrary to opinion, human appetite is not guided by instinct [13]. Individuals do not instinctively select a diet that meets their body's nutrient requirements, no matter how much they may anticipate the food. The view that cravings for certain foods signify physiological need for specific nutrients provided by those foods has not been substantiated. The amount of overweight in this country bears witness to the fact that appetite is an unreliable guide to the amount of food needed. Nor is appetite an infallible guide to the *kinds* of food required.

There is evidence that certain animals, when confronted with a variety of sub-

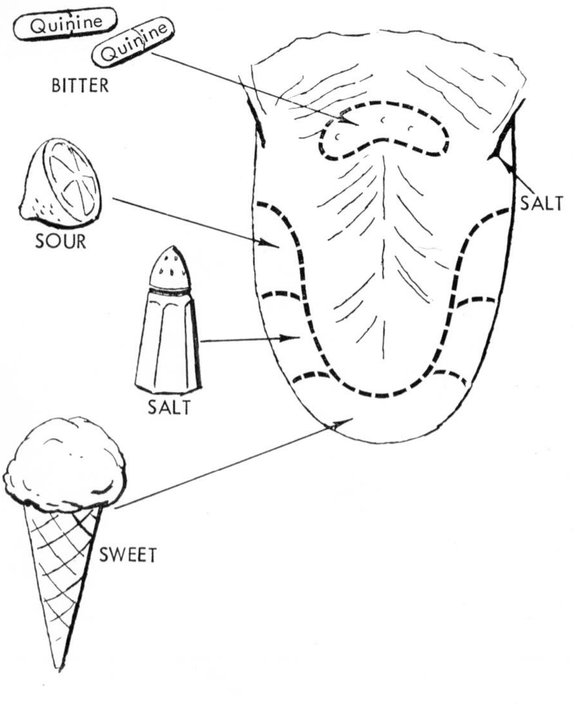

Fig. 1.1 Location of taste buds in the Tongue. (Adapted from *Today's Health*, published by the American Medical Association.)

stances under prescribed conditions, have the ability to select those elements which are lacking in their diets [13]. Some investigators have suggested that the same may hold true for children. No proof is available to support this suggestion. Once children have eaten a variety of foods, they develop taste preferences based on factors entirely unrelated to nutritional values. Personal preferences would thus tend to override any instinct to choose foods wisely, even if instinct did perform a basic function in this respect. Obviously the same conclusion applies to adults. People accustomed to high-fat or high-sweet diets, for example, have a strong appetite for and enjoy foods of this type, even though these may be the very foods they should avoid.

» GUIDING THE FOOD HABITS OF CHILDREN [14]

Food habits begin at birth. Therefore, the sooner a child is surrounded with influences that encourage good food habits, the better are his chances to develop a normal eating pattern. Basic influences, discussed earlier have application here.

The Beginnings

Infants react favorably to things about them that make them comfortable; unfavorably to those which make them uncomfortable. Food is a major consideration in both respects. Babies generate a friendly attitude toward food and the persons who feed them if they are fed when hungry in a relaxed atmosphere and with food that satisfies them. Food becomes the symbol for comfort, contentment, satisfaction, and security. This attitude remains, not only in later childhood, but throughout life. The child fortunate enough to have this introduction to food has the foundation for good food habits.

On the other hand, babies may develop negative attitudes toward food when they are held to rigid feeding schedules, are given formulae that do not satisfy their hunger, or are fed in an atmosphere of tension. Food may come to symbolize for them unhappiness, dissatisfaction, and conflict. These attitudes may also cling throughout life. As a child grows older, he may develop resentment toward and dislike for certain foods, particularly those which have been forced on him by oversolicitous adults.

Parental Guidance

A leading pediatrician has provided parents with the following "prescription" for helping a young child maintain a favorable attitude toward eating after infancy: attractive food, small servings, some freedom to choose his own foods, some freedom to eat his own way, adequate play and sleep, and relaxed parents. This simple approach continues the favorable influences and environment of infancy. It does not imply license for a child to eat whatever and whenever he chooses. It assumes the quiet, guiding hand of a parent in encouraging a positive interest in food and eating.

Living Schedules

The daily pace at which many children of school age live affects their food habits. Hurried meals, especially breakfasts and lunches, are usually eaten under pressure. Both quantity and quality of such meals are sacrificed. With a sketchy breakfast, or no breakfast at all, a child usually tries to compensate with a snack, en route to school or at recess. The snack is often a concentrated sweet, which in no way takes the place of the breakfast items he has missed. If the sweet is eaten at recess, it may interfere with his appetite for lunch. From any viewpoint, therefore, the hasty, neglected meal is a threat to good food habits.

Other health practices may have equal impact. Too little sleep and too little outdoor life diminish the desire for food. Inadequate sleep, if it becomes a habit, results in a nervous, irritable child who develops a finicky attitude toward his meals. Homework and a multitude of distractions lead to late bedtimes; a late bedtime leads to a late rising time. Thus the inevitable crowded morning routine and daily cycle of poor food habits repeat themselves.

A Realistic Picture of Children's Diets

What do all of these influences add up to in terms of children's food habits? Regional nutrition studies in the United States show that children up to 12 years of age, *on the average,* have diets reasonably adequate in most nutrients. From 13 to 20 years of age, boys, *on the average,* continue to obtain enough of most of the nutrients, but girls in this age range have diets seriously low or borderline in all but 3 nutrients [15]. (The adequacy of children's diets with respect to specific nutrients is discussed in Section Two.) Dietary data are necessarily reported in terms of *average* practice. Individual food habits are thereby obscured. But behind each average we find low as well as high values. Studies of individual diets of children show that low nutritive values reflect slighted breakfasts, inadequate lunches, too small amounts of milk, vegetables and fruits, and that sweets, and soft drinks predominate as snacks. Thus averages may lead to overoptimism—a feeling that there are no inadequacies. Those concerned with helping children to improve their food habits must, therefore, look behind averages to obtain a realistic picture of the needs of individual children.

» GUIDING THE FOOD HABITS OF ADULTS

Ideally, one should reach adulthood with a wide acquaintance with common foods and at least a tolerant attitude toward most of them. This situation would undoubtedly exist if all the influences affecting a child's food habits were favorable. As an adult, he would meet new foods in a spirit of adventure and would seriously try to adapt to new flavors.

This is a day when cosmopolitan food habits are in order. People in this country eat away from home frequently, often in the homes of friends from foreign countries or in restaurants that feature foreign foods. It is also a day of international travel and residence abroad, with unfamiliar foods as the regular fare. Adaptable adults can widen their horizons with respect to foods; the less venturesome adhere to familiar and conventional patterns of eating.

Conservatism in Adults

Adult food habits are usually not easily altered, especially if they fall into a limited, set pattern. If habits are of long standing, and the individual has known no other way of eating, he is particularly resistant to change. Adults clamor for variety and complain of monotony, particularly when meals planned by others are served them in institutions. This holds true from college dormitories to retirement homes, and often when the meals are well balanced and reasonably varied. This is an anomaly because, left to themselves, these same individuals usually revert, day after day, to meals consisting of the same core of foods to which they are accustomed.

Many factors may enter into the dissatisfactions expressed with institutional meals, but it seems likely that the real complaint, in many cases, is not with monotony, but with the fact that the foods and meal plans are *different* from the usual eating patterns. This desire for the familiar reveals a built-in conservatism, existent to some degree at all ages. For some people, clinging to well-known foods provides a feeling of security when they are experiencing other changes; for others, it may offer a way of asserting their individuality and independence.

When To Attempt Habit Modification

When should food habit modifications be attempted? Only after a careful study indicates that the present diet is nutritionally inadequate, and when the bases for present habits and the beliefs that support them are fully understood. The African situation discussed earlier is a case in point [1]. The tribe was convinced of the dietary importance of increasing the milk consumption of their women, as pointed out to them by the team of health specialists who served them. But this influence was not strong enough to overcome the tribal taboo. Painstaking analysis of the basis for the taboo and patience in developing a plan to circumvent it eventually paid off. Since the barrier to milk consumption lay in the link between milk and the specific herd from which it came, presumably the barrier could be removed if a source of milk were introduced from outside the community. The practical solution was powdered milk. The tribe accepted the powdered milk because it did not originate with cows belonging to its own people. The new milk was made available to members, and they were shown how to use it. As the habit grew and the benefits were apparent to the tribe, the women in a few families even began to use milk from family herds. Thus, a well-established habit finally grew strong enough to override the original taboo.

The same general principles govern the approach to food habit modification in any group. First one should ask: Is there need for a change—is the present diet inadequate? Second: What are the bases for present habits and what are the beliefs that support them? The adequacy of the present diet should be judged on its known nutritional content. If it includes unfamiliar foods, their food values must be determined and appraised. So far as feasible, customary foods should be retained and their use encouraged. They often form the foundation on which to add foods to make the diet adequate. When the foods needed to make the diet adequate have been ascertained, it is time to plan a course of action. Perhaps milk heads the list of foods required. In the case of the Italian family whose school-age children had soft drinks as a beverage with meals, you would want to know how to substitute milk. But you first need to find out what prompted the family to take up the soft drinks. What is the children's attitude toward milk? What would influence the mother to buy more milk? This type of analysis lays the groundwork for an effective educational approach in solving the problem of getting more milk into family meals.

The Possibilities for Improvement

Even deeply entrenched food habits can be altered, as has been shown. In this country, U.S. Department of Agriculture data indicate a considerable shift in eating habits in the past 50 years [16]. (See Fig.

1.2.) There has been a steady decline in the use of potatoes and cereal grains and an increase in the consumption of milk, vegetables, fruits, and meat. This does not mean that everyone has changed his eating practices. Again we are dealing with averages. The greatest change has taken place in the diets of children and young adults; the diets of older people have undergone the least change. Young homemakers tend to adopt new meal patterns. As the purchasing agents for the household, they are encouraging their families in new eating habits. When young homemakers were questioned on how they knew how to plan meals, many reported that they learned it in school [8]. Nutrition education of adults may start in elementary school classrooms. The younger the child, the more readily does he accept change.

Every time an adult is deprived of his accustomed way of eating, he is in a situation that calls for adjustment. If he is adaptable, he may accept the diet or some part or it. If his habits are rigid, he may merely endure the new until he can return to the old. What happens, for example, when young men join the armed forces [17]? In the mess hall, little effort can be made to cater to the individual likes and habits of recruits from various sections of the country. The extent to which the men accept the new and make it a part of their permanent eating pattern probably varies widely with individuals. Those who make some lasting changes in their way of eating are contributing to the gradual lessening of regional differences in food habits that is taking place in the nation today.

It should be emphasized that food habits that differ from our own are not necessarily poor or need to be changed. The elements of an adequate diet can be obtained from many sources. Meals that look and taste different from our own or are served on a different time schedule than ours may be entirely adequate nutritionally and suit perfectly those who eat them. For example, a meal-in-one stew, available at

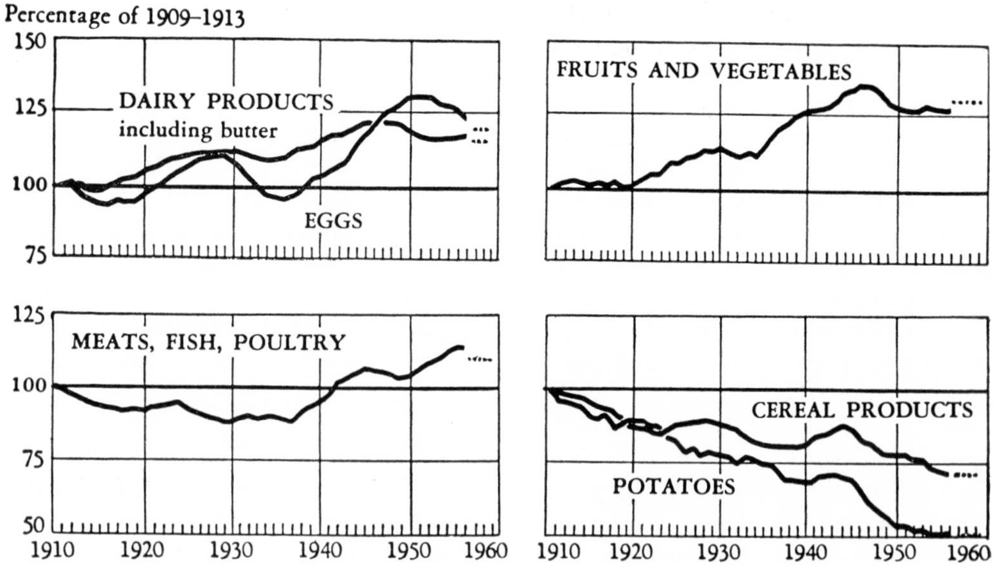

Fig. 1.2 Trends in Our Eating Habits. Five-year moving average centered. Data shown for year 1958. Per capita civilian consumption, United States (using 1947–1949 retail prices as weights). (U.S. Department of Agriculture.)

all hours of the day to a tribal family, can be as nutritious as our own separate meals, providing the necessary ingredients are included in the stew and each member of the family gets the amount he needs.

Even when food habits are poor they are not all bad. The majority of people have relatively few things wrong with their diets. But it is sometimes as difficult to make the small adjustments as it is to make the larger ones. As indicated, many diets are deficient not because of the complete omission of needed foods, but because of the inadequate quantities used, as in the case of milk, fruits, and certain vegetables.

Begin with familiar foods. An individual's present diet should be the point of departure for improvement, irrespective of the type or extent of poor food habits. The strongest prospect for success in effecting permanent modifications is in building on a nucleus of familiar and well-liked foods. By gradually adding certain foods to this nucleus, increasing the quantities of some and decreasing the quantities of others, a satisfactory adjustment may ultimately be effected without radically changing the eating pattern. Mark Twain's advice may well be heeded: "Habit is habit and not to be flung out the window by any man but coaxed downstairs a step at a time." It is always a temptation to "start from scratch," i.e., to display a recommended daily food pattern and to begin at the top to plan a brand new set of meals for the person to be helped. Those who have had the most encouraging results in improving food habits reverse the process—they work *up to* the pattern, not *down* from it.

The Need for Improvement

In the early 1930's, family food surveys showed that one-third of the diets in this country ranked as "poor." In the 1960's, probably 1 in 10 diets would be so classified [18]. This is progress, but a study of the records shows that most of these gains were achieved before 1948. Nutrient shortages that appeared in that year continue today, despite increased food supplies and higher incomes. In addition to the inadequacies noted in children's diets, older adults, groups in certain sections of the country, and people on restricted incomes in all regions are less well off nutritionally than the general population.

Influences for Habit Modification

Granted that changes *can* take place, what are the chief influences for alteration in adult diets, aside from those provided by new physical environments such as the armed forces and institutional living? These are some of the influences: formal class instruction in nutrition and related subjects, professional consultation, books, journals, magazines, pamphlets, lectures, television and radio programs dealing with the subject of nutrition at the adult level. The effect of these media on dietary habits depends on the extent of a person's exposure to them and the depth of his desire for change. Another, more insistent influence, is commercial food advertising.

Advertising Television, radio, newspaper, and magazine advertising are the chief avenues for announcing new forms of common foods, new combinations of well-known ingredients, new processing methods, and new ways of serving familiar dishes. Acceptance of advertised products may not signify the adaptability of the family palate so much as it suggests the response of the homemaker to new and short-cut methods of serving foods already favorably known. Sales figures show that advertised food products *do* sell. In a sense, the eating pattern is thereby broadened. The extent to which this is a desirable change, from the standpoint of nutrition, depends on:

> *Whether the foods advertised are needed to increase the nutritional adequacy of the family diet.* If they are nonessential foods or ones already used in quantities beyond need, advertising may encourage an undesirable excess.
>
> *Whether the cost is in proportion to the food value received.* If products are too expensive in relation to nutrient yield, it may mean that other foods needed to make the diet adequate are omitted or curtailed.
>
> *Whether the advertiser's promises of nutritional content are reliable.* If he promises too much and the consumer depends on the foods advertised for nutritive qualities they do not possess, the family diet may be nutritionally inadequate as a result.

Motives for Modifying Food Habits [19,20]

There is no sure way to motivate people to alter their food habits. But helping adults to help themselves through better understanding of the reasons why they accept or reject foods offers promise. Taking action after group discussion and decision has proved effective. If an adult analyzes his own food habits objectively, identifies his own eating problems, recognizes the origin of his prejudices, and faces the advantages to himself of making necessary adjustments, there is some hope for success, providing he sincerely wishes to change. Without doubt, the key to the outcome is the strength of his urge to make the adjustment.

Specific Motivations A driving urge to attain a concrete goal constitutes strong motivation for habit change. This may be the case in weight reduction, for example. Motives will vary with the sex, age, and state of health of the dieter. They may range from the desire for a trim appearance to the need for lowering blood pressure. The motive may be strong enough for the person to accept a diet that requires a sharp reversal in present eating practices. A similar situation may exist in the control of an illness, such as diabetes. The motive in this case is direct and compelling. Its intensity may be increased by fear of serious disability, or even death. The cause-and-effect relationship is clear cut. When an individual is so motivated, the diet change involved is accepted, even though it may be radical.

Specific motivations are usually strong, or can be made so. The objectives are well defined. The individual chiefly needs guidance in proper methods of application, such as adequate diets in weight reduction, and in reasonable goals, such as moderate weight losses.

General Motivations Goals for good, general nutrition are less tangible and the rewards are more remote. Motives are understandably weaker. Setting out at the age of 20 on a new pattern of eating that will insure reaching the age of 80 in good health is a worthy aim. But people are more concerned with concrete objectives, near at hand. Nutrition in the abstract has little appeal. They are interested in nutrition only as it can be translated into specific benefits, and they want those benefits now. The success of nutrition education, therefore, hinges on whether these personal aims are identified and used effectively.

Just why adults are not more actively concerned with the over-all health benefits to be derived from good general nutrition is an unsolved puzzle. Even though many profess to believe that nutritional well-being and physical fitness are essential to practically every human accomplishment, their words are not always translated into deeds. Contributing reasons for this inconsistency have been discussed in this chapter—emotions, prejudices, taboos, and prestige symbols, to name only a few [21]. They suggest that the individual, himself, and his personal opinions and urges with respect to food often supersede knowledge, judgment, and even experience in their effect on his eating practices. It has been said that a person is rational with respect to his own food habits only when he understands *himself* in relation to those habits.

Part of this understanding process is acceptance of the fact that the "laws" of nutrition apply to all: to himself as well as to other persons. His food habits often belie this point of view. He proceeds as though unaware that effect follows cause—as if, somehow, he is endowed with a special immunity to the consequences of poor nutrition. Chapter 2 seeks to show the weakness of this position. It examines the ways in which the human body, at all ages, responds to the conditions created by good and poor nutrition.

REFERENCES

1. Cassel, J., "Social and Cultural Implications of Food and Habits," *Am. J. Public Health,* 47 (June 1957) pp. 732–40.
2. National Research Council, Committee on Food Habits, *The Problem of Changing Food Habits,* Bull. 108. Washington, D.C.: National Academy of Sciences, Oct. 1943.
3. Tarulli, M. A., *Personal Communication.* Chicago: Infant Welfare Society, 1962.
4. Eppright, E. S., *Food Habits and Preferences—A Study of Iowa People of Two Age Groups,* Research Bull. 376. Ames: Agricultural Experiment Station, Iowa State College, 1950.
5. Van Riter, I. G., "Acceptance of Twenty-six Vegetables," *J. Home Economics,* 48 (Dec. 1956) pp. 771–73.
6. Breckenridge, M. E., "Food Attitudes of Five- to Twelve-year-old Children," *J. Am. Dietet. Assoc.,* 35 (July 1959), pp. 704–709.
7. Schuck, C., "Food Preferences of South Dakota College Students," *J. Am. Dietet. Assoc.,* 39 (Dec. 1961) pp. 595–97.
8. Young, C. M., Waldner, B. G., and Berresford, K., "What The Homemaker Knows about Nutrition: 4. Her Food Problems, Shopping Habits and Sources of Information," *J. Am. Dietet. Assoc.,* 32 (May 1956) pp. 429–34. (See reference list to article for Nos. 1, 2, and 3 in this series.)
9. Williams, R. J., *The Human Frontier.* New York: Harcourt, Brace & World, Inc., 1946.
10. Kare, M. R., and Halpern, B. P. (Eds.), *Physiological and Behavioral Aspects of Taste.* Chicago: University of Chicago Press, 1961.
11. Brozek, J. (Ed.), *Symposium On Nutrition and Behavior.* New York: National Vitamin Foundation Inc., Nutrition Symposium Series, No. 14, 1957. (For the same articles, see *Am. J. Clinical Nutrition,* 5, 1957.)
12. Wohl, M. G., and Goodhart, R. S. (Eds.), *Modern Nutrition in Health and*

Disease. 2nd ed. Philadelphia: Lea & Febiger, 1960. (Chap. 4, "The Psychology of Appetite.")

13. National Research Council, Committee on Food Habits, *Manual for the Study of Food Habits*. Bull. 111. Washington, D.C.: National Academy of Sciences, Jan. 1945, p. 64.
14. Martin, E. A., *Roberts' Nutrition Work with Children*. Chicago: University of Chicago Press, 1954. (Chaps. 5, 7.)
15. Morgan, A. F., *Nutritional Status U.S.A.* Bull. 769. Berkeley: California Agricultural Experiment Station, University of California, Oct. 1959.
16. Burk, M. C., "Pounds and Percentages," *Food—The Yearbook of Agriculture*. Washington, D.C.: U.S. Department of Agriculture, 1959. p. 591.
17. Pilgrim, F. J., "What Foods Do People Accept or Reject?" *J. Am. Dietet. Assoc.*, 38 (May 1961) pp. 439–43.
18. Stiebeling, H. K., "Food in Our Lives," *Food—The Yearbook of Agriculture*. Washington, D.C.: U.S. Department of Agriculture, 1959. p. 1.
19. Norman, C., "Group Discussion in Changing Food Habits," *J. Am. Dietet. Assoc.*, 34 (Nov. 1958) pp. 1187–89.
20. Schindler-Raimon, E., "Telling is Not Teaching," *J. Am. Dietet. Assoc.*, 37 (Aug. 1960) pp. 118–20.
21. Pumpian-Mindlin, E., "The Meanings of Food," *J. Am. Dietet. Assoc.*, 30 (June 1954) pp. 576–80.

READINGS

American Medical Association, *The Wonderful Human Machine* from *Today's Health*, 38 (May 1960) pp. 59–62.

Babcock, C. G., "Food and Its Emotional Significance," *J. Am. Dietet. Assoc.*, 24 (May 1948) pp. 390–93.

———, "Attitudes and the Use of Food," *J. Am. Dietet. Assoc.*, 38 (June 1961) pp. 546–51.

Dudley, D. T., Moore, M. E., and Sunderlin, E. M., "Children's Attitudes Toward Food," *J. Home Economics*, 52 (Oct. 1960) pp. 678–81.

Fathauer, G. H., "Food Habits—An Anthropologist's View," *J. Am. Dietet. Assoc.*, 37 (Oct. 1960) pp. 335–38.

Food Habits of Various Peoples:

J. Am. Dietet. Assoc.

Peru: vol. 30, 1954, p. 856; vol. 39, 1961, p. 126; Greece: vol. 31, 1955, p. 269; Gold Coast: vol. 31, 1955, p. 685; Thailand: vol. 35, 1959, p. 1143; Nigeria: vol. 39, 1961, p. 467; Angola: vol. 39, 1961, p. 585; Israel: vol. 40, 1962, p. 125; Southwest U.S.: vol. 40, 1962, p. 218.

Am. J. Clin. Nutrition

Southwest U.S.: vol. 7, 1959, p. 224; Puerto Rico: vol. 7, 1959, p. 349; Haiti: vol. 7, 1959, p. 538.

Galdston, I., "Nutrition from The Psychiatric Viewpoint," *J. Am. Dietet. Assoc.*, 28 (May 1952) pp. 405–409.

Lantis, M., "The Child Consumer," *J. Home Economics*, 54 (May 1962) pp. 370–75.

Lowenberg, M. E., "Food Preferences of Young Children," *J. Am. Dietet. Assoc.,* 24 (May 1948) pp. 430–34.

Queen, G. S., "Culture, Economics and Food Habits," *J. Am. Dietet. Assoc.,* 33 (Oct. 1957) pp. 1044–52.

Stiebeling, H. K., and Dreis, T. A., "Habits—and More," *Food—The Yearbook of Agriculture.* Washington, D.C.: U.S. Department of Agriculture, 1959. p. 631.

Tinsley, W. V., "As the Twig is Bent," *Food—The Yearbook of Agriculture.* Washington, D.C.: U.S. Department of Agriculture, 1959. p. 636.

Venable, T. C., "Nutrition Education—What is The Problem?" *J. Am. Dietet. Assoc.,* 33 (June 1957) pp. 600–601.

CHAPTER 2

Does nutrition make a difference?

Does nutrition really make a difference to individuals and to peoples in the way they develop and in what they achieve in terms of physical, mental and emotional behavior? This is a practical question of vital concern to everyone. The answer must be gleaned from a variety of sources, including planned research, population surveys, observations under known nutritional conditions, and statistical analyses of health data. Collectively, the findings provide an affirmative answer; regarded individually, they offer varied and interesting supporting information. The findings are grouped here for discussion under 4 topics that deal with nutrition in relation to body performance, body structure, body size, and to length of life. Since performance imposes the most severe test on any mechanism, it receives first consideration.

» NUTRITION AND BODY PERFORMANCE

The term "performance" refers here to the various ways the body behaves—how it expresses itself—under contrasting conditions of good and poor nutrition. Differences in performance are discussed in terms of mental application, nervous stability, motor efficiency, and the ability of the body to resist the inroads of infection. A few representative studies are reviewed briefly in each category.

Mental Application

It appears from the evidence that intelligence or mental capacity is not affected by nutritional status. On the other hand, in the case of poor nutriture, mental *performance* may be measurably inferior due to depleted energy, inability to concentrate, and fatigue associated with undernutrition. This type of deterioration in mental performance was demonstrated in young men during World War II. Conscientious objectors, who served as non-combatants in the armed forces, were subjects in an important experiment. The purpose of the experiment was to determine the effects on human beings of subsistence for long periods on substandard rations such as those prevailing in certain allied nations and in prisoner-of-war camps. According to the plan of the experiment, the young men lived for about six months on a diet considerably lower in calories than the one to which they had been accustomed. During this period their mental performance, as measured by various intelligence tests, did not deteriorate importantly as the period of undernutrition continued. Significantly, however, there was a sharp decline in spontaneous mental effort and in the capacity for sustained mental application and achievement, which only gradually returned to normal when the diet was restored to adequacy [1].

It should be pointed out that while the men in the experiment were living on a so-called "semistarvation diet," they were actually receiving about 1500 calories daily and adequate amounts of food nutrients. The diet was so labelled because it represented only about one-half the calories allowed the men during the control period when they had enough food to cover fully their estimated energy and nutrient needs. Thus the conditions simulated in this study are probably more favorable than those which often exist when people are compelled to eat less than they need or when they voluntarily cut down their intake, as on some reducing diets.

Following World War I German school children reacted much as did the armed forces personnel. The children had lived for many months on an extremely meager diet. Teachers complained of the pupils' inability to concentrate, of their slowness of comprehension, poor memory, and inattention. There was also a lowering of of the standard of school work in comparison with prewar records. The number of children who failed to pass to the next grade was about doubled. Only half as many children were doing superior school work, and the number doing inferior work increased as much as 30 percent [2].

The effect of nutrition on scholastic attainment and on attitude toward school work was shown more recently in a study of teen-age boys that noted their performance during one period when they had a good breakfast and during another when they had no breakfast. The majority of the boys had a much better attitude and an improved scholastic record when they ate breakfast than when they did not do so. Some of the boys were reported to be careless and inattentive during the late morning hours when breakfast was omitted. When they had eaten breakfast, the late morning performance of the same boys showed recognizable improvement, especially in scholastic attainment [3].

These studies suggest that the person whose dietary needs are fully satisfied can be expected to exert greater effort to take advantage of his intellectual opportunities than the person who is inadequately nourished. Raising the level of a child's nutriture may therefore offer one way of improving the quality of his school work. Bringing a malnourished adult up to a good state of nutrition may restore the initiative required to accomplish mental tasks.

Nervous Stability

The same young men of the armed forces who were tested for mental performance, as described earlier, exhibited various other behavioral changes while living for six months on their restricted diet [1]. Periods of restlessness and irritability were alternated with periods of apathy and seeming loss of will power. Some of the men became sullen and obstinate. They were moody, introspective and uncooperative. When the men were tested on the Minnesota Multiphasic Personality Inventory, important deviations from normality were observed. The personality changes during the calorie deficiency were labelled by the investigators as "semistarvation neurosis." In the refeeding period that followed, some of the manifestations returned to normal in about three months' time; others, among them a feeling of depression, responded less promptly.

The malnourished German children were restless and unruly in school. This restlessness was attributed to nervous instability caused by general undernutrition [2]. Although these hyperirritable children were the ones of which the teachers complained, about 20 percent of the children were of the dull phlegmatic type. Alertness and high spirits are usually observed in well-nourished children. They are not only buoyant in appearance and manner, but they have the best chance of possessing those personality traits which mark them as confident, well adjusted, and emotionally stable.

The nervous system also shows marked susceptibility to specific types of dietary deficiencies. Pronounced nervous symptoms, for example, are well-recognized accompaniments of the diseases beriberi (thiamine deficiency; see Chap. 7) and pellagra (niacin deficiency; see Chap. 7).

Motor Performance

As would be expected, strength, speed, and endurance also vary with nutritional status. The young men of the armed forces on the restricted diet were subjected at intervals to a battery of motor tests [1]. Deterioration was shown in all of the tests, but the amounts varied considerably. By the end of the experiment about one-third of the men's original strength was lost, as measured by a grip test (Fig. 2.1) and by a lifting test. The largest loss (80 percent) was shown in an endurance test that involved running on an inclined treadmill to exhaustion (Fig. 2.2). Performance involving the central nervous system, as in speed tapping tests, showed only about a 5 percent loss; tests requiring eye-hand coordination registered about a 16-1 percent increase in error during the period of the poor diet.

In another study, tests were applied to several age groups in the late morning hours during 2 experimental periods—one when the subjects had eaten breakfast, the other when they had not. The groups consisted of boys 12–14 years of age; women 22–27 years; women 18–25 years; men 21–28 years; and men 25–35 years of age. Maximum *work rate* was measured only in the group of school boys. The findings obtained by the use of a bicycle ergometer (Fig. 2.3) showed that the boys did significantly better following a basic breakfast consisting of fruit, cereal, cream, toast, butter, and nearly 1 pt of milk than when breakfast was omitted [3]. Maximum *work output* for all groups was measured on the same device. They all did significantly more work in the late morning hours following a basic breakfast than when the morning meal was omitted.

Several studies on industrial workers have shown poor food habits to be associated with fatigue, physical inefficiency, and decreased work output. A recent test of the effect of the coffee break as a factor in productivity in reality points up the importance of breakfast. The productivity of men and women office and factory workers was measured on a bicycle ergometer. All of the subjects did significantly more work in the late morning hours when they started the day with a grood breakfast than when breakfast was omitted. A midmorning snack added nothing to their productiveness if they had had a good breakfast. A midmorning snack that replaced breakfast, compensated for lack of breakfast for only about half of the subjects in the amount of work they accomplished [4].

In another concept of performance, absenteeism from the job was studied in relation to illness of the worker, and illness in turn, to the adequacy of his diet [5]. In general there appears to be a positive relationship between a well-nourished person

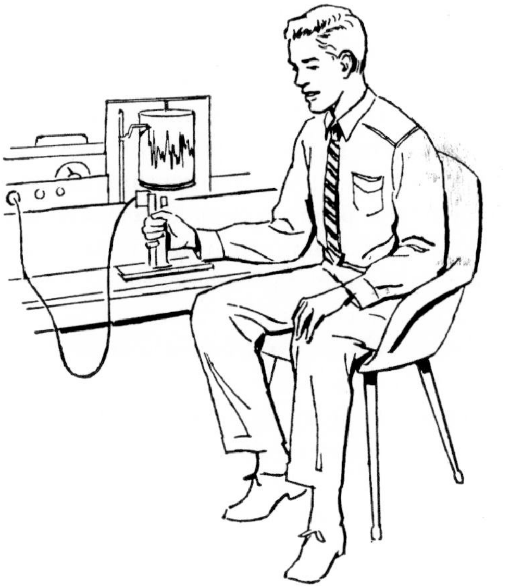

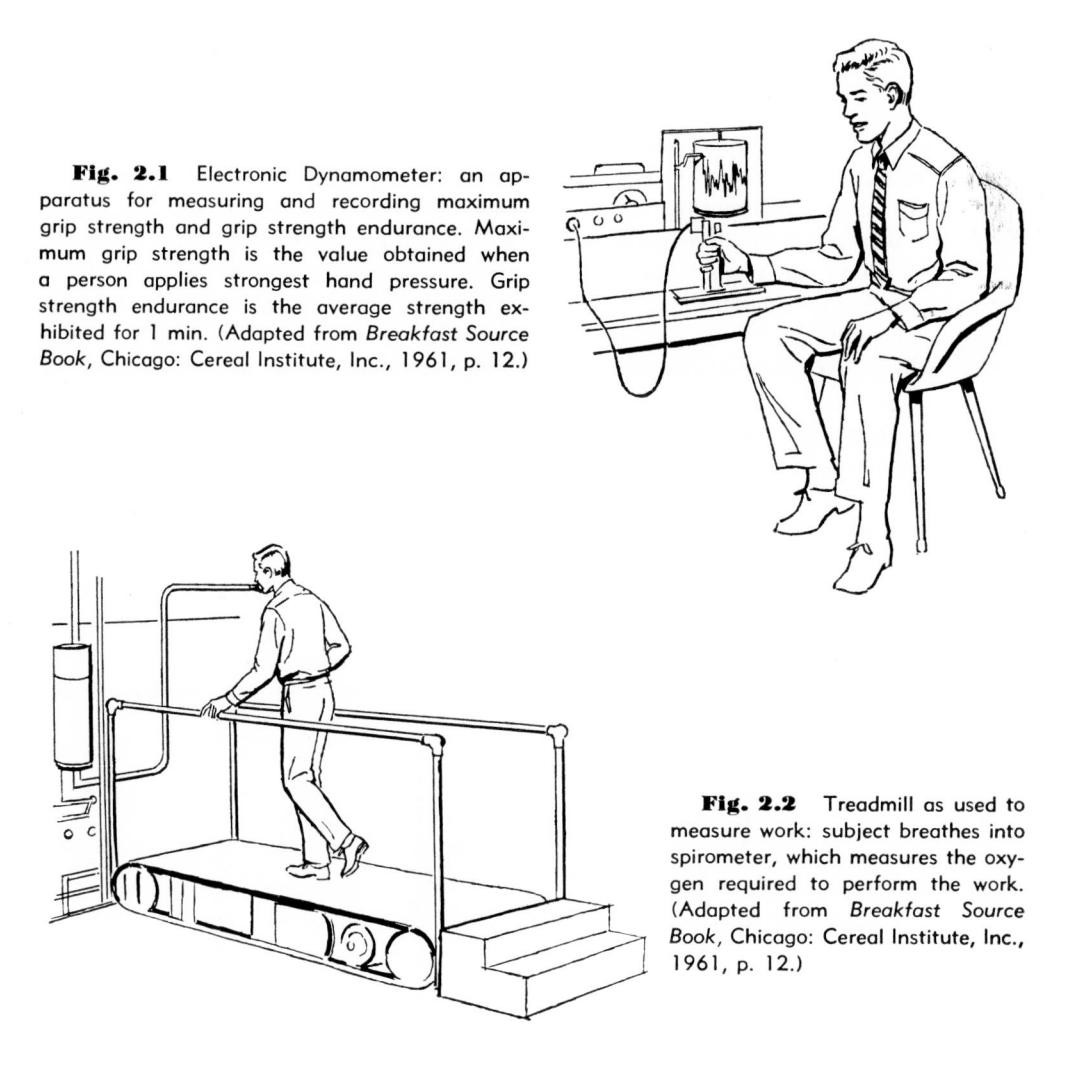

Fig. 2.1 Electronic Dynamometer: an apparatus for measuring and recording maximum grip strength and grip strength endurance. Maximum grip strength is the value obtained when a person applies strongest hand pressure. Grip strength endurance is the average strength exhibited for 1 min. (Adapted from *Breakfast Source Book*, Chicago: Cereal Institute, Inc., 1961, p. 12.)

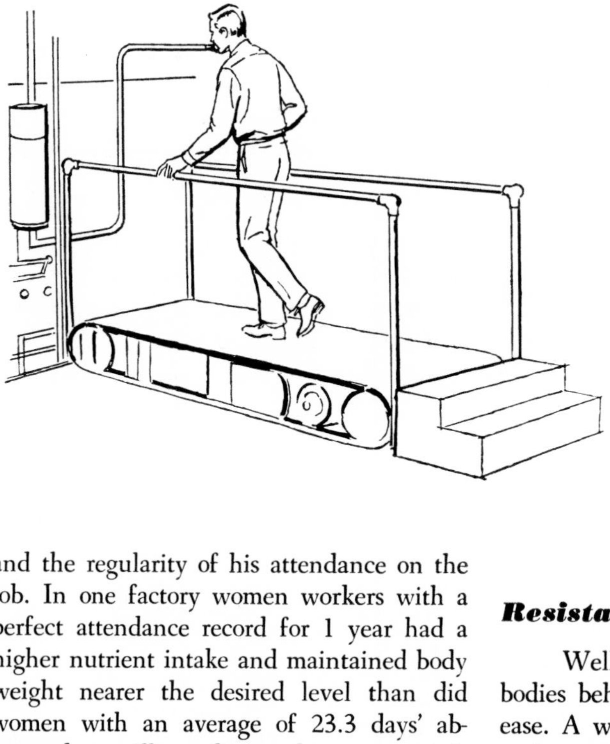

Fig. 2.2 Treadmill as used to measure work: subject breathes into spirometer, which measures the oxygen required to perform the work. (Adapted from *Breakfast Source Book*, Chicago: Cereal Institute, Inc., 1961, p. 12.)

and the regularity of his attendance on the job. In one factory women workers with a perfect attendance record for 1 year had a higher nutrient intake and maintained body weight nearer the desired level than did women with an average of 23.3 days' absence due to illness during the same period. The cause and effect relationship is not proved, but the fact remains that the poor diet paralleled the high absentee record, and absenteeism is obviously an important factor in productivity.

Resistance to Disease

Well-nourished and poorly-nourished bodies behave differently in relation to disease. A well-nourished body tends to resist and overcome infections; a poorly-nourished body tends to be susceptible to disease and to delay the process of recovery. Thus, good nutrition offers a measure of protection in dealing with disease.

There are many laboratory, clinical,

and field observations which show that malnutrition and the existence and severity of infections go hand in hand. Malnutrition predisposes the body to infections, and infections create the conditions for poor nutritional status. These relationships are clear cut in the populations of developing countries where malnutrition and infections are both rampant; the relationships may be masked or completely obscured where people are relatively well nourished [6].

The mechanisms by which resistance to infectious diseases can be lowered by malnutrition are not fully understood. Many explanations have been offered. One school of thought holds that the poorly nourished body lacks the capacity to form the antibodies necessary to overcome infections. Research has supported this theory in cases of human beings and laboratory animals suffering nutrient deficiencies, notably of protein. For example, severely malnourished human subjects have shown a diminished antibody response to diphtheria toxin and to typhoid vaccine [6].

Other schools of thought have proposed that malnutrition acts in other ways to invite the onset or progress of infections. One group maintains that various nutrient deficiencies tend to diminish a nonspecific bactericidal effect possessed by blood serum and other body tissues; yet another group believes that malnutrition, particularly a deficiency of vitamin A, lowers barriers to bacterial invasion by weakening the epithelial tissues. (Medical and public health aspects of disease control are considered later in this chapter.)

What may be said of the relationship between comparatively moderate malnutrition, as encountered in our own country, and diseases such as tuberculosis, commonly

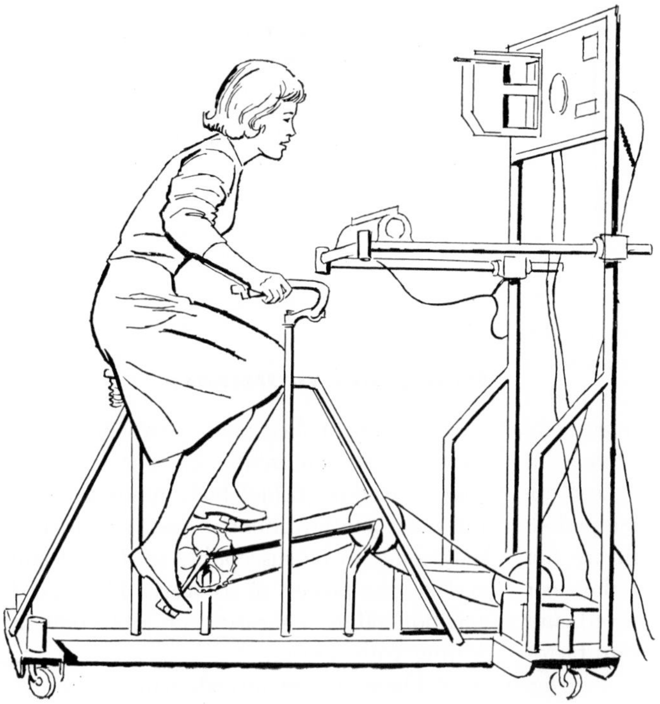

Fig. 2.3 Bicycle Ergometer: a stationary bicycle that measures maximum work rate and maximum work output. The work output is that from riding the bicycle at maximum effort for 1 min. The maximum work rate is determined from the 1-min output record. (Adapted from *Breakfast Source Book*, Chicago: Cereal Institute, Inc., 1961, p. 12.)

associated with nutritional status? Malnourished individuals fall easy prey to tuberculosis. The rising incidence of the disease under conditions of World War II is cited as evidence. The rise was greatest in overseas areas where food shortages were most acute. In this country, where food supplies remained relatively normal, the steady decline in the death rate from tuberculosis continued.

The death rate from all forms of tuberculosis in the United States has dropped from 201.9 per 100,000 population in 1900 to approximately 8 per 100,000 at the present time [7]. In general, the decline corresponds to a rising standard of living with improvement in food habits and advances in our knowledge of treatment of the disease. The decline is less marked in the late teens and in adult life. This situation has also been linked to nutrition; teen-age diets are notably inadequate, and it is believed that they may be a major contributing factor [8]. Antibiotics have done much to speed recovery from tuberculosis but they have not displaced nutritious food as a factor in prevention and treatment.

The impact of nutrition in dealing with disease is evident. Its negative implications are more easily demonstrated than its positive ones and they are more dramatic when extreme malnutrition exists. (See protein deficiency, Chap. 5.) Adults are sometimes skeptical of the nutrition-disease relationship when they cannot readily detect health benefits following an improvement of their own diets. It should be pointed out that amplifying an already adequate diet should not be expected to produce noticeable results. On the other hand, bringing a mediocre or borderline diet up to nutritional adequacy cannot fail to bolster the body's defenses. There is increasing evidence that this is the case even though the benefits are sometimes difficult to measure.

» NUTRITION AND BODY STRUCTURE

Can good nutrition make a difference in the structure of the body itself? Is the body a sturdier, better developed, and more effective mechanism as a result of good nutrition? Answers supplied by research apply both to the skeleton and to the soft tissues which, together, compose the body's foundation.

The Bony Framework

The progress of a child's developing bones can be followed by periodic X-rays. Usually the status of the bones of the wrist and hand is regarded as typical for the skeleton. To gauge the level of development at any one time, comparisons are made with representative X-ray pictures of the hands and wrists of children of similar age [9]. Minor variations from them may be meaningless, for there is increasing awareness of a wide normal range in skeletal development in children. However, wide divergence below the norm can indicate retardation that has delayed the maturing process.

What relation does this maturing process in bone bear to nutrition? A number of studies have shown that rate of bone calcification is influenced by the diet of the child. In these studies, improvement in skeletal development was achieved in various ways: by providing children with better school lunches; by supplementing their diets with plain milk, vitamin D milk or cod-liver oil. All children who received the improved diets showed greated progress in skeletal development than did the controls.

The retarding effect of prolonged undernutrition has been shown dramatically

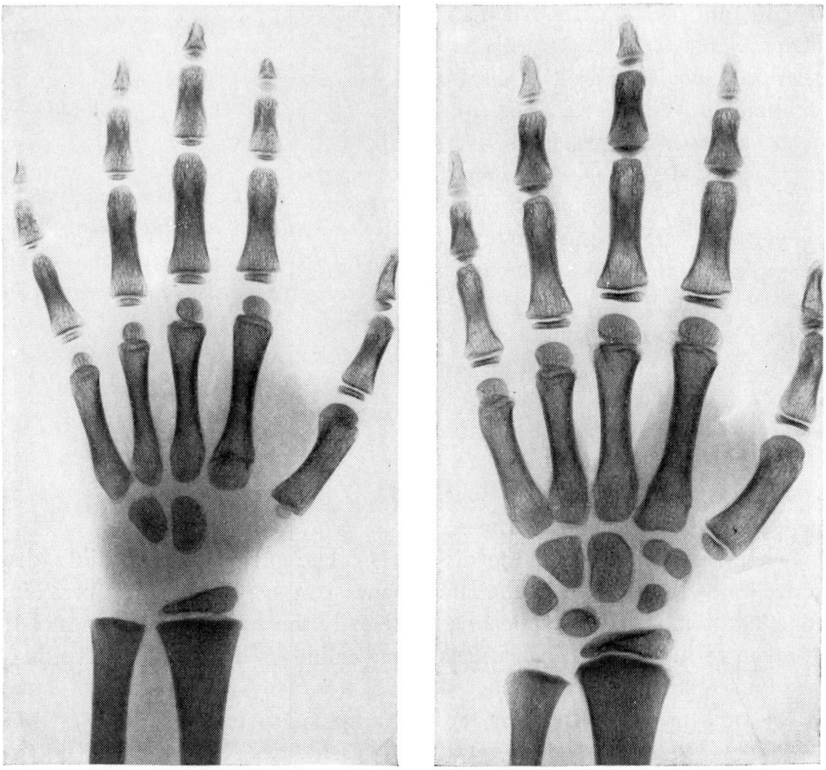

Fig. 2.4a and b Effect of known undernutrition (left) and known adequate nutrition (right) as shown by X-rays of hand skeletons of two 7-year-old boys. The X-ray on the left shows only 2 carpal centers; the one on the right, 7. The latter is regarded as normal for children of this age. (*Human Biology*, 30 [Dec. 1958], p. 258. Courtesy Samuel Dreizen, D.D.S., M.D.)

in a study of the development of the bones of the hands and wrists of several hundred children. In every poorly nourished child of both sexes there was delay in the development of the bones compared with those of well-nourished children of corresponding ages. Figure 2.4 demonstrates typical differences in the wrists of two 7-year-old children: the X-ray on the left shows the wrist of a poorly-nourished child in the study, the one on the right, the wrist of a child known to be well nourished. At the age of these children, about 7 carpal centers should be present. Only 2 are apparent in the wrist of the undernourished child. All 7 appear in the wrist of the well-nourished child [10].

Skeletal development as a measure of good and poor nutrition is also apparent in a study of native- and American-born Japanese children that is discussed later in this chapter. The larger and better fed American-born Japanese were consistently more advanced skeletally than those born and reared in Japan.

Teeth Teeth are a part of the bony structure of the body. Nutrition acts in two ways as a determining factor in susceptibility to tooth decay: by affecting the structure of the teeth and supporting tissues during their development, and by affecting the environment of the teeth after they have erupted. These relationships between nutrition and teeth have been established by well-controlled research on laboratory animals [11].

Similar studies can be carried on with human beings only when they are living under regulated dietary conditions for a considerable period of time. Such an opportunity presented itself in certain European countries during World War II when there was government-imposed food rationing. In general the rations then available differed from the usual food supplies in that sugar and other refined carbohydrates were reduced, with proportionate increases in whole-grain flours and vegetables, and a milk distribution plan was introduced that provided satisfactory amounts of milk for children and pregnant women.

The investigators in each country approached the problem differently, but the major findings were similar. In Norway detailed data were collected [12]. They showed that caries incidence in children decreased gradually during the rationing program in that country and that maximum reduction occurred 5–6 years after the start of the program (Fig. 2.5). This was the length of time needed for the development of the permanent teeth, prior to eruption. It was apparent that planned wartime rations played an important part in building teeth resistant to decay.

Following the war, even after food rationing had ceased, a low caries incidence continued for a time. Eventually it began to rise; the increase in caries apparently was related to postwar dietary changes (Fig. 2.5). Children and mothers were once more on free-choice diets. Sugar consumption rose, milk intake decreased, and highly milled, unenriched cereals were again available. It is believed that these postwar diets contributed not only to the development of caries-susceptible teeth but to the actual increase in caries in these vulnerable teeth, after they had erupted. (See Chap. 6 for further references to teeth and dental health.)

The Soft Tissues

The thickness of the layer of tissue that lies directly below the skin reflects developmental status in childhood [13]. This subcutaneous tissue is a repository for body

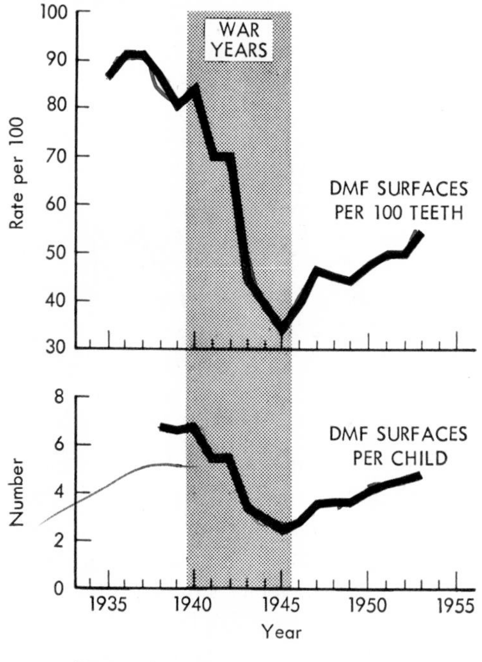

Fig. 2.5 Decrease in dental caries during war years when the diet of mothers and children was improved; increase in dental caries with the return of the usual diet. The figure shows the rate per 100 of carious surfaces in permanent teeth of first-grade children (7 years of age) in Oslo for the school years 1935–1936 through 1953–1954. War years include 1939–1940 through 1944–1945. (Adapted from Fig. 42, Toverud series on the teeth of children, *Milbank Memorial Fund Quarterly*, vol. 35.)

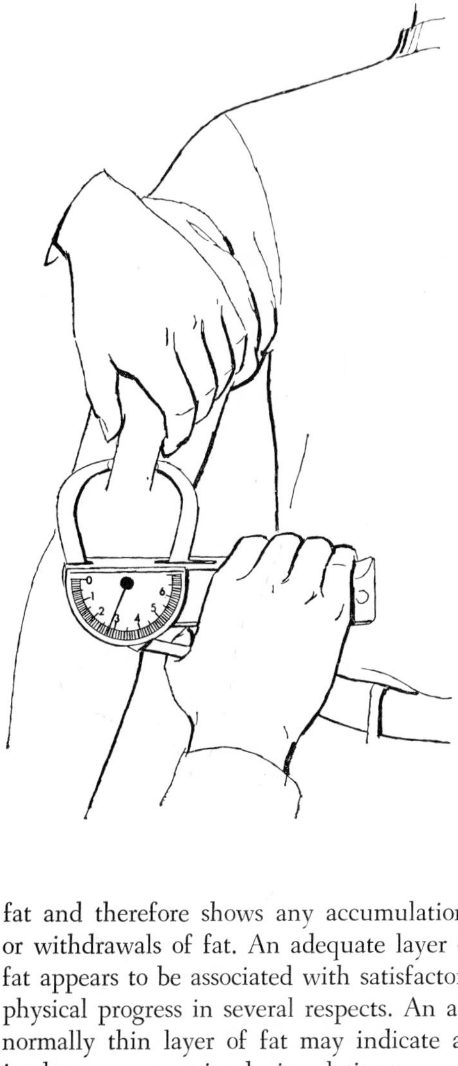

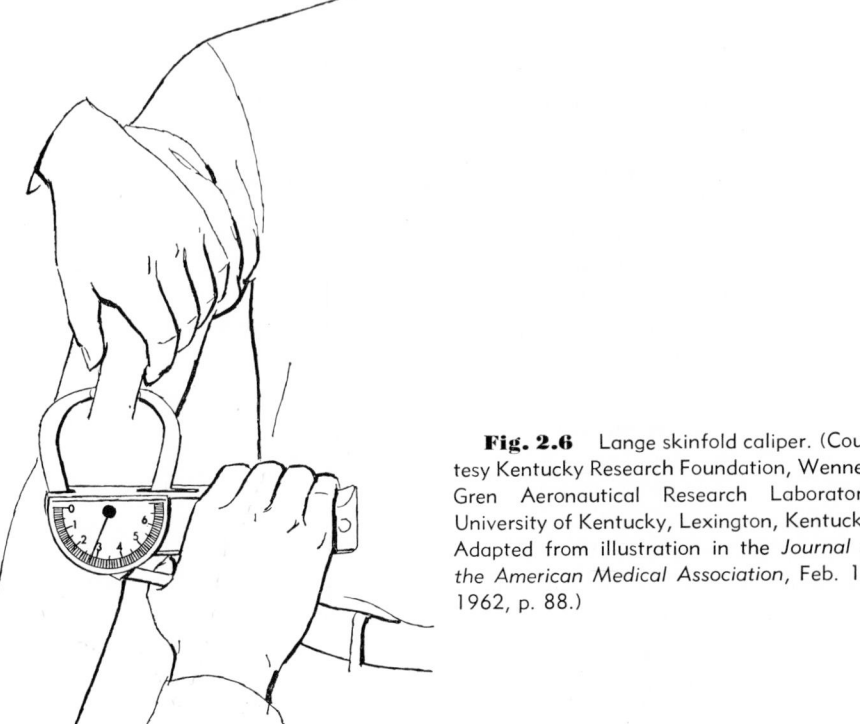

Fig. 2.6 Lange skinfold caliper. (Courtesy Kentucky Research Foundation, Wenner-Gren Aeronautical Research Laboratory, University of Kentucky, Lexington, Kentucky. Adapted from illustration in the *Journal of the American Medical Association*, Feb. 17, 1962, p. 88.)

fat and therefore shows any accumulations or withdrawals of fat. An adequate layer of fat appears to be associated with satisfactory physical progress in several respects. An abnormally thin layer of fat may indicate an inadequate energy intake in relation to need, which makes it impossible to store fat desirably. A very thick layer of fat, on the other hand, may indicate an oversupply of energy-producing foods in relation to energy expenditure.

A physician uses his thumb and index finger to take a rough measure of an individual's padding of fat. The same measure (skinfold thickness) is made more precisely in designated body areas with a caliper, a pincer-like instrument designed for the purpose (Fig. 2.6). X-rays offer still another method. They are used to record on film the thickness of the fat layer at specified points on the body [14]. Some progress has been made in developing norms for the second and third methods of measuring subcutaneous tissue. Their application would make it possible to discover how a person ranks with other individuals of the same age and sex with respect to thickness of the fat layer directly underneath the skin.

The size and firmness of muscles are also indications of nutriture. An adequate diet, especially one plentiful in muscle-building nutrients, contributes to well-grown, strong muscles, coordinated in action (See Chap. 3).

The nutrient content of the blood may be said to *reflect* the adequacy of the diet and to *forecast* the body's state of nutrition. This is because the blood is the carrier of nourishment to body parts [15]. The blood can nourish the tissues only to the extent that the diet provides the sources of the nourishment. A low concentration of a nutrient of the blood, such as ascorbic acid (vitamin C), may be evidence that the body is malnourished with respect to vitamin C. If the shortage is severe and continuous, outward evidences of vitamin C deficiency will eventually appear. (See Chap. 7.)

The Structure as a Whole

These elements of body structure—bones, teeth, fat, muscles, and blood—are thus separate symbols of the nutritive state of the body as a whole. Taken together, their status determines how the individual looks, acts, and feels. A person in excellent nutriture from infancy, for example, can expect to have a well-developed skeleton, with straight arms and legs, well-formed teeth and jaws; to exhibit a moderate padding of fat over bones and muscles that gives the body a suitably rounded contour, with neither too much nor too little body fat; to have firm, well-coordinated muscles that contribute to rhythmic movements and good posture; and finally, to have a blood supply that nourishes the cells and gives a healthy color to the skin and lips. It is safe to predict that most persons with these basic evidences of good nutrition will also have about them an air of buoyancy, alertness, and confidence that is unmistakably associated with excellent nutrition and vigorous health.

► *As a basis for class discussion, collect pictures of persons about your own age who, in your estimation, are examples of good and of poor nutriture.*

Use a mirror to roughly evaluate your own outward signs of good and of poor nutriture.

» NUTRITION AND BODY SIZE

Two chief factors determine the rate at which a person grows and the size which he attains: his inborn capacity to grow, and various environmental conditions, important among which is nutrition. The 2 are interdependent in the sense that heredity limits the final size a person may become; nutrition largely determines whether an individual achieves this limit. This concept has been aptly paraphrased: the blueprint is in the chromosomes, but the bricks and mortar are in the market basket.

There is considerable evidence to show that children are growing larger in this country, and that adults are attaining greater size. Data of the latter type are available from studies on comparable groups in successive generations [16].

Size Increases of Adults [17]

An increase in the size of adults has been demonstrated in college freshmen in this country. Entering students in 2 men's colleges were found to be 3 in. taller on the average in 1957 than freshmen three-quarters of a century earlier. During the same period their average weight increased about 20 lbs. Five percent of the freshmen were 6 ft tall and over in 1880; in 1955, 30 percent were in that height classification. During approximately the same period, freshmen in 2 women's colleges showed 2-in. increases in average height and 7-lb increases in average weight.

Similarly, comparisons of the heights of United States recruits for World Wars I and II showed the men to be on the average 67.5 in. tall and about 68.5 in. tall, respectively. In a comparative study of U.S. civilians for the period 1885–1908 and for the year 1955, both men and women in 1955 averaged at least 2 in. taller than those in the prevoius generation and they reached that height several years earlier.

Thus adults have gradually increased in size in this country. This should not be interpreted as meaning that larger size in itself is necessarily a desirable objective. However, it is a usual accompaniment of improved diet and better living conditions, which serve as measures of progress. The often-expressed fear that we will become a race of giants, if size increases continue, appears to be without foundation. A recent study of growth records shows that increases in average stature in successive generations of a population become progressively smaller as more individuals in the population attain what appears to be their full growth limits set by heredity [18].

Size Increases of Children

Children living under favorable economic conditions are almost always taller, heavier, and better developed at a given age than children living under poor conditions. In an analysis of studies conducted between the years 1873 and 1950, it was found that North American boys from poor homes were more than 2 in. shorter and 5 lbs lighter at a given age than those from wealthy homes. In Britain, at the completion of growth, the industrial group is 2 in. shorter than the professional group [19]. Diets poor in quality and quantity are more common at the low than at the high income level. Thus, inferior growth in children is associated with poor diet and economic status.

An Ohio Experiment Station report compares physical measurements of Ohio school children in the years 1939 and 1951 [20]. It indicates that even in as short a period as 12 years, children became larger, on the average (Fig. 2.7). For example, in 1951 boys and girls 9 years old were as large as 10-year-olds in 1939. Increases in height tended to be proportional to those in weight—that is, the 9-year-olds had about the same body build as the 10-year-olds, but the former grew at a faster rate. In 1951, relatively few of the children had what would be considered very poor diets. Undoubtedly this situation represents a gradual betterment in diet over the years as the

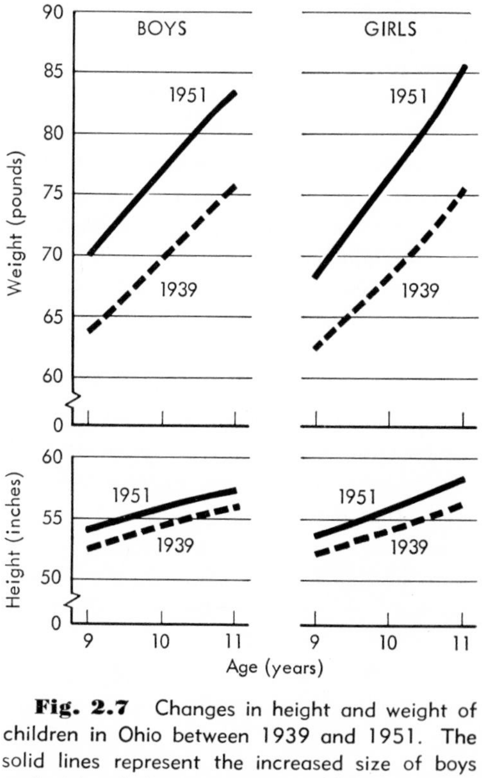

Fig. 2.7 Changes in height and weight of children in Ohio between 1939 and 1951. The solid lines represent the increased size of boys and girls of the same age in 1951. (Adopted M. B. Patton *et al.*, "Growth Patterns of Ohio School Children," *J. Am. Dietet. Assoc.*, 35 [May 1959], p. 459, Fig. 1.)

quality of the national food supply has been improved. And the improved diet has apparently helped children to attain more nearly the size set by heredity.

Sizes of Racial Groups

The small size of certain peoples has been popularly considered a racial characteristic, based on heredity. Thoughtful observers, however, have suggested that the effect of retardation of growth may be cumulative. Smaller size may appear to be an inherited trait, when, instead, it is the result of poor environmental conditions over successive generations. The soundness of this theory has been demonstrated in a recent study on Japanese children. It offers a rare opportunity to isolate hereditary and environmental influences and to evaluate them separately.

Japanese Children A comparison was made of the relative growth progress and development of Japanese children born and reared in their homeland and those born and reared in the United States [18]. Data were collected on nearly 900 American-born Japanese boys and girls 6–19 years of age living in the San Francisco Bay Area of California. These records were compared with those of children of the same sex and age in present-day Japan. The California Japanese children were found to be taller and heavier than the children of Japan. At every age considered in the study, the stature of the American-born Japanese boys exceeded that of the native-born Japanese boys by an amount (1.5–5 in.) greater than the increase that had taken place in the stature of boys in Japan during the preceding 53 years (1–2 in.). A similar superiority of stature was shown by American-born Japanese girls up to 14 years of age. Thereafter, although still considerable, this superiority was somewhat lessened, perhaps because of the relatively greater increase since 1900 in the average stature of Japanese women as compared with that of men.

Fig. 2.8 shows the height curves for boys born in California (highest), those born and reared in Japan in recent times (medium position), and those born in Japan about 50 years ago (lowest). It reveals that considerable progress was made in raising height levels in Japan in the past half century. But despite that increase, heights and weights of Japanese boys born and reared in this country are strikingly greater. Thus, heredity would seem to be ruled out as a limiting factor in the heights of Japanese people. The investigator believes the difference is due "rather to a more limited diet and to other less favorable environmental conditions existing in Japan" [18]. Another investigator has pointed out that during the period of improved growth in Japan, total

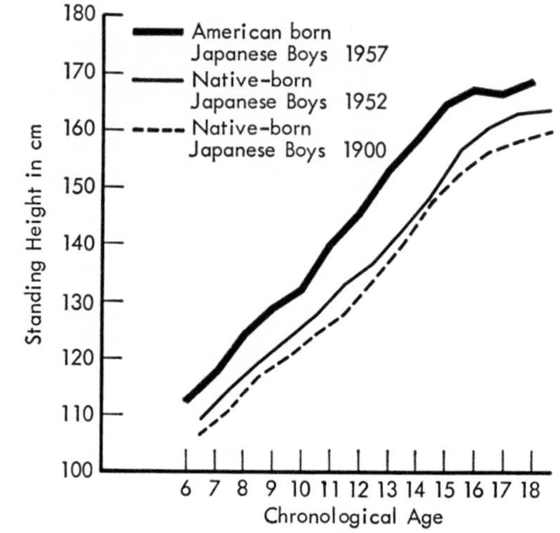

Fig. 2.8 Average standing height of American-born Japanese boys compared with that of boys in Japan, in 1900 and 1952. (Adapted from W. W. Greulich, "Growth of Children of the Same Race under Different Environmental Conditions," *Science*, *127* [March 7, 1958], p. 515, Fig. 1. Reprinted from *Science* by permission.)

protein consumption has increased about 10 perecent and that intake of animal protein has almost doubled [21].

Better Growth with Planned Dietary Improvements

Another way of showing the nutrition-growth relationship is by demonstrating an improvement in growth rate when additions are made to the diet. An adequate diet has been defined as one which is not susceptible of improvement as judged by growth and other signs of development. When growth can be improved by dietary supplementation alone, it may be assumed that the original diet was inadequate and that the supplement was responsible for the growth improvement.

There are many examples of this type of experimentation. A study in a British boarding school for boys was among the first of such inquiries [22]. The boys were housed on the cottage system. One cottage group served as the control while each of the others received a different supplement to the same basic diet. The chief food supplements were milk, cress, sugar, margarine or butter; each supplement yielded about 335 calories. There were other aspects of this experiment. But a primary finding was that any addition to the basic diet produced some improvement in growth (Fig. 2.9). The boys who received 1 pt of milk daily as a supplement had the greatest growth acceleration. On their original basic diet they made annual gains of 3.85 lbs in weight and 1.84 in. in height. These gains

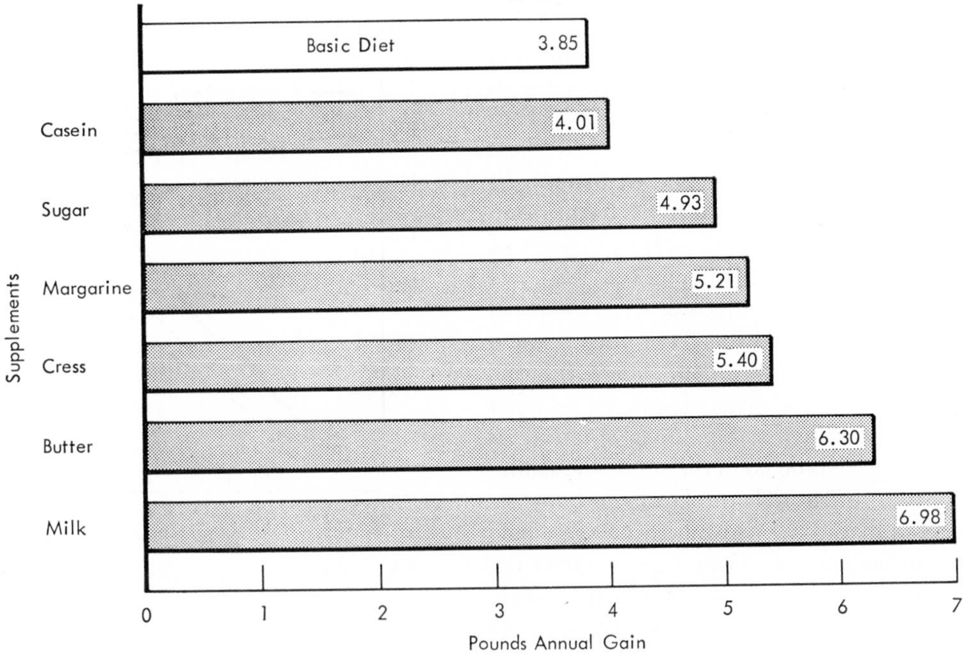

Fig. 2.9 Annual gains in weight made by British school boys with various dietary supplements, each added to the school diet of a different group. (Adapted from C. H. Mann, *Diets for Boys during the School Age*. London: Medical Research Council Special Report Series No. 105, 1926.)

increased to 6.98 lbs and 2.63 in. annually after the milk was added.

Many studies in this country and abroad have shown that practically any food added to existing diets of children can produce improved growth. These studies have been organized on different bases and many foods and food combinations have been tested, among them: figs, oranges, bananas, wheat germ, milk (in different quantities and kinds including whole and skim milk), biscuits, and sweet sandwiches. The amount of extra gains for which the supplements were responsible depended on the deficiency of the original diet and on the extent to which the supplements supplied the needed calories and missing nutrients.

Similar observations have been made, on a broad scale, on population groups. The children of western Europe, for example, showed measurable declines in growth progress during the period of diet deprivation of World War II. When food supplies were again ample, growth was resumed if starvation had not been prolonged.

A Fully Adequate Diet

The results obtained in studies with single food additions suggested the desirability of a study in which the diets of children were supplemented with all foods needed to meet generally accepted standards of dietary adequacy. Such a study was conducted in a boarding school for children, 2–14 years of age, by nutritionists at the University of Chicago [23]. The original institutional diet contained some of all the essential foods but not enough of them. Foods were added to make the diet fully adequate. Comparisons of the rate of gain in height and weight of the children were made before, during, and after the diet was improved. The beneficial effects were clear cut: in the period before improvement of the diet the group on the whole averaged 61 percent of its expected gain in weight; in the supplementation period this average rose to 140 percent; and gains continued at a high level in the period subsequent to the supplementation. The gains in height followed a similar pattern (Fig. 2.10). The children who had had the benefits of the improved diet regularly for a year showed better gains, by every basis of comparison, than did the children whose attendance was irregular and of shorter duration.

» NUTRITION AND LENGTH OF LIFE

Statistics show that people in this country are living longer now than at any time in history. A male 1 year of age in 1900 could expect to live 48 years; in 1956, he could expect to live 67 years. Comparable figures for women are even more favorable. In 1900, a female 1 year of age could expect to live 51 years; in 1956, nearly 74 years. Table 2-1 bears out these facts and provides additional information on the life expectancy of men and women, calculated at 50 and at 70 years of age.

TABLE 2-1

RELATIVE LIFE EXPECTANCY OF WHITE MALES AND FEMALES IN THE UNITED STATES (in years)*

Year of Life	1900 Males	1900 Females	1956 Males	1956 Females
1	48.2	51.1	67.2	73.7
50	20.8	21.9	23.1	27.7
70	9.0	9.6	10.3	12.2

* Adapted from Food—*The Yearbook of Agriculture.* Washington, D.C.: U.S. Department of Agriculture, 1959. p. 178.

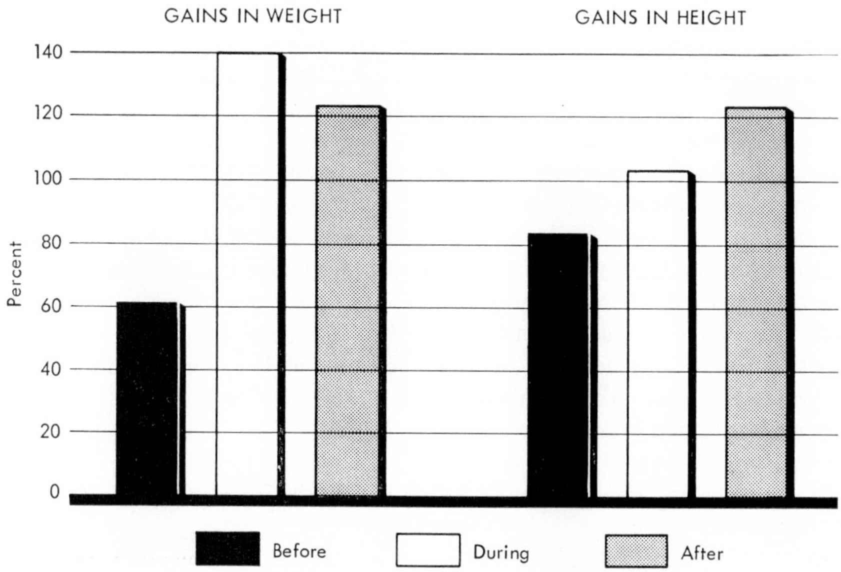

Fig. 2.10 Percentage of expected gains in weight and height made by children in a boarding school—on the regular institutional diet (before), during the time the diet was supplemented to make it nutritionally adequate, and after the experiment was terminated. (Adapted from Blair *et al.*, "Results of Providing a Liberally Adequate Diet to Children in an Institution," *J. of Pediatrics*, 27 [Nov. 1945].)

Has nutrition entered into this picture of lengthened life in the United States? Does nutrition make a difference in how long life will last? A full answer to these questions calls for examining the data and exploring the possible causes for the present favorable picture.[1]

A closer look at Table 2-1 will show that the greatest gains in life expectancy have been made in the earliest years of life. This is due to the drastically reduced death rate at this early age level. There are many reasons for the drop. Major among them is success in dealing with infectious diseases. Factors contributing to this success include advances in medical knowledge, improvements in sanitation, better medical care, and public health facilities. It is impossible to assess the exact proportionate role of nutrition in relation to other environmental factors in controlling the death rate in children. It is undoubtedly an important factor under all conditions—an overriding one in severe malnutrition. This relationship was suggested earlier in the discussion of the place of malnutrition in lowering body barriers to infectious disease. In countries where malnutrition and infectious disease continue severe, average life expectancies are as low as 35–45 years.

Table 2-1 shows that relatively small gains were made between 1900 and 1956 in life expectancy in this country in the ages above childhood. At 50 years of age the average woman gained about 6 years of life;

[1] National actuarial life expectancy tables are prepared at 10-year intervals from population and official statistics on birth and death by the National Office of Vital Statistics in the U.S. Department of Health, Education and Welfare.

at 70 years, she made a gain of less than 3 years. These minor increases are in sharp contrast to the nearly 23-year gain made in the life span at 1 year of age. The failure of the death rate to continue its rapid decline of early childhood into the mature years is responsible for this contrast. This situation leads to a consideration of the chief causes of death in middle and later lfe and the possibilities that exist for conquering diseases common at these periods. Obviously a striking drop in death rate in the mature years could lead to a significant increase in life expectancy for the average older person.

Chronic degenerative diseases are leading causes of death in adults. Heart diseases head the list [7]. In several of these conditions, the root of the disability lies in the arteries which undergo deteriorative changes, thus impairing their usefulness. There is some reason to believe that artery changes of this character are linked importantly to diet. (See Chap. 3.) If research now in progress confirms such a relationship it may also point to specific ways of preventing or reversing such changes. Thus, new discoveries in nutrition could be the means of adding many years to life.

Effective Living

Even at the present rate of life expectancy, older people make up a steadily growing segment of the population. They are confronted with the problem of maintaining a level of health that will enable them to remain productive and to enjoy those extra years. Merely adding length to life is not enough. Added years may actually be a burden unless they bring with them vigor and independence. Forming good food habits at any age helps, but the person who has been well nourished throughout life has the best prospect of sustaining this high nutritional level into the late years. A well-known figure in nutrition and public health fields has associated diet, health, and longevity, as follows: "Diet is one of the most important factors in determining how long an individual lives . . . even though you never suffer from acute malnutrition, years and years of improper eating will add up to various kinds of damages to your body that will eventually shorten your life. . . . While a good diet can't guarantee that you will be in good health, you can't be in the best of health unless you live on a good diet" [24]. (See Chap. 9 for diets for older people.)

» SEEING IS BELIEVING

Examples of the benefits of good nutrition have been confined here, as far as possible, to human beings because of their unquestioned applicability. This chapter would be incomplete, however, without referring to the backlog of research on animals that substantiates the human studies. Much of the most convincing data showing that nutrition is a positive factor in achieving good health is based on animal experimentation.

It is a matter of common knowledge that pets, laboratory animals, and farm animals all rely for health, strength, growth, biological performance, general appearance, and vigor on diets that are suitable and adequate for each species. To those who dismiss such information with the statement that animal needs are different from those of people and that research in one species does not apply to the other, this should be said: needs of the species do differ, physiological responses to individual nutrients may vary considerably, and specific findings are not always transferable, but both experimentation and careful observation of animal feeding and its results have demonstrated without a doubt a nutrition-health relationship that applies to man.

There are several advantages to animal research: short life span of animals, brief growth period, pure strains, and opportunity to feed highly restricted diets. Underfeeding of animals can result in gross body changes and in impairment of function, which makes irrefutable the nutrition-health relationship. For obvious reasons, this relationship cannot be as clearly demonstrated in people.

There is no more effective way of convincing children that nutrition makes a difference than with simple animal feeding demonstrations. Almost every sign of good and poor nutrition that we have considered in this chapter can be produced in a period of a few weeks by feeding two groups of laboratory-type animals on contrasting diets. Children can see for themselves that the well-fed animals have smooth, glossy coats and bright eyes; that they are lively, alert, and friendly; are strong, healthy, and active; that they grow rapidly in length and weight, and eat with good appetite and obvious enjoyment. Children can also see that the response of the poorly-fed animals is the opposite in appearance, behavior, growth, and attitude toward their food. These contrasts provide children with strong motivations for eating the foods that produced the favorable results.

» NUTRITION IS A SCIENCE

It is apparent from Chapters 1 and 2 that nutrition has its roots in the research of many fields, including medicine, physiology, chemistry, anthropology, and psychology. Out of this broad background has grown a body of knowledge that is the basis for the modern science of nutrition. But nutrition is not static. It is a growing science that changes and expands with the findings of research on which it feeds. The study of nutrition, therefore, is never completed; the problems are never all "settled." It constantly brings into focus new and old findings and raises new questions. Applied to everyday living, this concept of change in nutrition is a never-ending source of interest and challenge. The chapters that follow in Section Two introduce the study of nutrition as it is concerned with the nutritional needs of the human body and how to meet them, in light of *current* understandings.

REFERENCES

1. Keys, A., Brozek, J., Henschel, A., Mickelsen, O., and Taylor, H. L., *The Biology of Human Starvation.* Minneapolis: University of Minnesota Press, 1950. Vols. I, II.
2. Blanton, S., "Mental and Nervous Changes in the Children of the Volksschulen of Trier, Germany, Caused by Undernutrition," *Mental Hygiene,* 3 (July 1919) pp. 343–86.
3. Tuttle, W. W., Daum, K., Larsen, R., Salzano, J., and Roloff, L., "Effect on School Boys of Omitting Breakfast: Physiologic Responses, Attitudes and Scholastic Attainments," *J. Am. Dietet. Assoc.,* 30 (July 1954) pp. 674–77. (See Reference Nos. 1, 2, and 3 to article for reports of other age groups.)
4. Tuttle, W. W., and Herbert, E., "Work Capacity with No Breakfast and a Mid-morning Break," *J. Am. Dietet. Assoc.,* 37 (Aug. 1960) pp. 137–40.

5. Peel, R. M., and Dodds, M. L., "Nutritive Intake of Women Factory Employees," *J. Am. Dietet. Assoc.*, 33 (Nov. 1957) pp. 1150–53.
6. Scrimshaw, N. S., Taylor, C. E., and Gordon, J. E., "Interactions of Nutrition and Infection," *The Am. J. Medical Sciences*, 237 (March 1959) pp. 367–403.
7. National Office of Vital Statistics, *Mortality from Selected Causes—1959*. Vital Statistics—Special Reports, National Summaries, Vol. 54, No. 4, May 17, 1961. U.S. Department of Health, Education and Welfare, Public Health Service.
8. Johnston, J. M., *Nutritional Studies in Adolescent Girls and their Relation to Tuberculosis*. Springfield, Ill.: Charles C. Thomas, Publisher, 1953.
9. Greulich, W. W., and Pyle, S. I., *Radiographic Atlas of Skeletal Development of the Hand and Wrist*. 2nd ed. Stanford, Calif.: Stanford University Press, 1959.
10. Dreizen, S., Snodgrasse, R. M., Webb-Peploe, H., and Spies, T. D., "The Retarding Effect of Protracted Undernutrition on the Appearance of the Postnatal Ossification Centers in the Hand and Wrist," *Human Biology*, 30 (Dec. 1958) pp. 253–63.
11. Wohl, M. G., and Goodhart, R. S. (Eds.), *Modern Nutrition in Health and Disease*. 2nd ed. Philadelphia: Lea & Febiger, 1960. (Chap. 20, "Nutrition in Relation to Dental Medicine.")
12. Toverud, G., *The Milbank Memorial Fund Quarterly:*
    - I. "The Influence of War and Post-war Conditions on the Teeth of Norwegian School Children—Eruption of Permanent Teeth and Status of Deciduous Dentition," 34 (Oct. 1956) pp. 354–430.
    - II. "Caries in the Permanent Teeth of Children Aged 7–8 and 12–13," 35 (April 1957) pp. 127–96.
    - III. "Discussion of Food Supply and Dental Condition in Norway and Other European Countries," 35 (Oct. 1957) pp. 373–459.
13. Garn, S. M., and Haskel, J. A., "Fat Thickness and Developmental Status in Childhood and Adolescence," *Am. J. Diseases of Children*, 90 (June 1960) pp. 746–51.
14. Garn, S. M., "Roentgenogrammetric Determinations of Body Composition," *Human Biology*, 29 (Dec. 1957) pp. 337–53.
15. Morgan, A. F., *Nutritional Status U.S.A.*, Bull. 769. Berkeley: California Agricultural Experiment Station, University of California, Oct. 1959. ("Blood Composition, Relation to Diets," p. 46.)
16. Hathaway, M. L., *Heights and Weights of Children and Youth in the United States*. Home Economics Research Report No. 2. Washington, D. C.: U.S. Department of Agriculture, Oct. 1957.
17. ———, "Trends in Heights and Weights," *Food—The Yearbook of Agriculture*. Washington, D.C.: U.S. Department of Agriculture, 1959. p. 181.
18. Greulich, W. W., "A Comparison of the Physical Growth and Development of American-born and Native Japanese Children," *Am. J. Physical Anthropology*, 15 (Dec. 1957) pp. 489–515.
19. Leitch, I., and Boyne, A. W., "Recent Change in the Height and Weight of Adolescents," *Nutrition Abstracts and Reviews*, 30 (Oct. 1960) pp. 1173–86.
20. Patton, M. B., and Hunt, F. E., "Growth Patterns of Ohio School Children," *J. Am. Dietet. Assoc.*, 35 (May 1959) pp. 457–61.
21. Mitchell, H. S., "Nutrition in Relation to Stature," *J. Am. Dietet. Assoc.*, 40 (June 1962) pp. 521–24.

22. Mann, C. H., *Diets for Boys During the School Age.* London: Medical Research Council Special Report Series No. 105, 1926.
23. Blair, R., Roberts, L. J., and Greider, M., "Results of Providing a Liberally Adequate Diet to Children in an Institution: II. Growth in Height and Weight," *J. Pediatrics,* 27 (Nov. 1945) pp. 410–17.
24. Sebrell, H. W., "What to Eat to Live Longer," *U.S. News and World Report,* April 11, 1960, p. 90.

READINGS

Breakfast Source Book. Chicago: Cereal Institute, Inc., 1961.

Brozek, J., "Experimental Studies on the Impact of Deficient Diet on Behavior," *Review of Nutrition Research,* 20:6 (Nov.–Dec. 1959). New York: The Borden Company.

———, "Nutrition and Performance," *Nutrition News,* 21 (Dec. 1958) p. 13. Chicago: National Dairy Council.

Cowgill, G. R., "Evaluating Body Composition," *Review of Nutrition Research,* 19:6 (Jan.–Feb. 1958) New York: The Borden Company.

"Dairy Products and Dental Caries," *Nutrition Reviews,* 18 (Feb. 1960) 49–51.

Eppright, E. S., "The Power of Good Nutrition," *Food and Nutrition News,* 32 (June 1961) p. 1. Chicago: National Livestock and Meat Board.

Everson, G. J., "Bases for Concern About Teenagers' Diets," *J. Am. Dietet. Assoc.,* 36 (Jan. 1960) pp. 17–21.

Greulich, W. W., "Growth of Children of the Same Race under Different Environmental Conditions," *Science,* 127 (March 7, 1958) pp. 515–16.

Hathaway, M. L., "Heights and Weights of Adults in the United States," *Nutrition News,* 24 (April 1961) p. 5. Chicago: National Dairy Council.

Heath, B. H., Hopkins, C. E., and Miller, C. D., "Physiques of Hawaii-born Young Men and Women of Japanese Ancestry, Compared with College Men and Women of U.S. and England," *Am. J. Physical Anthropology,* 19 (June 1961) pp. 173–84.

Hill, M. M., "Nutrition Activities Promote Dental Health," *Nutrition Committee News,* (Jan.–Feb. 1961). Washington, D.C.: U.S. Department of Agriculture.

Hundley, J. M., "Statistics of Health," *Food—The Yearbook of Agriculture.* Washington, D.C.: U.S. Department of Agriculture, 1959. p. 175.

Martin, E. A., *Roberts' Nutrition Work With Children.* Chicago: The University of Chicago Press, 1954. ("Effects on Physical Growth," pp. 164–74.)

Patton, M. B., Tyrrell, D., Carver, A. F., Hunt, F. E., and Thornbury, M., *Nutrition of a Group of School Children in Ohio with Improved Diets.* Research Bull. 887. Wooster: Ohio Agricultural Experiment Station, July 1961.

Scrimshaw, N. S., "Nutrition and Infection," *Food and Nutrition News,* 31 (May 1960) p. 1. Chicago: National Livestock and Meat Board.

Weiss, R. L., and Trithart, A. H., "Between-meal Eating Habits and Dental Caries Experience in Preschool Children," *Am. J. Public Health,* 50 (Aug. 1960) pp. 1097–1104.

SECTION TWO

The Science of nutrition

This section presents certain fundamentals of the science of nutrition. It is not intended as an exhaustive treatment of the subject. A primary aim is to help students attain a degree of independence in applying their learnings in nutrition. And a functional knowledge is based on experience. Experience in this situation results from actually handling some of the tools of the science of nutrition. It means knowing and applying dietary criteria and becoming familiar with the nutrient values of common foods. It means knowing how to calculate a simple dietary and to recognize wherein nutrient shortages lie. This method has proved effective in demonstrating that food selection makes a difference in dietary adequacy.

Persons who analyze their own food habits and their own food intakes, as suggested in Sections One and Two, are known to be motivated to improve their patterns of eating. It is therefore urged that students follow this procedure whenever possible. However, for those classes too restricted by the time limits of the course to do so, exhibits are provided in the text. These include specimen food lists, meal records, weight charts and calculated diets to be used as bases for class discussions.

CHAPTER 3

How food nourishes the body

It is evident from Section One that the kinds and amounts of foods you eat from day to day largely determine whether you are well or poorly nourished. Common foods provide those substances which form the structure of your body, keep it running smoothly, and furnish the energy for everything you do. It is literally true that the meat, vegetables, fruits, milk and cereals you eat miraculously become a part of you. And how well they succeed as builders of bone, muscle, and blood depends on how well you choose what you eat. Wise choice of foods depends on knowing about the substances foods provide and how they nourish you.

Nutrition begins with food. And you are most familiar with foods as you eat them at breakfast, lunch, dinner, and as snacks. If you were to recall what you ate yesterday the record might look something like the sample at the top of page 42.[1]

It is apparent that your meals may include as many as 20 different food items during the day. (Refer to your own 3-day meal record, Chap. 1.) However, each of those items fits naturally into a grouping with other foods, similar in composition and use. Thus the separate food items may be classified into a small number of food groups, as shown in the list at the top of page 42.

A similar analysis of many menus would yield essentially the same results. You would merely have different examples of food items classified under the same few main headings. Obviously such groupings are a convenience for checking meals for variety in selection. But, more important, they are helpful in the initial planning of nutritionally adequate meals. Each food group makes distinctive contributions to the total food for the day and the complete assortment of the foods you choose determines the quantity and quality of your food intake.

» A WORKING KNOWLEDGE OF NUTRITION

To acquire a working knowledge of nutrition, foods are studied from 2 standpoints:

As *"wholes"*—the foods themselves, which fit together in good tasting, satisfying, nutritionally adequate meals

As "parts"—those individual dietary substances which, in varying amounts and combinations, constitute the "whole" foods (It is in terms of these

[1] This sample diet is not intended as a model in any sense; see footnote 2, Chapter 4.

Breakfast	Lunch	Snack	Dinner	Snack
Fruit juice	Baked beans	Soft drink	Hamburger	Cupcake
Breakfast food	Celery		Potato	
sugar	Apple sauce		Green beans	
milk	Gingerbread		Cabbage slaw	
Toast	Milk		Rolls	
Jelly			Lemon meringue pie	
Coffee				

Food Groups	Examples of Food Items on the Menu
Milk group	Milk
Meat group	Hamburger, baked beans
Vegetable group	Celery, potato; green beans, cabbage
Fruit group	Fruit juice, apple sauce
Bread-cereal-group	Breakfast food, toast, gingerbread, rolls
Fats group	Spread for bread, fat for potato and other vegetables
Sweets group	Sugar, jelly, soft drink, pie, cake

specific substances that daily human nutritional requirements have been established.)

The individual dietary substances—the "parts"—will be considered in the present Section, as background to an understanding of foods, as "wholes" in Section Three of this text.

» THE PARTS OF FOODS: THEIR COMPOSITION

There are some 50 known nutrients—separate chemical substances in foods, each known by a different name. Fortunately, similarity of content and function makes it possible to narrow down this long list of nutrients to 6 classes as follows:

Nutrient Classes:

Proteins	Mineral elements
Fats	Vitamins
Carbohydrates	Water

Proteins, fats, carbohydrates, and water are by far the most abundant nutrients in foods. They account for almost the total weight of the nutrients in the diet. The mineral elements as a class, although in much smaller quantity, rank next. The vitamins, so important nutritionally, occur in amounts too small to be demonstrated quantitatively except by special methods in the laboratory. The kinds and assortments of mineral elements and of vitamins present in foods are more important than total quantities of either nutrient class.

Each nutrient has its own specific functions but no nutrient acts independently of other nutrients. Examples of the ways nutrients are dependent on each other and work together to achieve results will be cited throughout this section.

Most foods are composed of more than one nutrient class. It is customary to identify foods loosely according to their quantitative contributions of proteins, fats, and carbohydrates. For example, when a food contains more protein than carbohydrate or fat it is usually known as a *protein* food; one with more fat than protein or carbohydrate is often called a *fat* food; one with more carbohydrate than protein or fat is referred to as a *carbohydrate* food. This rule holds in spite of the fact that there are many exceptions, some of which are cited in the following discussion of these classes. There are obvious limitations to any plan that does not take into account all of the nutrient classes in foods or the fact that some foods supply significant amounts of all three nutrients under consideration—proteins, fats, and carbohydrates. Nevertheless, there is need to know and to understand the basis for a terminology widely applied in nutrition.

The bar graphs a, b, and c in Fig. 3.1 showing the percentages of protein, fat, carbohydrate, mineral elements (total ash), and water in a few typical foods illustrate how the composition of a food qualifies it, in most cases, to be labelled as a protein, a fat or a carbohydrate food. Food values pertain to forms of the foods as they are purchased in market.

Protein Foods (Fig. 3.1a)

Lean meats, fish, poultry, and eggs can obviously be considered protein foods because they yield more proteins than they do fats or carbohydrates. However, there are exceptions to the rule in so classifying foods. Dry legumes (dry peas and beans) are included in the protein class even though their carbohydrate content is higher than their protein. This exception is made because their protein contribution is a significant one—much higher than that of other vegetables—and dry legumes provide inexpensive alternates for the meat group. Nuts, particularly peanuts, are also classified as proteins for essentially the same reasons, in spite of the fact that they contain more fats than proteins.

Milk and cheeses are usually classed as protein foods even though whole milk has slightly more carbohydrate and fat than protein, and commonly used hard cheeses, such as cheddar, have more fat than protein. Both foods may provide a significant amount of protein in the daily diet. A child of early school age, for example, may obtain half his daily requirement of protein from a quart of milk. When cheese is eaten in quantity (2 oz) as the main dish of a meal, the protein yield is also significant.

Certain meats, such as ham (not shown on the chart), are higher in fat than in protein. Nevertheless, if the lean of such meats is the part chiefly eaten, they qualify as protein foods. Meats are distinctive in that fat which is cooked out of them may not be used, and edge fat is often cut off and discarded.

Fat Foods (Fig. 3.1b)

Fats, oils, fat spreads, oil dressings, and meats composed largely of fat, such as salt pork, belong to the class of fat foods. Cooking fats and salad and cooking oils are 100 percent fat. Butter and margarine contain negligible amounts of protein and carbohydrate. Bacon has proportionately more of these two nutrients, particularly protein, as shown in Figure 3.1b. Crisp, drained bacon may lose a large part of its fat in preparation. Even so, the relatively smaller amount of protein in a serving of bacon prevents it from qualifying as a full alternate to lean meats as a source of protein. Salad dressings are made from several ingredients and vary in content. However, mayonnaise is predominantly fat and French dressing is sufficiently higher in fat than in other nutrient classes to qualify for this

Fig. 3.1 Composition of Foods. Percent of protein, fat, carbohydrate, water, and ash.

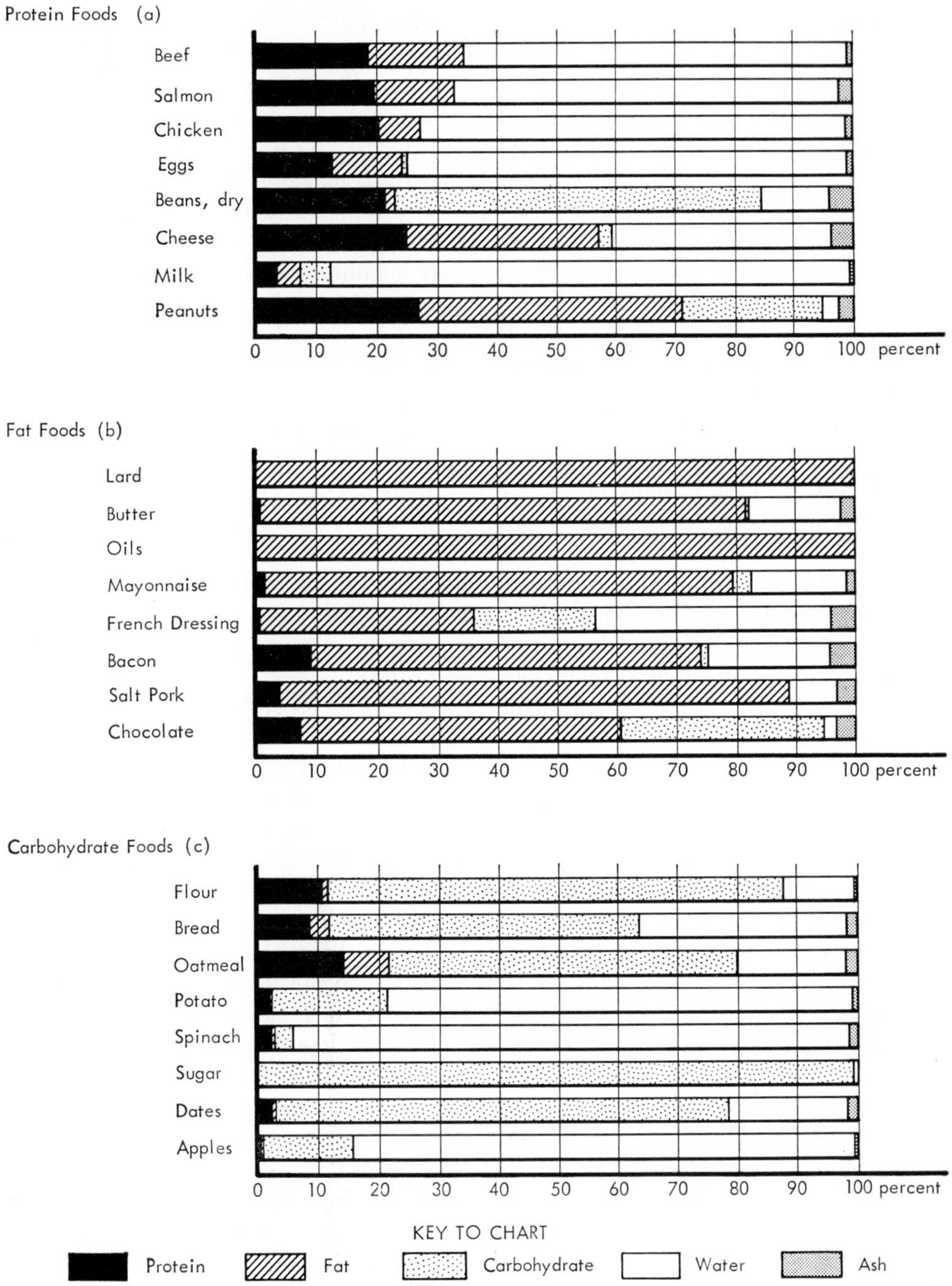

Data From Table 1, Agriculture Handbook No. 8, U.S. Department of Agriculture

grouping. Bitter chocolate is a concentrated food with fat making up more than half its content.

Carbohydrate Foods (Fig. 3.1c)

Flours, breads, cereals, and sweets are classed as carbohydrate foods. Almost all foods shown in Figure 3.1c are composed of distinctly more carbohydrates than of other nutrients. Sugar is the only food shown that is virtually 100 percent carbohydrate. Honey, jellies, jams, and candies are other sweets that rank high as carbohydrate foods.

Vegetables as a whole are higher in carbohydrates than in proteins and fats, but proportions vary greatly. Potatoes, for example, are concentrated sources of carbohydrates in comparison with leafy vegetables of higher water content, such as spinach. Essentially the same situation exists with respect to fruits; dates, which are relatively concentrated, are regarded as carbohydrate-rich, whereas juicy fresh apples are a more dilute source.

Figure 3.1 and the accompanying discussions show that most basic foods can be grouped loosely under 1 of these 3 nutrient classes—proteins, fats or carbohydrates. This system of classifying foods arose because these nutrient classes were the first to be recognized, and because, quantitatively, they overshadow the mineral elements and vitamins. That it is a useful system of classification will be apparent as this section develops. Such grouping, however, should not obscure the total concept of body nourishment, which includes a variety of mineral elements (represented in the figure as ash), and a large number of vitamins, each almost infinitesimal in quantity. Practically all foods contain mineral elements and vitamins of varying kinds, amounts, and proportions. As we proceed, it will be evident that many foods *within* the protein, fat, and carbohydrate classifications, are best known for their distinctive contributions of certain mineral elements and/or vitamins.

Nutrients from the 6 classes occur in different amounts and in different associations in foods, thus making nutritionally different even those foods which seem on the surface to be alike. You will want to know first the nature of these nutrients and what changes they must undergo before they can be useful to your body—before they can become a part of you.

» HOW THE BODY "PROCESSES" FOOD FOR ITS OWN NOURISHMENT [1]

Nutrients are taken into the body in complex assortments in the foods you eat. The nutrients must then be separated and simplified before your body can put them to work. Foods are "brought into the nutritional service" of the body by the intricate processes of digestion, absorption and assimilation. A thorough understanding of these processes requires a background in chemistry and physiology. The brief résumé that follows does not consider the subject in depth. It will merely help you to understand the relationship of the food you eat to the ultimate nourishment of your body and to appreciate the fact that you cannot expect to be well nourished unless the nutrients you need are present in adequate amounts in the foods you select.

Digestion of Foods

The word "digestion" refers to the processes by which nutrients are changed into their simplest forms and become liquids, ready for absorption from the lower part of the digestive tract. The digestive tract is composed of the mouth, stomach, small intestine, and large intestine (Fig. 3.2). At various points in this tract, foods are broken down by chemical and mechanical means, which work together. They are broken down chemically when then are acted upon by digestive juices (enzymes). They are broken down mechanically when moved along the digestive tract by different types of muscular contractions and waves, which mix and churn the food mass.

Absorption and Utilization of Nutrients

Absorption and utilization of the simple liquid forms of the nutrients begin when digestion is completed. Absorption of nutrients into the blood takes place largely through the walls of the small intestine. In the lining of the intestinal walls are large folds with tiny hairlike structures called "villi." These villi are constructed of blood and lymph channels, which carry the digested, liquefied material into larger vessels for passage throughout the body. With the blood stream serving as the conveyor, nutrients are carried to every cell in every tissue of the body. The chemical process that takes place in cells to build tissue or release energy is called metabolism. It is at this point that the adequacy of the diet meets its real test. Does the diet provide all of the nutrients in the amounts the body cells require? Or, are there shortages which, if continued, will result in poorly nourished cells and, eventually, in a poorly nourished person?

Although all nutrients undergo the same general processes, they differ in the sections of the tract where they are digested, in the particular digestive enzymes that act on them, in their final digestive products, and in the specific pathways they take to reach the body parts to be nourished. As will be seen, whether all the required nutrients are present simultaneously at the point of need is an important consideration. A brief review of individual nutrient classes will clarify the ways in which nutrients are made serviceable to the body.

Digestion and Disposition of Carbohydrates [2]

All carbohydrates are of 2 general kinds—*starches* and *sugars*. These are similar in structure, and their breakdown in the body follows the same general pattern: both are reduced in digestion to the same simple forms, ready for absorption and use.

Starches are actually only complex forms of sugar. When starch is eaten, a digestive enzyme in the saliva of the mouth mixes with the starch and begins the digestive process. As the food is swallowed, this step continues in the stomach. Starch is now being converted to sugars. In the small intestine, digestive enzymes from the pancreas and from the walls of the intestine itself complete the process. The final products are single sugars. We have a similar transformation when sugar replaces starch in the ripening of fruits. Cellulose, a starch-like carbohydrate present in bulky vegetable tissues, is not digested by humans. It is important in the mechanics of the digestive process, however, because it provides bulk and thus aids in discarding residues of digestion.

When sugars are eaten they are in 1 of 2 forms: *single* sugars, which is the simplest form, ready for body use, or *double* sugars, which must be broken down by digestive enzymes into 2 single sugars. An example of a double sugar is the ordinary table variety made from cane or beet juice. Digestion of double sugars takes place in the small intestine, as described in the pre-

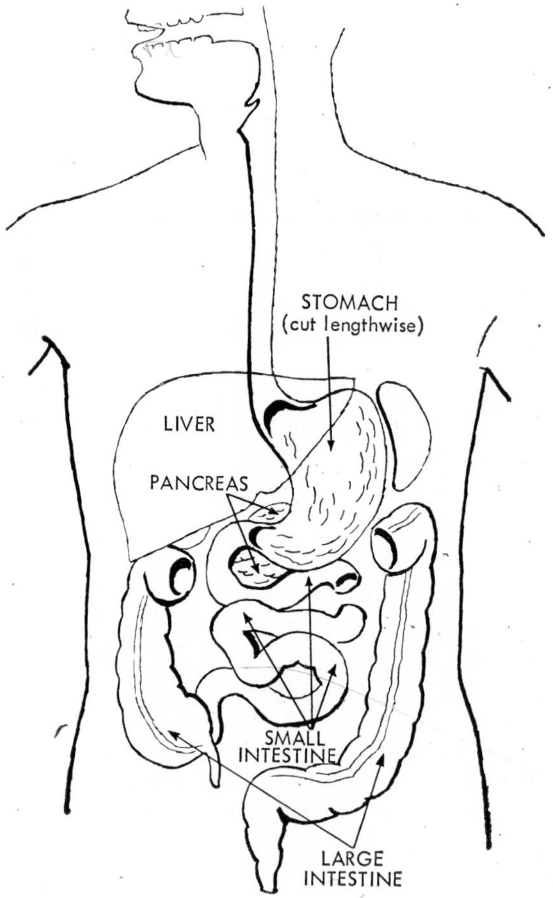

Fig. 3.2 Diagram of the digestive tract. (Adapted from *Today's Health*, published by the American Medical Association.)

ceding paragraph. Single sugars are not commonly eaten, as such. They are found chiefly as ingredients of fruits and vegetables. They need no digestive action and they reach the small intestine ready for absorption.

Single sugars, chiefly in the form of glucose, are now ready to be of "nutritional service" to the body, whether they have been eaten as starch or as sugar. They are absorbed through the walls of the small intestine and enter the circulation through the portal vein. They pass through the liver and on to other body parts. As the blood flows to the tissues, glucose is taken out to carry on the work of the muscles (exercise) and the internal work of the body.

Only a very small amount of carbohydrate is stored as such; about two-thirds of it is stored in the muscles as glycogen, known as animal starch; about one-third is stored in the liver as glycogen; and a small but essential amount is retained in the blood as glucose—blood sugar. The glucose level of the blood normally remains stable. When in use, muscles have their carbohydrate needs replenished by glucose from the blood. The blood sugar, in turn, is replenished by glycogen from the liver, which has been changed back to glucose. Glucose can be provided by fats and proteins as well as by carbohydrates. Likewise, excess carbohydrates can be converted to fat in the body and used as such, or stored as body fat (Table 3-1).

Digestion and Disposition of Fats [3,4,5,6]

Digestion of fats takes place chiefly in the small intestine. Here, the emulsifying action of bile from the liver assists in bringing the fat into contact with fat-splitting digestive enzymes from the pancreas and from the intestinal walls. The final products of these actions are two simpler forms of fat: fatty acids and glycerol. These are absorbed through the walls of the small intestine. During the passage, some of them are believed to be reunited and to enter the circulation as microscopic droplets of fat. The droplets of fat are not in true solution in the blood but are in suspension, much as the fat of homogenized milk. Transportation may be either via the portal vein or via the lymph vessels and thoracic duct. The end products of fat digestion are carried by the blood directly to the body tissues. Here, as with glucose, the fat is used to carry on the work of the muscles and the internal activities of the body.

Fat that is not needed immediately is stored as body fat. When needed, it is moved into the blood stream again and is drawn upon by the tissues. Since carbohydrates and proteins can be converted into fat in the body, all foods are potential sources of body fat (Table 3-1). The amount of stored fat, therefore, reflects the total amount of food that has been eaten in excess of immediate energy needs. About one-half of the body fat is stored directly under the skin; other stored fat serves as a protective covering for internal organs.

Fatty acids, end products of fat digestion, fall into two groups: *saturated* and *unsaturated.* Saturated fatty acids predominate in fats that are solid at room temperature. The name is derived from the fact that they contain as much hydrogen as their carbon atoms will hold—they are "satisfied" or saturated. Unsaturated fatty acids predominate in fats that are liquid at room temperature. They are *un*satisfied or *un*saturated because 2 or more hydrogen atoms are missing. They may become saturated by hydrogenation (adding hydrogen), thus changing a soft fat into a solid one. Methods have been developed recently whereby a liquid fat, rendered semisolid, may retain a considerable amount of its *un*saturated fatty acids. The terms *vegetable* fat and *animal* fat are not definitive terms with respect to their degree of saturation. Beef and pork fats, for example, are relatively low in unsaturated fatty acids; poultry fat is relatively high. Most vegetable oils, on the other hand, are high in unsaturated fatty acids; coconut oil is low.

Certain unsaturated fatty acids are known as *essential* fatty acids. They are so named because they must be provided by foods—that is, they cannot be synthesized by the body—and because they have specific body functions. The amount of linoleic acid, an essential fatty acid, in foods is indicative of their total essential fatty acid value. Figure 3.3 shows the percentage of linoleic acid in a wide variety of fats from plant and animal sources.

A deficiency of essential fatty acids has long been linked with certain types of skin disorders. More recently, essential fatty acids have been associated with the occurrence of the fatlike substance, cholesterol, and its level in the blood. It appears possible that diets rich in unsaturated fatty acids may help to keep fatty deposits, high in cholesterol content, from forming in the linings of the arteries, whereas diets rich

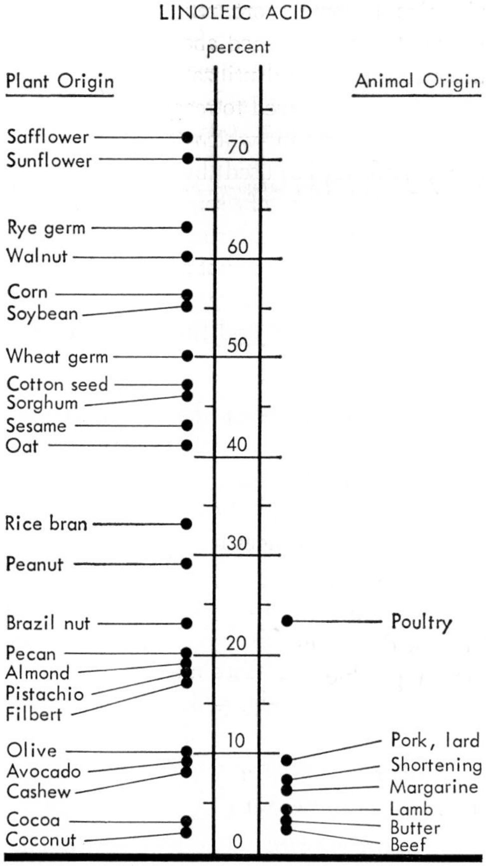

Fig. 3.3 Percentage of linoleic acid in fats and oils of plant and animal origin. (C. M. Coons, "Fatty Acids in Foods," *J. Am. Dietet. Assoc., 34:3* [March 1958], p. 242.)

in saturated fatty acids may fail to do so. The significance of these observations lies in the relationship of the artery deposits to obstruction of the blood flow and the possible onset of a coronary thrombosis if the obstruction occurs in the coronary artery. It should be emphasized that research on this problem continues and that findings to date are incomplete. Other nutritional factors, including excess total fat intake and body overweight, are believed to be involved in the cause of coronary artery disease. In view of the preliminary nature of the findings of research, major changes in the present concept of an adequate diet for healthy persons, with respect to fats, are not indicated [3].

Digestion and Disposition of Proteins

Digestion of proteins begins in the stomach, where they are acted upon by gastric juice (hydrochloric acid and digestive enzymes), and continues in the small intestine, where intestinal and pancreatic juices complete the process [1]. Amino acids are the final products of protein digestion. They are the simplest forms—the fragments—to which proteins are reduced. Amino acids, in watery solution, are absorbed through the walls of the small intestine into the blood stream. They are carried via the portal vein to the liver and thence to the tissues and organs of the body. The tissues and organs have the capacity to select from the amino acids in the blood the ones they need for building, sustaining, and repairing their own structures. In so doing, the amino acids are regrouped into combinations needed for new and rebuilt tissues, or for making certain active compounds, such as hormones. If the diet fails to provide proteins that yield the amounts and kinds of amino acids required for these functions, the body stands to suffer the consequences eventually.

Amino acids differ from the final products of carbohydrate and fat digestion chiefly in that they provide nitrogen *in addition to* carbon, hydrogen, and oxygen. It is in this respect that proteins are distinctive, for nitrogen is essential to the development, maintenance, and life of every cell of the body, and thus to life itself. But the contribution of amino acids (proteins) to the energy needs of the body should not be overlooked. When, in the regrouping process described above, there are amino acids left over, they are returned to the liver. Here the nitrogen is removed and excreted from the body. The carbon, hydrogen, and oxygen that remain can be used for energy, just as when they are supplied by carbohydrates and fats. If the energy is not needed at once, body fat is formed and stored for future use (Table 3-1).

Absorption and Disposition of Other Classes of Nutrients

Mineral elements, vitamins, and water are not acted upon by digestive juices as are proteins, fats, and carbohydrates. They are absorbed practically as they occur after being freed from foods during the digestive process.

Mineral Elements Most mineral salts are easily soluble in water. They are absorbed through the walls of the small intestine into the blood stream and are carried to the tissues where they are used as needed. The absorption of certain minerals is handled differently. These variations are covered in Chapter 6, which discusses mineral elements in some detail. Unlike most other nutrients, mineral elements are not "used up" in the body. Nor do they provide energy for body work. When they have discharged their building and regulatory functions in the tissues, they are discarded. A regular supply of mineral elements in the diet is thus essential in order to make good their constant turnover and loss.

Vitamins There is little exact information about the absorption of vitamins from the digestive tract. It is believed that the water-soluble vitamins enter the blood along with other water-soluble nutrients, such as amino acids and glucose. And fat-soluble vitamins probably accompany the fats. As chemical methods for detecting vitamins become more reliable, more will undoubtedly be learned about pathways for their absorption and utilization in the body. Vitamins are believed to reach the tissues in the same form in which they enter the body, and to be used by the tissues as needed. Excesses of some vitamins are stored; excesses of others are discarded from the body. Vitamins are not sources of energy for work, but they serve in multiple ways in the development and functioning of the body.

Water Water is the chief solvent of all the nutrients. As pointed out earlier, nutrients are reduced to a liquid state in digestion, in preparation for absorption. Water brings the digestive enzymes into the digestive tract and carries the products of digestion through the intestinal wall into the blood, which is largely composed of water. The blood distributes nutrients to the cells of the body, which are bathed in water. And finally, some of the waste products from the cells are removed from the body in the urine, which is largely water.

Food Additives The above discussion of the "processing" of foods in the body assumes that the nutrients—the separate chemical substances—occur naturally in the foods. This section would be incomplete without brief reference to those chemical additives, or food additives, which become a part of foods and food mixtures through intentional or incidental inclusion. Several hundred different substances come under the heading of *intentional* food additives. They are added purposely to better the product in some way or to enhance its use. Examples of additives used to improve the nutritive value of foods are: iodine added to salt to make iodized salt, vitamin A, which is added to margarine, and vitamin D, which is added to milk. Such additives will be referred to and explained at appropriate points in the text. Chemicals that are added to foods to improve appearance, texture, and keeping qualities include: stabilizers, preservatives, colorings, sweeteners, and flavorings. The manner in which the body "processes" each food additive depends on the chemical make-up of the individual additive.

Incidental additives are those which become a part of foods unintentionally. This may occur at different stages in the growing, harvesting, or marketing of foods. Residues from pesticide sprays, used in the growing of vegetables, are an example of undesirable incidental additives. The public is protected from harmful food additives of any type by federal law, administered by the Federal Food and Drug Administration [7, 8,9].

In a broad sense, radioactive materials in the atmosphere become incidental additives to food. They are always present in the air and soil to some degree, but after atmospheric tests of nuclear weapons the amounts are increased. Food and water become carriers as the result of fallout. Certain of the radioactive substances are potentially dangerous to health when they are concentrated in the body. Designated federal agencies have the responsibility for regularly assaying food and water supplies for their content of specified radioactive materials, for establishing limits beyond which the intake of such materials may be harmful, and for undertaking measures to curtail intakes when it seems desirable to do so [10].

» THE SERVICES PERFORMED BY NUTRIENTS

The 6 classes of nutrients, which we may now assume are available in usable form, serve the body in three ways:

For growth, and to sustain its own structures: proteins, mineral elements, vitamins, water

To control and coordinate its internal processes: vitamins, mineral elements, amino acids, water

To provide energy for its activities, and heat to keep it warm: fats, carbohydrates, proteins

As indicated, all nutrient classes serve in one or more capacities. But there is greater overlapping in function and there are more interrelationships between the actions of nutrients than was once thought. Nutrients are therefore grouped here under their main functions merely for convenience in discussion. It must be understood that each—alone, and with other nutrients—contributes in many and intricate ways to the nourishment of the body.

For Growth and to Sustain Body Structure

Proteins, mineral elements, vitamins, and water nourish the bones, muscles, organs, and blood, which make up the body. There is no more dramatic demonstration of their contribution than that of a child's increase in size from infancy to fully developed adulthood. This increase in bulk is evidence of the gradual enlargement during the growth process of bones, organs, and muscles, and of the increased volume of blood. We have only to consider the inferior physiques of peoples who have been deprived of proper nourishment to appreciate the importance of adequate nutrient intakes throughout life.

The bones (skeleton) and teeth form the rigid foundation of the body. They are made hard and strong by certain mineral elements deposited on a delicate framework that is composed chiefly of proteins. If bones grow normally they acquire more and more of the mineral elements. Figure 3.4 illustrates normal increases in the mineral content (calcium) of bones with increases in age and size. Average amounts of body calcium present at various ages are indicated for boys between infancy and 20 years of age.

A normal young adult acquires through the years some 40 times the amount of calcium he had in infancy. He has, indeed, grown in calcium. Only to the extent that daily meals supply the kinds and amounts of mineral elements needed do the bones grow to desirable size and become hard and strong.

Surrounding and covering the bones are the soft tissues—muscles, tendons, and skin. Bones are principally held in position and supported by the muscles. And body protein is the chief constituent of muscles. As a child grows, there must be an increasing deposit of protein in his muscles if he is to become steadily stronger. Figure 3.5 illustrates protein growth from 1 to 10 years of age; it supplies data on the average daily excretion of creatinine at different ages. Creatinine excretions are an index of the protein content of the body; thus, increment in excretion is a measure of the growth of body musculature.

Increasing need for muscle strength is demonstrated when a baby advances from the crawling stage to an upright position. Good muscle texture is required if the change is to be made without undue strain and if posture is to remain good. As a child grows older, increasing demands are made on his muscles. Weak, sagging muscles may result from inadequate protein intake. Drooping posture and fatigue stance may be an outcome.

The blood that carries nutrients to bones and muscles is likewise built and nourished by proteins, mineral elements, and other nutrients. And the quality of the blood

Fig. 3.4 Body growth in calcium from infancy to adulthood.*

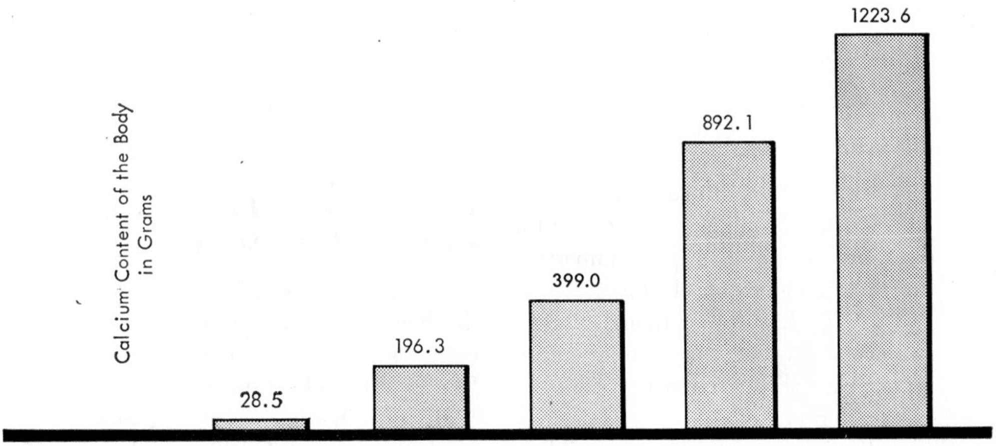

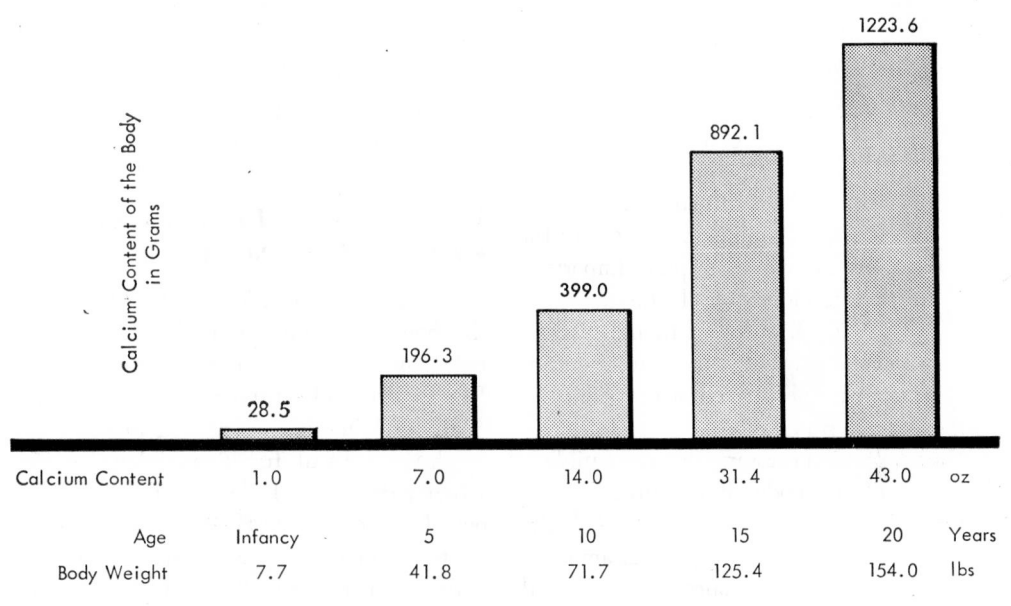

Calcium Content	1.0	7.0	14.0	31.4	43.0	oz
Age	Infancy	5	10	15	20	Years
Body Weight	7.7	41.8	71.7	125.4	154.0	lbs

*Adapted from Table 3 in I. Leitch and F. C. Aitken, "The Estimation Of Calcium Requirement: A Re-examination," Nutrition Abstracts and Reviews, 29 (April 1959), pp. 393-411.

Fig. 3.5 Body growth in protein: children 1–10 years of age.*

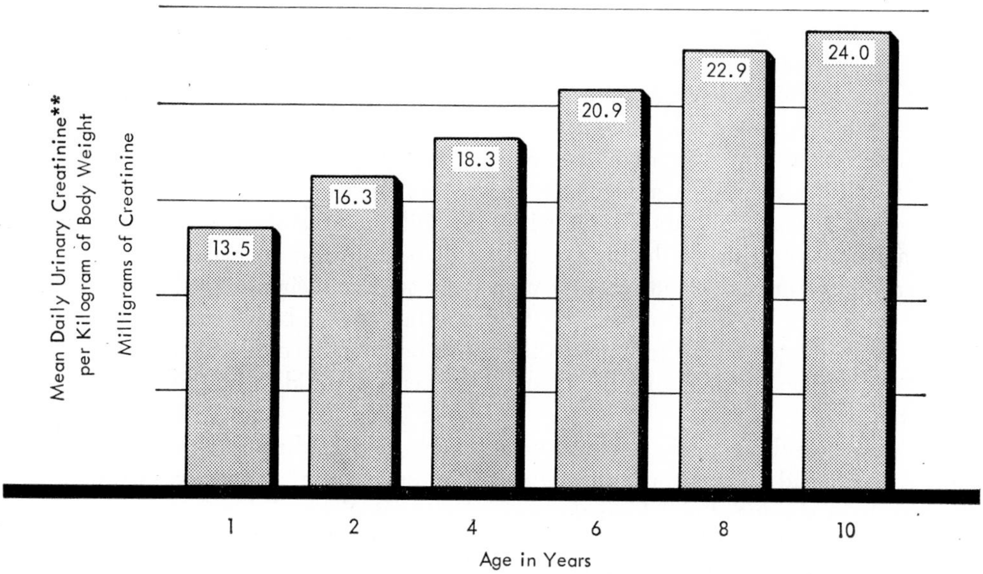

*Adapted from Table 1 in G. Stearns, K. J. Newman, J. B. McKinley, and P. C. Jeans, "The Protein Requirements of Children from One to Ten Years of Age," Annals of the New York Academy of Science, 69 (Jan. 10, 1958), pp. 857–868.

**"In the normal person the amount of creatinine excreted in 24 hours is an excellent measure of quantity of skeletal musculature".

determines in large measure the vitality and vigor of the individual. Obviously, proper choice of blood-building nutrients is essential to good nutrition

Vitamins have many functions in the building process. Vitamins are necessary for growth. Certain vitamins play important roles in the development of the teeth, in the building of healthy epithelial tissues, and, in conjunction with bone-building mineral elements, help to construct bone of good strength and quality.

Water is necessary to all building functions in the body. It constitutes about two-thirds of the weight of the adult body. Water is present in greater or lesser amounts in every tissue. Even bones are composed of about one-third water. Body fluids are the most obvious carriers of water. Five to 10 qts of blood circulate constantly in the adult body, and digestive secretions probably make up a similar amount.

To Control and Coordinate Internal Processes

The same nutrient classes that build the body—vitamins, mineral elements, proteins (amino acids), and water—also regulate and control its internal processes. Practically all vitamins are related in some way to the successful functioning of the body when eaten in sufficient quantity, and to poor functioning when the supply in inadequate. In many cases vitamins are associated with other nutrients in their coordinative activities. Certain mineral elements control such vital functions as the clotting of the blood and muscular contractions, including the beat of the heart. (See Chap. 6.)

Proteins and their amino acids also take part in many regulatory processes. These include the actions of protein-containing hormones, provided by the glands of internal secretion. Thyroxin from the thyroid gland, for example, is a regulator of energy metabolism. Enzymes in digestive juices are proteins with the highly specialized function of preparing nutrients for use by the body. Hemoglobin, a protein in the blood, carries oxygen from the lungs to the tissues and carbon dioxide from the tissues to the lungs.

Water regulates body temperature. Heat is eliminated by means of evaporation of water from the lungs and from the surface of the skin. Probably as much as one-half of the water available to the body daily is disposed of from the skin surface. The amount of water loss through the skin is increased in hot weather through sweating. As water evaporates from the skin there is a sense of cooling.

To Provide Energy for Activities, and Heat to Keep the Body Warm

Assuming that nutrients are available to build and maintain the body, there must still be nutrients to make it "go." Proteins (divested of their nitrogen), carbohydrates, and fats are the body's sources of energy for this purpose. To create the capacity to work, nutrients are said to be "burned" in the tissues. These 3 sources of energy are interchangeable in the sense that the body can use them, alone or together, in widely varying proportions. Table 3-1 shows the ultimate use of proteins, carbohydrates, and fats. Each is a source of energy to meet current needs; each is a potential source of body fat. Energy needs of the body and the ways in which energy-yielding nutrients meet these needs are discussed in the next chapter.

TABLE 3-1

BODY USE OF CARBOHYDRATES, FATS, PROTEINS

	Burned to Yield Energy	Other Functions	Stored As	Excess Changed To
Carbohydrates	√		Glycogen	Fat
Fats	√	Formation of Tissue Fats	Fat	Carbohydrate (possibly some)
Proteins	√ (after losing Nitrogen)	Build, repair protein tissue; formation certain hormones and enzymes	Protein (in new tissue	Carbohydrate Fat

REFERENCES

1. *The Heinz Handbook of Nutrition.* New York: McGraw-Hill Book Company, Inc., 1959. (Chaps. 2, 3.)
2. Harper, A. E., "Carbohydrates," *Food—The Yearbook of Agriculture.* Washington, D.C.: U.S. Department of Agriculture, 1959. p. 88.
3. Food and Nutrition Board, *The Role of Dietary Fat in Human Health.* Pub. 575. Washington, D.C.: National Academy of Sciences-National Research Council, 1958.
4. Brewer, W. D., and Arnrich, L., "The Role of Fat in the Diet," *J. Am. Home Economics Assoc.,* 50 (April 1958) pp. 269–73.
5. Coons, C. M., "Fats and Fatty Acids," *Food—The Yearbook of Agriculture.* Washington, D.C.: U.S. Department of Agriculture, 1959. p. 74.
6. Goddard, V., and Goodall, L., *Fatty Acids in Food Fats* (A tabulation). Home Economics Research Report No. 7. Washington, D.C.: U.S. Department of Agriculture, March 1959.
7. *Food Additives—What They Are/How They Are Used.* Washington, D.C.: Manufacturing Chemists Association, Inc., 1961.
8. *What Consumers Should Know about Food Additives.* Leaflet No. 10. Washington, D.C.: U.S. Department of Health, Education and Welfare, Food and Drug Administration, 1961.
9. Food and Nutrition Board, *The Use of Chemicals in Food Production, Processing, Storage and Distribution.* Pub. 887. Washington, D.C.: National Academy of Sciences-National Research Council, 1961.
10. ———, *Radionuclides in Foods.* Pub. 998. Washington, D.C.: National Academy of Science-National Research Council, 1962.

READINGS

Agricultural Research Service, *Protection of Food and Agriculture Against Nuclear Attack.* Handbook No. 234. Washington, D.C.: U.S. Department of Agriculture, 1962.

Darby, W. J., and Lam, G., *Food and Science . . . Today and Tomorrow.* New York: Public Affairs Pamphlets, 1961.

Dunning, G. M., "Foods and Fallout," *Review of Nutrition Research,* 23:1 (Jan.–Mar. 1962). New York: The Borden Company.

McCollum, E. V., "Today's Knowledge of Nutrition," *Today's Health,* 35 (Oct. 1957) pp. 18–21.

Nasset, E. S., *Your Diet, Digestion and Health.* 2nd ed. New York: Barnes & Noble, Inc., 1962. (Chaps. 1–5.)

The Wonderful Human Machine. Chicago: American Medical Association, 1961. ("The Digestive System," p. 45.)

CHAPTER 4

Foods supply energy to meet body needs

Energy is released whenever food is burned, and heat is a by-product of the energy. This fact was demonstrated dramatically some years ago, when dry milk was used as fuel to drive a locomotive. The powdered milk was burned in the fire box to provide the energy to drive the engine, and heat was given off.

» CALORIES

The energy generated when food is burned is measured in terms of calories [1]. A calorie is the unit of heat that will raise the temperature of 2 qts of water 1°F. A calorie is not, itself, a nutrient. It serves as a convenient measure of the energy (calorie) yields of the nutrients—proteins, fats, and carbohydrates. The energy values of separate nutrients and of many food mixtures have been determined by measuring the calories of heat given off when they were burned in equipment specially designed for the purpose. The objective of such efforts has been to discover relative calorie values of foods as potential sources of energy for the body. Two methods of measuring calories have been used, one direct and one indirect.

Direct Measurement of Heat in a Bomb Calorimeter

In this method, a weighed sample of a food is placed in a capsule or bomb filled with pure oxygen. The bomb is immersed in a container holding a known amount of water (Fig. 4.1). The food in the bomb is burned completely when an electric spark ignites a fuse. As the food burns, sensitive thermometers register the rise in temperature of the surrounding water. This rise indicates the amount of heat generated by burning the specified amount of the food [2]. From the temperature reading the calorie yield is calculated.

Indirect Measurement of Heat in an Oxycalorimeter

In this method, the amount of oxygen required to burn a weighed sample of food is measured. The energy yield of the food is then obtained by using standard factors established with the bomb calorimeter to convert the known volume of oxygen to calories. The dried food—a single food or a mixture of foods—is ignited and burned in a stream of nearly pure oxygen in a closed circuit.

The original work in establishing calorie values was done with the bomb calorim-

Fig. 4.1 Parr Oxygen Bomb Calorimeter (cross-section). Food contained in the bomb is burned, thereby releasing heat which raises the temperature of the water surrounding the bomb. The number of calories of heat released by a given weight of food sample is computed from the rise in temperature of the water and the heat capacity of the apparatus. (Courtesy the Parr Instrument Co., Inc.)

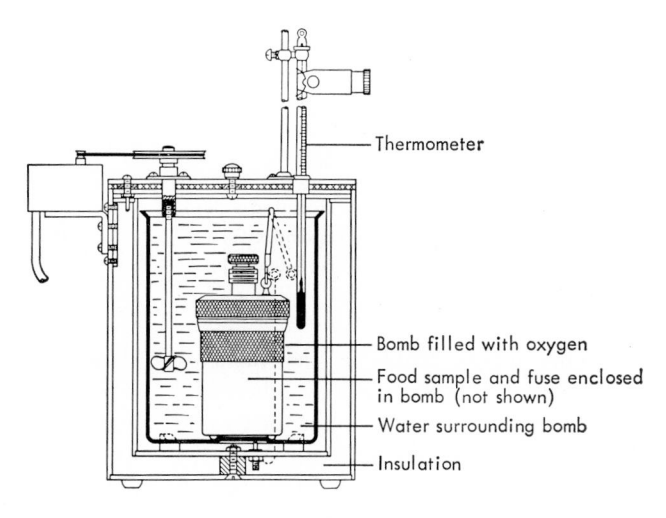

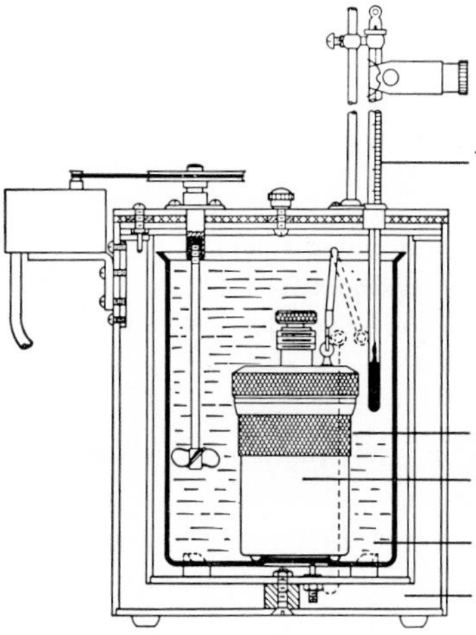

eter using weighed amounts of pure fat, pure carbohydrate, and pure protein. In this way it was possible to arrive at average energy values for a specified weight of each. It was soon discovered that certain corrections were necessary when calculating energy values for human diets, because the body handles foods somewhat less efficiently than does the calorimeter. Extensive experimentation showed that the adjoining rounded figures were suitable for practical use in calculating calorie values of the usual mixed diets eaten in this country:

1 gram of pure carbohydrate yields	4 calories
1 gram of pure fat yields	9 calories
1 gram of pure protein yields	4 calories

Once such calorie values were established it was possible to calculate the energy yield of a given weight of any food if its percentage composition of protein, fat, and carbohydrate were known. This process is demonstrated below in the calculation of the energy value of one egg.

This process may be carried a step

CALORIE VALUE OF 1 EGG

Weight of 1 egg: 50 g (1.8 oz) (without shell)

	Protein	Fat	Carbohydrate
Composition of egg	12.8 percent	11.5 percent	0.7 percent
In 1 g of egg	0.128 g	0.115 g	0.007 g
Energy factors	×4	×9	×4
Calories, 1 g of egg	0.512	1.035	0.028

0.512	
1.035	
0.028	
1.575	Total calorie value of 1 g of egg
×50	Weight of 1 egg in grams
78.75	Calories, the energy value of 1 egg (see Appendix G) (weight of 1 egg in shell, 1.9 oz)

further by combining a series of single foods in a recipe such as that for custard:

Calorie Value of
One Serving of Custard

½ egg	40 cal	(from calculated value)
½ cup milk	83 "	(from Appendix G)
⅓ tbsp sugar	17 "	(from Appendix G)
	140	

This recipe could be elaborated to apply to custard pie or to any other food combination for which the ingredients and their calorie values are known. When an entire recipe is calculated—as for a pie—the calorie value of one portion is determined by dividing the total calories by the number of servings. It is apparent that servings of food combinations may vary widely in calorie value, depending on the ingredients used and their proportions. And it is only by knowing exactly what ingredients enter into a recipe and how much is used of each that its calorie value can be calculated with certainty. The size of servings, which is also a very important factor in determining the calorie value of portions, is discussed later in this chapter.

In studying calorie values of foods, one soon learns that fat-rich foods are concentrated sources of energy, and that small servings of such foods have the same calorie value as much larger servings of foods low in fat and/or high in water content and bulk. One gram of fat yields more than twice as much energy as one gram of either carbohydrate or protein. The comparison in the next column illustrates this point.

Foods Yielding Approximately 100 Calories

1 tbsp mayonnaise	high fat
⅔ cup whole milk	low fat, high water
4½ cups raw cabbage	low fat, high water, high bulk

Removal of fat from food reduces its calorie content dramatically. A glass of skim milk, for example, from which much of the fat (cream) has been removed, furnishes about 90 calories, but a glass of whole milk gives about twice that number. Composition figures tell the story. That the difference lies in fat content is shown by the comparison at the bottom of this page.

The difference between pork chops with fat and with the fat trimmed off is equally striking. One cooked pork chop with both lean and fat, yields 260 calories; the same chop with the fat removed yields one-half this amount. (See top next page.)

Thus calorie values of foods vary greatly, and fat content is an important cause of such variations. But calories themselves do not vary in value; one calorie of heat represents exactly the same amount of energy as every other calorie. Therefore no food can be said to be more "fattening" than any other food. Calories merely count up faster in a concentrated food, high in fat.

» CALORIE VALUES OF COMMON FOODS

The calorie values of hundreds of foods are available today. These data largely emanate from the U.S. Department of

	Protein percent	Fat percent	Carbohydrate percent	Calories per cup
Skim milk	3.5	0.1	5.1	90
Whole milk	3.5	3.9	4.9	165

Cooked Pork Chop	Protein Percent	Fat Percent	Carbohydrate Percent	Calories per Chop
Lean only	31	16	—	130
Lean and fat	26	32	—	260

Agriculture. They represent average calorie values based on the composition of individual foods as determined in many scientific laboratories. These average values have been derived and published periodically by the Department of Agriculture since 1896. Calorie values of mixtures of foods, as found in "made" dishes, are usually calculated from the known content of protein, fat, and carbohydrate in each of the separate food ingredients (such as egg in custard). The same information can be derived by burning dried samples of such mixtures in an oxycalorimeter. As pointed out earlier, calorie values of food mixtures can vary widely except when they are based on typical recipes. This fact must be kept in mind in applying such information.

Appendix G gives the calorie values of some 400 single foods and prepared combinations of foods, such as main dishes, soups, and puddings.[1] They are presented in familiar measures such as cups, tablespoons, and teaspoons, and, as far as possible, in practical serving sizes. A "serving," of course, may have a different connotation for each person who uses the term. The serving denominations applied are those used rather generally, such as 3 oz cooked meats, ½ cup cooked vegetables, 1 slice of bread, and individual units of fruits. When necessary the amounts can be divided conveniently into smaller units, or multiples can be arrived at easily.

[1] Appendix G also presents nutrient values for the same foods. The discussion with respect to origin of data, determination of servings, and visualization of given quantities of foods applies to nutrients as well as to food energy.

It is important to learn to visualize servings of common foods as they ordinarily appear at the table. There are several ways to do this. You can measure foods at home —½ cup servings of cooked vegetables, for example—and then form a mental image of how that amount looks on a plate or other serving dish. Members of the class can cooperate by each bringing in a few measured foods to make a collection for class viewing and discussion; food models which represent exact measures of foods, can be used for part or all of the foods to be studied. When equipment is available for preparing foods, the class may assemble and arrange displays in laboratory sessions. If an accurate scale is available, certain foods, notably meats and units of fruits, may well be weighed in order that the class learn to recognize such servings as 3 oz of cooked meat, a "large" banana, or a "small" apple.

How To Use Appendix G

You can use the table as a dictionary of information to be drawn upon when needed. But you can also derive from its contents practical tools for routine use. Two approaches are suggested:

First, grouping foods similar in use, physical characteristics, composition, and energy value

Second, concentrating on the relatively few foods that are representative of your routine meals

Grouping Similar Foods The grouping method is useful if *approximate* calorie values are acceptable. It calls for assigning a single calorie value to a small grouping of similar foods. It involves classifying the major food items in Appendix G into the food groups listed in Chapter 3: milk, meat, vegetables, fruits, bread-cereals, fats, and sweets. Although there is a considerable range in calorie yield of the foods within each group, there are also striking similarities between them. It is the similarities that form the basis of the proposed plan. In the vegetable group, for example, several of the dark green leafy vegetables range in calorie value from 20 to 40 calories per ½ cup serving. This suggests that 30 calories might serve as the single value for ½ cup of any of the "greens." A similar grouping could be made of the root vegetables. In the fats group, most fats and oils provide about 100–125 calories per tablespoon. Sweets, on the other hand, furnish about half that number—50 calories per tablespoon. This type of condensation can be applied throughout the food groupings. It is reasonably satisfactory for *estimating* calorie values of meals, particularly if one's selection of foods within food groups is sufficiently varied to justify using such approximations. It not only provides a practical interpretation of the factors that determine calorie values but makes calorie estimation an easy process once the simplified system has been developed.

► *Classify the foods from Appendix G in groups, as suggested in the preceding paragraph. Assemble subgroups, such as different types of vegetables, to establish similarities in energy values of servings of foods. Students may work in committees on the different food groups to see what can be done to condense and coordinate information on calorie values.*

Concentrating on Representative Foods It is estimated that the average family uses about 50 different food items in a week's time. Your own 3-day meal record (Chap. 1) will reveal to some extent your own food range. The list of foods in Table 4-1 was compiled from 3-day food records of 100 university students as the foods from which their meals were usually drawn. Thus, while each ate meals that looked and tasted differently from those of his classmates, they all drew upon this relatively small number of basic foods for the nucleus of their meals. There are 50 different food items in Table 4-1. They are divided among the food groups as follows: milk, 5; meat, 12; vegetables, 12; fruits, 11; bread-cereals, 5; fats, 3; and sweets, 2.

With repeated use of a limited number of foods such as this, one can gradually become familiar with the calorie values of a sizable core of common foods. Such a method should in no sense narrow the scope of nutrition for students, nor suggest that a limited selection of foods is desirable. It should be regarded rather as a familiar base to use as a point of departure. It serves somewhat the same purpose as learning a few common words and phrases in beginning the study of a new language.

It will be noted that the items in Table 4-1 are confined largely to individual foods. The exceptions are those foods which are commonly bought as mixtures, such as breads and luncheon meats. The only feasible way of confining the list to a minimum number is to follow such a plan. When values of individual foods are established they can be combined as needed: milk on cereal, butter on bread, sugar on fruit, etc. For the relatively few intricate recipes used in daily meals, Appendix G offers a source of information. If a certain few of such food mixtures are daily items of diet, they should be included on your representative food list. There are obvious advantages in a student's making his own representative list. It offers an opportunity to include regional foods and personal favorites that help to give the activity practical significance.

► *Make your own representative food list, beginning with the foods on your 3-day meal record. Enlarge it as seems indicated, but, for practical considerations in handling, confine it, if possible, to 30 to 40 foods. If desired, individual lists may be pooled to make a representative food list for the class.*

These 2 methods of developing a practical knowledge of calorie values are not mutually exclusive. There are advantages in each and it is desirable that both be adopted, if possible. The grouping method applies only to the energy values of foods. The second method applies to all nutrients. Therefore, if only one method is employed,

TABLE 4-1

SPECIMEN REPRESENTATIVE FOOD LIST CLASSIFIED BY FOOD GROUPS: CALORIE VALUES IN SINGLE SERVINGS

Food*	Weight or Approximate Measure†	Calories
Milk Group		
Cheese, cheddar	1 ⅛ cube	115
Cheese, cottage, creamed	¼ cup	60
Cream, coffee	1 tbsp	35
Milk, fluid, skim (buttermlik)	1 cup	90
Milk, fluid, whole	1 cup	165
Meat Group		
Beans, dry, canned	¾ cup	250
Beef, pot roast	3 oz	245
Chicken	¼ small broiler	185
Egg	1 medium	80
Frankfurter	1 medium	155
Haddock	1 fillet	135
Ham, luncheon meat	2 oz	170
Liver, beef	2 oz	120
Peanut butter	1 tbsp	90
Pork Chop	1 chop	260
Salmon, canned	½ cup	120
Sausage, salami	1 slice	135
Vegetable Group		
Beans, snap, green,	½ cup	15
Broccoli	½ cup	20
Cabbage, shredded, raw	½ cup	10
Carrots, diced	½ cup	20
Corn, canned	½ cup	85
Lettuce leaves	2 large or 4 small	5
Peas, green	½ cup	55
Potato, white	1 medium	90
Spinach	½ cup	20
Squash, winter	½ cup	50
Sweet potato	1 medium	155
Tomato juice, canned	½ cup (small glass)	25
Fruit Group		
Apple, raw	1 medium	70
Apricots, dried, cooked	½ cup	135
Banana, raw	1 medium	85
Cantaloup	½ melon	40
Grapefruit	½ medium	50
Orange	1 medium	70
Orange juice, fresh	½ cup (small glass)	60
Peaches, canned	2 halves with juice	90
Pineapple juice, canned	½ cup (small glass)	60
Prunes, dried, cooked	5 with juice	160
Strawberries, raw	½ cup	30
Bread-Cereal Group		
Bread, white, enriched	1 slice	60
Cornflakes, fortified	1 ⅓ cup	110
Macaroni, enriched, cooked	¾ cup	115
Oatmeal, cooked	⅔ cup	100
Rice, cooked	¾ cup	150
Fats Group		
Bacon, crisp	2 slices	95
Butter or fortified margarine	1 tbsp	100
Oils, salad or cooking	1 tbsp	125
Sweets Group		
Beverages, kola type	6 oz	80
Sugar, granulated	1 tbsp	50

* Foods on this list are in forms ready to eat. All meats and vegetables are cooked unless otherwise indicated.

† See Appendix G for further identification of these foods. On that comprehensive list, all foods are described more fully and both weights and measures are included.

it is suggested that the second one be chosen because representative foods will serve as the basis for class activities throughout Section Two. If not even the second method is feasible, the specimen list of representative foods in Table 4-1 can become the focal point for class discussions.

► *Enter your representative foods on 3- by 5-in. cards or on slips of paper, 1 food to a card or slip. For each food add description, measure, weight, calorie value, and nutrient values, from Appendix G, as follows:*

Hamburger, beef, cooked
1 patty: 3 in. dia
weight: 3 oz

Calorie value	Protein g	Calcium mg	Iron mg
245	21	9	2.7

Vitamin A IU	Thiamine mg	Riboflavin mg	Ascorbic Acid mg
30	.07	.02	—

Sort the cards by food groups. You may also wish to make a listing of the foods with their calorie values as on Table 4-1.

Choose a typical day's meals from the three you recorded earlier (Chap. 1). Enter the meals on the diet record form used in Appendix B.[2] Add the calorie value of each food and the totals as called for on the form.

It is urged that you enter only calories on the diet record at the present time. The purpose of the activity is to coordinate study and discussion with actual dietary situations. It is intended that the various nutrients be entered on the meal record as each is considered in the text.

» ENERGY NEEDS OF THE BODY

It may be easier for you to visualize what happens when nutrients provide energy for the body if you remember that foods outside the body can actually burn when they are ignited. The engine driven with dry milk provides evidence that food can be used for fuel, that energy is released in the process, and that heat is generated by the action. When a comparable process takes place in the cells of your body it is referred to as oxidation. The body heat generated is indication that oxidation is taking place.

In the oxidation process, oxygen unites slowly with the end products of digestion of the food you eat. The operation goes on largely in the muscle cells. It consists of the chemical union of oxygen breathed *in* with the carbon and hydrogen yielded by the assimilated food nutrients. The carbohydrates, fats, and proteins oxidize because they are composed of carbon and hydrogen, both of which can unite with oxygen. They all yield carbon dioxide and water when oxidized. The chemical action releases energy, which makes it possible to do work, and heat, which helps to maintain a constant body temperature [1,2].

Evidence that the body's source of heat is internal is the fact that body temperature does not normally fluctuate, irrespective of the temperature of the room. Wearing heavier clothing in cold weather helps

[2] The specimen diet, Appendix B, provides calorie and nutritive values for the sample meals given in Chapter 3. This diet purposely does not meet accepted dietary standards in all respects; it is not intended as a model. It is referred to throughout the text to suggest how nutritive requirements are met, or fail to be met, because of the food choices that are made. In this chapter particular attention should be given to the *calorie* values of the foods and meals in the specimen diet. If class members do not record their own meals, the specimen diet may be subjected to the same type of analysis proposed in this and later chapters for personal meal records.

to hold *in* the heat already there—it does not *warm* the body. Wearing lightweight clothing in a warm room merely facilitates release of the heat that has been generated by the body.

Measurement of Body Energy Needs [1,2]

Scientific proof that oxidation in the body produces energy and heat has been provided by experiments with two types of equipment—one called a respiration calorimeter, the other a respiration apparatus.

The Respiration Calorimeter measures heat output directly. It consists, in essence, of an airtight chamber that can house one or more persons. Body heat given off by the subjects is measured as fast as it is produced by recording the rise in temperature of a current of cold water piped through the chamber. The amount of heat is then computed in terms of calories.

The Respiration Apparatus measures heat output indirectly. This apparatus consists of a closed circuit from which a subject breathes oxygen-enriched air through his mouth (Fig. 4.2). A nose clip prevents taking in air through the nostrils. The oxygen consumed in a specified length of time is a measure of the amount of oxidation going on in the body during the same period. By a series of calculations, based on the number of calories represented by a given amount of oxygen consumed, oxygen consumption is translated into calories of heat.

Data obtained from both direct and indirect methods have demonstrated the relation of energy expenditure by the body to its heat output. This has been done by testing subjects when completely at rest as

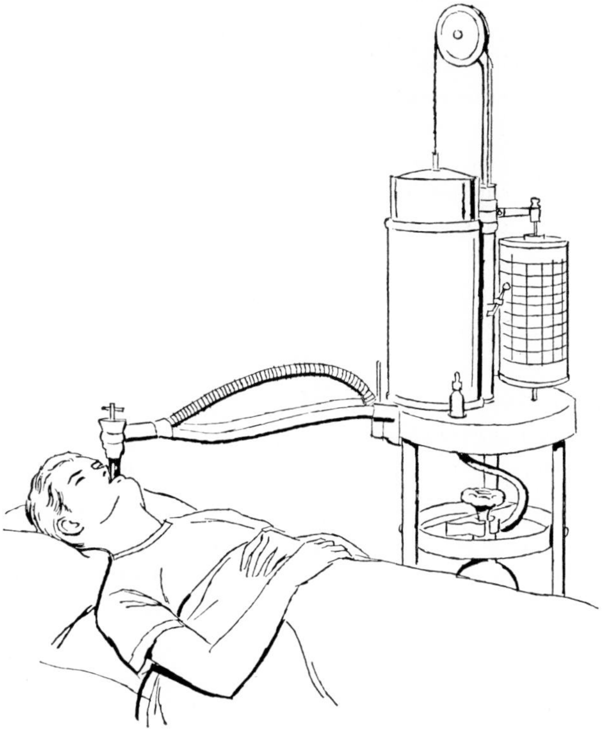

Fig. 4.2 Benedict-Roth Metabolism Apparatus as used to measure basal metabolism. With a respiration apparatus it is possible to determine the energy expenditure of an individual in a given period of time. The amount of oxidation going on in the body is indicated by the amount of oxygen used in a specified time. Oxygen consumption is translated into calories of heat by the application of a formula. (Courtesy Warren E. Collins, Inc.)

well as when performing many different types of activities. Such data make it possible to estimate the daily calorie needs of people carrying on similar activities.

It should be made clear that the word *energy* as used here applies to the ability to perform work as a result of an adequate supply of body fuel. The same word is often used when the reference is to a feeling of fitness or "pep." Energy in the true sense refers to food energy that precedes and makes possible physical activity. On the other hand, a feeling of "pep" and vigor, often largely psychological, frequently follows and can be the result of physical activity.

» HOW THE BODY USES ENERGY

The body uses energy in 3 ways:

1. For *internal* activities: those basic, involuntary processes such as heart beat, breathing, and circulation
2. For *external* activities: every voluntary move that requires even the slightest effort or the most extreme exertion
3. For *storage* of energy-yielding materials, chiefly during childhood and pregnancy

Energy for Internal Body Activities

The energy level required to keep the internal mechanisms of the body functioning is called *basal metabolism.* The term "basal" implies the minimum. It is descriptive of the relatively constant, internal energy needs for sustaining life at lowest ebb. Never—day or night, awake or asleep—do the behind-the-scenes activities cease—activities that are concerned with keeping the body alive, with chemical changes in the cells, and with processes involved in the oxidizing of nutrients that serve as body fuels. Never is there even a brief letup in the need for the more obvious activities, such as breathing or heart beat, over which the individual has no control.

Basal Metabolism [1,2,8] One's basal energy requirement is determined with a respiration apparatus (Fig. 4.2). The findings may be translated into calories of heat that represent the amount of energy needed for internal activities for a period of 1 day. The basal metabolism is measured when a person is resting quietly, awake, in a comfortably warm room, 12–15 hours after eating.

Norms have been developed for persons of different size and age from data accumulated on healthy individuals. One's basal metabolism is regarded as satisfactory if it falls within the limits for normality, which have been established at each age level. An adult's basal energy rate is relatively constant from day to day, but gradually decreases, a few calories annually, beginning at about the age of 20 years. At 75 years of age, the reduction may be as great as 10–15 percent below that at 35 years. The basal metabolism of children fluctuates somewhat as the growth rate varies. It is higher during infancy and adolescence, for example, periods of accelerated growth. A number of conditions cause variations from the normal in basal metabolism, notably high or low levels of thyroxin, the hormone secreted by the thyroid gland. An overproduction of thyroxin causes a rise in the energy rate; an underproduction causes a fall.

Data on the basal energy metabolism of large numbers of normal people have helped to identify some of the physical factors that determine basal metabolic rate. And this information has made it possible to devise ways of *estimating* basal metabolism. One simple procedure for making a rough estimate is on the basis of energy need per unit of body weight. The findings are reasonably satisfactory, assuming there are no upsetting factors such as an abnormal secretion of thyroxin. It has been found, for example, that a normal young adult expends basal energy at the rate of about 1 calorie every hour for each 2.2 lbs (1 kg) of his body weight. For an adult weighing 125 lbs (57 kg) the basal energy expenditure in 24 hours, therefore, would be 1368 calories ($1 \times 24 \times 57$). A saving of about 10 percent of basal energy during sleep reduces the final figure slightly. To illustrate: if a person sleeps 8 hours a day, he may deduct 46 calories ($0.1 \times 57 \times 8$), thus bringing his basal metabolic rate for the 24 hours to 1322 calories ($1368 - 46$). He is now ready to consider the additional factors that determine his total daily calorie needs.

Energy for External Activities [1,2,8]

Muscular efforts of every type qualify as external activities. An activity may consist of such slight exertion as sitting up or standing after the basal metabolism test. Or it may involve the increasingly strenuous operations of walking, ironing, or playing tennis. As stated earlier, a considerable amount of data have been assembled on the energy required to carry on many different activities. This type of information has been classified by activities and occupations and is available for reference in tabular form. Such data should be used in calculating daily energy expenditures. In a given case, this would involve careful recording of activities—work and play, hour by hour throughout the day—and matching these activities to similar activities for which there is energy data.

Simpler methods have been devised for use when an *estimated* figure is sufficiently accurate. One such method has been devised by Taylor, Macleod, and Rose. They have characterized 6 types of days on the basis of their activity level, ranging from almost no activity on the first type day to very severe exercise on the sixth type day. Using this plan (Table 4-2), one can simply select the type of day most like his own.

TABLE 4-2

ESTIMATION OF CALORIES FOR ACTIVITIES FOR VARIOUS TYPES OF DAYS*

Type of Activity	Cal† per lb per hr
A. At rest most of day (sitting, reading, etc., very little walking and standing)	0.23
B. Very light exercise (sitting most of the day, studying, with about 2 hr of walking and standing)	0.27
C. Light exercise (sitting, typing, standing, laboratory work, walking, etc.)	0.36
D. Moderate exercise (tanding, walking, housework, gardening, carpentry, etc., little sitting)	0.50
E. Severe exercise (standing, walking, skating, outdoor games, dancing, etc., little sitting)	0.77
F. Very severe exercise (sports—tennis, swimming, basketball, football, running—heavy work, etc., little sitting)	1.09

* Adapted from C. M. Taylor, G. Macleod, and M. S. Rose, *Foundations of Nutrition*, New York: The Macmillan Company, 1956, p. 56.

† Exclusive of basal metabolism and the influence of food.

If, for example, one engages chiefly in light exercise, he may choose category C (0.36 cal per lb per hr). If moderate exercise characterizes his day, category D would be his choice. And if his level of activity seems to coincide with neither C nor D but is somewhere between the two, he may choose an intermediate figure (as 0.43 cal per lb per hr). To estimate his total energy expenditure for external activities he would merely multiply one of these calorie factors by his weight (125 lbs), and then multiply this result by the number of active hours (16) in his day (0.36 × 125 × 16), giving a total of 720 calories. This figure would represent the energy expenditure for external activity alone.

Influence of Food One additional item must be considered in estimating total daily energy need: increased energy expenditure due to the influence of food in the body. This increase has been referred to as a "tax" that is applied for handling the metabolic processes as the food nutrients are made available to the body. When the diet is almost exclusively carbohydrate, the tax is about 6 percent; when almost exclusively fat, the tax can be as high as 14 percent; and when the diet is almost exclusively protein, the tax is 30 percent or more. But, by mixing the nutrients as is the practice in everyday meals, the average energy increase is believed to be no more than 10 percent. This increase is accounted for in estimating the total calorie need for the day by adding 10 percent of the sum of the calories for basal energy metabolism and external physical activities (1322 + 720 = 2042 × 0.10 = 204).

Thus we have considered the separate components of the total energy metabolism of the adult—his basal energy need, the energy required for physical activity, and the amount to be added to account for the influence of food. You may wish now to estimate your own daily energy requirement by the simple method suggested below.

To Estimate Your Own Daily Calorie Need

A Short-cut Method

A. Weigh yourself; using your body weight as a basis, estimate your basal calorie need for 24 hours.
B. Keep a diary of your activities for a typical day. Decide from Table 4-2 in which category your day falls—A, B, C, D, E, or F. Calculate the calorie need for your activities, for one day.
C. Total your calorie needs, taking into consideration the 10 percent "tax" for influence of food.

Sample of Calculation

Assume: an adult weighing 125 lbs (57 kg)
a day with 16 hr of activity; 8 hr of sleep
category of activity: C, light exercise

1. Calories for basal metabolism (corrected for saving in sleep)	1322
Basal metabolism for 24 hr—1368 cal (1 × 57 × 24)	
Saving in sleep, 8 hr— 46 cal (0.1 × 57 × 8)	
1322	
2. Add calories for activity (0.36 × 125 × 16)	720
	2042
3. Add calories for the influence of food (10 percent of 2042)	204
4. Total estimated calories needed for the day	2246

► *How does your own estimated daily calorie need compare with the total calories recorded on your personal meal record? If they differ widely, how do you explain the discrepancy? (Add your estimated daily calorie need to the meal record form for ready comparison with the calorie value of your day's diet.)*

Recommended Dietary Allowances Another way to discover your approximate daily calorie need is to refer to the recommended daily dietary allowances [3,4]. The fifth column of Table 4-3 presents the daily calorie allowances for categories of people of different age, sex, size, and condition. Merely by identifying yourself properly on Table 4-3 you may read from the table the recommended calorie level for the group into which you fall. The values are based on the knowledge that groups similar in physical characteristics and in activity have similar energy needs.

Although only the daily calorie allowances will be considered at this point, it should be noted that daily allowances are also proposed for protein, 2 minerals, and 6 vitamins at various age levels from infancy through adult life. (The complete allowance table, with footnotes, is provided in Appendix C.) These allowances will be referred to repeatedly throughout the text. Allowances have been established for only a fraction of the total number of nutrients known to be useful to the body. It is believed, however, that if meals provide these few nutrients in quantities to meet the specified allowances, they will also provide adequate amounts of the nutrients for which allowances have not been established.

The allowances were first presented in 1941 by the Food and Nutrition Board of the National Academy of Sciences-National Research Council [5]. They were based on nutrition research, applicable to quantitative human needs. Since that time, adjustments have been made as new research has dictated the need for change and revised editions have been issued at intervals of 5 years or less. From the first, the Food and Nutrition Board has used the term *allowances* to convey the idea that they are not hard and fast *standards*. Neither do they represent final judgments. They are expected to hold only until reconsidered in the light of newer research findings. The Board has conceived of the allowances as designed "to maintain good nutrition in healthy persons in the United States under current conditions of living and to cover nearly all variations of requirements for the population at large. They are meant to afford a margin of sufficiency above minimal requirements and are therefore planned to provide a buffer against the added needs of various stresses and to make possible other potential improvement of growth and function" [3].

Application of Daily Calorie Allowances The calorie allowances apply to individuals usually engaged in moderate physical activity. For persons who take very little exercise, they are excessive. If, for example, you lead a sedentary life, you probably will find that the allowances are above your daily calorie intake or your estimated energy need, particularly if you are shorter and lighter than the height and weight given for your age group in Table 4-3. Or the reverse may be true if you are very active and you are taller and heavier than the average.

The Food and Nutrition Board provides for systematic adjustment of calorie allowances for age, body size, climate, activity, pregnancy, lactation, rate of growth, and activity. For example, adjustments for age should be made by a 3-percent reduction in calorie allowance for each decade from age 50–70 years, and a further decrease of 10 percent for ages 70–80. It is important that such adjustments be made if a precise calorie allowance is sought. If an *estimate* is

TABLE 4–3

FOOD AND NUTRITION BOARD, NATIONAL RESEARCH COUNCIL RECOMMENDED DAILY DIETARY ALLOWANCES, REVISED 1958 [3]

Designed for the Maintenance of Good Nutrition of Healthy Persons in the United States

	Age Years	Weight kg (lb)	Height cm (in.)	Calories	Protein g	Calcium mg	Iron mg	Vitamin A IU	Thiam. mg	Ribo. mg	Niacin mg equiv.	Asc. Acid mg	Vitamin D IU
Men	25	70 (154)	175 (69)	3200	70	800	10	5000	1.6	1.8	21	75	
	45	70 (154)	175 (69)	3000	70	800	10	5000	1.5	1.8	20	75	
	65	70 (154)	175 (69)	2550	70	800	10	5000	1.3	1.8	18	75	
Women	25	58 (128)	163 (64)	2300	58	800	12	5000	1.2	1.5	17	70	
	45	58 (128)	163 (64)	2200	58	800	12	5000	1.1	1.5	17	70	
	65	58 (128)	163 (64)	1800	58	800	12	5000	1.0	1.5	17	70	
	Pregnant (second half)			+300	+20	1500	15	6000	1.3	2.0	+3	100	400
	Lactating (850 ml daily)			+1000	+40	2000	15	8000	1.7	2.5	+2	150	400
Infants	0–1/12												
	2/12–6/12	6 (13)	60 (24)	kg × 120		600	5	1500	0.4	0.5	6	30	400
	7/12–12/12	9 (20)	70 (28)	kg × 100	4	800	7	1500	0.5	0.8	7	30	400
Children	1 – 3	12 (27)	87 (34)	1300	40	1000	7	2000	0.7	1.0	8	35	400
	4 – 6	18 (40)	109 (43)	1700	50	1000	8	2500	0.9	1.3	11	50	400
	7 – 9	27 (60)	129 (51)	2100	60	1000	10	3500	1.1	1.5	14	60	400
	10–12	36 (79)	144 (57)	2500	70	1200	12	4500	1.3	1.8	17	75	400
Boys	13–15	49 (108)	163 (64)	3100	85	1400	15	5000	1.6	2.1	21	90	400
	16–19	63 (139)	175 (69)	3600	100	1400	15	5000	1.8	2.5	25	100	400
Girls	13–15	49 (108)	160 (63)	2600	80	1300	15	5000	1.3	2.0	17	80	400
	16–19	54 (120)	162 (64)	2400	75	1300	15	5000	1.2	1.9	16	80	400

sufficient, some consideration should still be given to adjusting the calorie figure if the person involved varies greatly in size from the average dimensions given on Table 4-3 and if his activity is rated either above or below the moderate level. Comparison of the daily calorie allowance with actual calorie intake and estimated energy need should give some basis for adjustment.

► *What is your own calorie allowance, based on Table 4-3? (If you are between the ages of 20 and 25 years, use the 25-year level.) How does your calorie allowance compare with your estimated calorie need? With your calorie intake as shown on your personal meal record? (Enter your calorie allowance on your meal record form for ready comparison with actual calorie intake and calculated calorie need.)*

Body Weight and Calorie Requirement For practical purposes, an adult's daily calorie need is one which assures a body weight that is best for him [6,7]. It is well then to know how much you weigh, how your weight compares with the desirable range for your age and height, and how steadily your weight holds from week to week. To obtain such information:

1. Take your height and weight. Observe the following rules with respect to this and future weighings: Take height against a flat surface, with heels, buttocks, and head touching the surface, eyes looking directly ahead. Have a helper place a flat object such as a book atop your head; press the book straight back against the flat surface and mark the lower side to indicate your height. Measure the distance to the floor.
   Weigh yourself on a balance (platform) scale, if possible. Use the same scale each week. Weigh at the same time of day to minimize variations in weight resulting from bowel movements and food intake. Note suggestions for clothing, Appendix D.
2. Refer to Appendix D for desirable weights for men and women.
   Classify yourself as of small, medium, or large frame. Select the weight range that corresponds to your height. For example, if you are a woman of medium frame, 5 ft, 4 in. tall, your desirable weight is in the range of 113–126 pounds. (Desirable weights are considerably below *average* weights. The latter are based on data from a large number of individuals, many of whom are overweight [6,7].)
3. Draw up a form for your own weight chart. (See specimen chart, Appendix E.)
   Show your desirable weight range as a "zone" and allow sufficient space above and below the zone to indicate actual weight above or below the desirable and to permit the showing of gains or losses in the coming weeks. Keep the chart on a weekly basis as long as it has value as a guide to the proper calorie content of meals.

► *Does your actual weight in relation to the desirable weight zone shed any light on your calorie intake as shown on your personal meal record? On your estimated daily energy expenditure? On your calorie allowance as taken from Table 4-3? How do you account for discrepancies if they exist?*

Storage of Energy-yielding Material during Growth

During childhood, total energy needs include not only basal metabolism and muscular activity but they must take into account growth itself. Unless there is enough energy-yielding material to permit reserve during childhood, growth is curtailed. There is no way of knowing exactly what proportion of energy-yielding nutrients is used for the needed reserve and what is used for muscular exercise. It *is* known that the toll for activity is taken first. If a child does not have enough for both, growth suffers. Thus, a child with inadequate energy intake may be active at the expense of his growth.

Calorie allowances for children of different ages are presented in the fifth column of Table 4-3. Growth rate, size, and activity have been considered in arriving at these values. Nevertheless, it cannot be expected that the calorie needs of individual children will always coincide with those of the corresponding age ranges in the table. Larger, rapidly growing, extremely active children may require more calories; smaller, slower growing, inactive children may need fewer.

The recommended calorie allowance for any child can be considered satisfactory only if he is growing at what appears to be a normal rate for him. As with the adult, it is body performance that counts. In Section Three meal plans are presented to meet calorie allowances of children of different ages.

Pregnancy and lactation represent forms of growth. The additional energy needs at these periods are indicated on Table 4-3: 300 calories per day during the second half of pregnancy; 1000 calories per day for the lactation period. The higher energy needs of pregnancy are due to a higher metabolic rate, which begins about the fourth month. The increase is caused by the larger amount of protoplasmic tissue in the mother's body, resulting from the growth of her own uterine and mammary tissues and the body of the fetus. The basal metabolism of the mother may increase as much as 20 percent above the nonpregnant level. The fetus increases in weight threefold during the final trimester. The physician decides if and how much the energy value of the diet should be increased for the individual mother, and how much she should gain in weight. The daily calorie allowance will depend on her actual weight in relation to her desired weight at the onset of pregnancy.

The higher energy allowance for lactation is needed for milk production—the amount of additional energy to be commensurate with the actual amount of milk produced. The specified 1000 additional calories assumes the production of about 3½ cups of milk per day with a calorie value of about 130 per ½ cup.

» BUDGETING CALORIES

In the preceding pages we have considered normal energy needs and the energy values of foods that must satisfy these needs. Problems of achieving balance between energy needs and values, as related to weight control, is discussed in Section Three. Currently there is a tendency to emphasize certain nutrients in the diet—such as vitamins—and to regard calories as a necessary evil. It should be understood that the body's energy need is basic to all others. We cannot live and work without sources of energy, no matter how well the diet supplies vitamins.

Rather than discount the importance of calories for good nutrition, we should conceive of them as indispensable partners of the nutrients. This thought was forcefully expressed by M. S. Rose in the first edition of *Foundations of Nutrition* in 1927, and has been included in each succeeding edition: "Practically, our task is to learn first how many calories we need and then see how, by intelligent choice of foods which yield them, we may make them the carriers of every other dietary essential" [8]. Thus, we cannot do without calories, but we can make them serve us well.

It is this concept—that calories may be *good* or *poor* nutrient carriers—that has led to the use of the term "empty" calories when the nutrient yield of a food is poor or nil. When the nutrient yield is good, calories may be said to pay a bonus. Variation in the nutrient yield among foods accounts for the fact that foods of the same calorie value rarely have the same nutritive value as well. Trading one food for another on the basis of calorie value alone is obviously a dangerous practice.

A consideration of calories therefore merely lays the groundwork for an appreciation of the various nutrients that are available in varying amounts in the foods we eat daily. The succeeding chapters in this section point up the importance of these nutrients to good nutrition and show how "intelligent choice" of common foods assures an abundant nutrient intake.

REFERENCES

1. *The Heinz Handbook of Nutrition.* New York: McGraw-Hill Book Company, Inc., 1959. (Chaps. 5, 6.)
2. Swift, R. W., "Food Energy," *Food—The Yearbook of Agriculture.* Washington, D.C.: U.S. Department of Agriculture, 1959. p. 39.
3. Food and Nutrition Board, *Recommended Dietary Allowances.* Pub. 589. Washington, D.C.: National Academy of Sciences-National Research Council, 1958.
4. Leverton, R. M., "Recommended Allowances," *Food—The Yearbook of Agriculture.* Washington, D.C.: U.S. Department of Agriculture, 1959. p. 227.
5. Roberts, L. J., "Beginnings of the Recommended Dietary Allowances," *J. Am. Dietet. Assoc.,* 34 (Sept. 1958) pp. 903–908.
6. Lew, E. A., "New Data on Underweight and Overweight Persons," *J. Am. Dietet. Assoc.,* 38 (April 1961) pp. 323–27.
7. *Overweight–It's Prevention and Significance* (Statistical bulletin). New York: Metropolitan Life Insurance Company, 1960.
8. Taylor, C. M., Macleod, G., and Rose, M. S., *Foundations of Nutrition.* 5th ed. New York: The Macmillan Company, 1956.

READINGS

Eppright, E. S., and Swanson, P. P., "Distribution of Calories in Diets of Iowa School Children," *J. Am. Dietet. Assoc.,* 31 (Feb. 1955) pp. 144–48.

Hauck, H. M., "Food For Energy," *Today's Health,* 35 (Nov. 1957) pp. 22–25.

Leverton, R. M., Ellison, J. M., Childs, M. T., Carver, A. F., and Twardock, D., "Source of Calories in the Recorded Self-chosen Diets of Women," *J. Home Economics,* 51 (Jan. 1959) pp. 33–38.

Richardson, M., and McCracken, E., *Energy Expenditures of Women Performing Selected Activities.* Home Economics Research Report No. 11. Washington, D.C.: U.S. Department of Agriculture, Dec. 1960.

Robinson, M., and Scoular, F. I., "Calorie Value of Food Served in a Woman's Residence Hall," *J. Am. Dietet. Assoc.,* 33 (Dec. 1957) pp. 1270–73.

Todhunter, E. N., "Food Composition Tables in U.S.A. A History of 'Bulletin 28,'" *J. Am. Dietet. Assoc.,* 37 (Sept. 1960) pp. 209–14.

Weaver, E. K., and Elliot, D. E., "Factors Affecting Energy Expended in Homemaking Tasks," *J. Am. Dietet. Assoc.,* 39 (Sept. 1961) pp. 205–208.

CHAPTER 5

Proteins

Earlier in the text certain aspects of proteins were considered: that proteins, collectively, represent one of the 6 nutrient classes; that certain types of foods yield more proteins than they do other nutrients; and that the body prepares proteins in specific ways to enter its "nutritional service." Some of the important ways in which proteins nourish the body were also discussed. You are now ready to consider such practical matters as the relative importance of different food sources of proteins, how much protein you need daily, and what difference it makes to you whether or not you get the proteins you need.

» HOW PROTEINS ORIGINATE

Plants are the original source of all food proteins. Only plants can make their own proteins by combining the "raw materials"—nitrogen from soil or air, carbon dioxide from air, and water. Energy for the task is furnished by the sun. The animals you eat for food utilize mainly plant proteins in making their own body proteins. You, therefore, obtain your protein supply, ready-made, from both plant and animal sources [1].

» IMPORTANT SOURCES OF PROTEIN

Figure 3.1 will refresh your memory of some of the important types of foods regarded as protein sources. In this figure the foods are represented on a percentage basis. This does not tell you how much protein you can obtain from eating a serving of any of the foods charted. But from the percentage composition you can calculate the protein content of a serving of each food if you know its weight. For example, cooked lean beef yields about 26 percent protein (raw, about 18.6 percent), which means that every gram of cooked lean beef contains 0.26 g of protein. It follows that a 3-oz serving (85 g) of the beef furnishes about 23 g of protein (85×0.26). It is well to know that protein values can thus be determined by simple multiplication. However, making such calculations for many foods would be tedious and time-consuming. The protein contents of average servings of many foods have therefore been provided for you in Appendix G.

Comparative Protein Values

You need to become familiar with the amounts of protein in common foods in the portions in which they are usually served. One way to begin is to study the protein yields of your own representative foods. The arrangement of foods in Figure 5.1 suggests an approach to such a study. The foods in this figure are the identical 50 items that compose the specimen representative food list. (See Table 4-1.) The 50 foods, in average servings, are listed in Figure 5.1 in order of their quantitative importance as sources of protein. This arrangement reveals comparative protein values and offers a practical basis for associating levels of protein content with food sources.

Figure 5.1 provides the following assistance in studying comparative protein values of common foods:

The more concentrated sources of protein are immediately evident by their top position.

Foods with approximately the same protein value per serving can be associated in type and use.

Grouping the foods according to protein content makes it possible to characterize each group and to assign one approximate protein value to each. (Such approximations are valid when an *estimate* of total protein content of meals is sufficient.)

The list shows the types of foods that are *not* good sources of protein—the ones which cannot usually be counted upon for an adequate protein intake if they are the sole sources.

The bars signalize by their length the comparative protein values of the foods on the specimen representative list.

Excellent Sources

It is evident from Figure 5.1 that lean meats, fish, poultry, and baked beans are the foods that provide the most protein per portion when eaten in the size servings indicated. These foods are all easily identifiable with the *meat group*. The values per serving in this assortment range from 12 to 23 g of protein. Kinds and cuts of meat and varieties of fish vary somewhat in protein content, but the ones listed here are fairly typical of the entire group. The canned beans are representative of the different kinds of dried beans, prepared in various ways. If a value of 18 protein g per serving were assigned to all the foods represented by the items in this series, an estimate of the protein yield from these types of foods would be reasonably accurate, provided the selection of foods was a varied one.

Very Good Sources

The next best sources of protein on the list—milk, cheese, eggs, and lean sausages (salami and frankfurters)—also constitute a distinctive assortment. Eggs, cheese, and milk are often characterized as "meat alternates" with respect to protein and are associated in meal use with meats. The yield of protein per serving of these foods is about one-half that of the first series of sources. They are not rich sources but their total contribution to a day's meals can be considerable, as shown later in this chapter. The range of values for this second series is 6–9 g of protein per serving, with a value of 8 g fairly representative for all.

Serving size is a critical factor in determining position in Figure 5.1. This is particularly apparent in the two food series

Fig. 5.1 Servings of representative foods in order of their importance as sources of protein. (Each bar represents an approximate protein value for the series of foods listed below it.)

Food *	Weight or Approximate Measure **	Protein Grams
18 g		
Beef, pot roast	3 oz	23
Chicken	1/4 small broiler	23
Salmon, canned	1/2 cup	17
Haddock	1 fillet	16
Pork chop	1 chop	16
Ham, luncheon meat	2 oz	13
Liver, beef	2 oz	13
Beans, dry, canned	3/4 cup	12
8 g		
Milk, fluid, skim (or buttermilk)	1 cup	9
Milk, fluid, whole	1 cup	9
Cheese, cottage, creamed	1/4 cup	8
Cheese, cheddar	1 1/8" cube	7
Sausage, salami	1 slice	7
Egg	1 medium	6
Frankfurter	1 medium	6
4 g		
Bacon, crisp	2 slices	5
Macaroni, enriched, cooked	3/4 cup	4
Peanut butter	1 tbsp	4
Peas, green	1/2 cup	4
2.5 g		
Broccoli	1/2 cup	3
Corn, canned	1/2 cup	3
Oatmeal, cooked	2/3 cup	3
Potato, white	1 medium	3
Rice, cooked	3/4 cup	3
Spinach	1/2 cup	3
Apricots, dried, cooked	1/2 cup	2
Bread, white, enriched	1 slice	2
Cornflakes, fortified	1 1/3 cup	2
Squash, winter	1/2 cup	2
Sweet potato	1 medium	2
less than 2 g		
Banana, raw	1 medium	1
Beans, snap, green	1/2 cup	1
Cabbage, shredded, raw	1/2 cup	1
Cantaloup	1/2 melon	1
Carrots, diced	1/2 cup	1
Grapefruit	1/2 medium	1
Lettuce leaves	2 large or 4 small	1
Orange	1 medium	1
Orange juice, fresh	1/2 cup (small glass)	1
Pineapple juice, canned	1/2 cup (small glass)	1
Prunes, dried, cooked	5 with juice	1
Strawberries, raw	1/2 cup	1
Tomato juice	1/2 cup (small glass)	1
Apple, raw	1 medium	trace
Butter or fortified margarine	1 tbsp	trace
Cream, coffee	1 tbsp	trace
Peaches, canned	2 tbsp with juice	trace
Beverage, kola type	6 oz	....
Oils, salad or cooking	1 tbsp	0
Sugar, granulated	1 tbsp	0

*Foods are in forms ready to eat. All meats and vegetables are cooked unless otherwise indicated.

**See Appendix G for further identification of these foods. On that list all foods are described more fully and both weights and measures are indicated.

just discussed. For example, the reduction of a serving of baked beans from ¾ cup to ½ cup would move this food from the "excellent" to the "very good" category. On the other hand, doubling the portion of cottage cheese from ¼ cup to ½ cup would elevate it to the "excellent" category. In ranking foods on your own representative food list, you will want to adjust size of servings to your own food habits.

Good Sources

The third food series is a small one composed of macaroni, peanuts, peanut butter, green peas, and bacon. A check with Appendix G will show that the protein value for plain cooked macaroni is representative of values for the same amounts of such similar foods as spaghetti and noodles, and that green peas yield the same protein content as green lima beans. Both fresh green legumes are much higher in protein than other vegetables. Peanuts, which are legumes, are nearly twice as high in protein, weight for weight, as most other nuts. Peanut butter is similar to peanuts in protein value. Each food in this series yields approximately 4 g of protein per serving—about one-half the yield of the "very good" sources.

Fair Sources

The fourth series of foods in Figure 5.1 includes cereals in different forms, bread, potatoes, and certain vegetables. A narrow range of 2–3 protein grams, with an approximate value of 2½, characterizes this series. In the main, 3 g of protein per serving of oatmeal applies to other whole-grain cereals such as rolled wheat and shredded wheat; bakers' breads average about 2 g of protein per slice; flaked cereals yield 2 to 3 g per 1-oz serving. Milled cereals such as farina and grits, yield about 2 g of protein per serving. Although cereals and breads have relatively low yield of protein per serving, their total contribution to meals is large because of the amount eaten of such foods. You will find that in the specimen diet given in Appendix B, about 20 percent of the total day's protein comes from grains in various forms.

The vegetables in this series are, for the most part, the concentrated, starchy type: potatoes, corn and winter squash, and the dark green vegetables, spinach and broccoli. Spinach runs somewhat higher in protein per serving than other "greens," except collards and dandelion greens. Although none can be considered a protein-rich source, servings of the vegetables named furnish two to three times as much protein as those appearing lower on the list. Discussion later in the chapter will show that most proteins in the third series and below are lesser in quality, as well as in quantity per serving of food, than those in the first 2 series.

The remaining foods on the list—almost one-half the total number—fall below 2 g of protein per serving. These could be characterized as poor sources. They consist of fruits, many vegetables, fats, and sweets. They are negligible sources of protein in this country. The fruits and vegetables yield about 1 g of protein per serving. Fats and sweets provide little or no protein.

► *Arrange your own list of representative foods (sort cards) in order of their quantitative importance as sources of protein. Experiment with grouping the foods as in Figure 5.1 and assign approximate protein values to groups.*

Enter protein values on your personal meal record. Use exact data from your representative food list so far as possible. Supplement with values from Appendix G. Total the protein intake for the day.

Use your approximate group values to estimate the protein content of the foods on your meal record. How does the total for the day compare with that from using the more exact method?

Establish what percentage of your total daily protein intake is provided by lean meats, by milk, and by cereals.

» YOUR PROTEIN NEEDS [1,2]

The body's protein requirement is based on its building and upkeep functions—not on body work and exercise, even though some of the food protein is used for energy. Upkeep is not merely a matter of routinely making good the wear and tear on body protein. Protein is in a "dynamic state" in the adult body. Every cell constantly requires nitrogen to work over into living tissue and to construct enzymes, hormones, and antibodies. This situation exists throughout life. Body proteins are continuously undergoing a breaking-down and building-up process. As proteins are used up, nitrogen is excreted from the body and new sources are needed from the food supply.

The body's need for protein is determined by so-called "balance" experiments. In these experiments, the nitrogen is measured and the results translated in terms of protein. When the amount of nitrogen consumed in meals "balances" (is identical with) the amount excreted from the body on a daily basis, one is said to be in nitrogen equilibrium. When this condition exists in an adult, his protein intake is believed to be essentially satisfactory for good protein nutrition. However, nitrogen equilibrium is not a completely reliable gauge of protein requirement, because if protein intake is deficient, body tissues can compensate for a time by supplying the nitrogen needed to achieve "balance."

A person who is in *positive* nitrogen balance is excreting less nitrogen than he is taking in; therefore, he is storing protein. This situation should exist when new tissues are being formed, notably in childhood and in pregnancy, and when milk is being formed in lactation. A person is in the reverse position when he is in *negative* nitrogen balance, i.e., is excreting more nitrogen than he is acquiring. This happens when the diet is deficient in protein and fails to meet the body's needs. Adults, on the average, maintain nitrogen balance on a minimum of about 0.5 g of protein per 2.2 lbs (1 kg) of body weight per day. On this basis, an adult weighing 125 lbs (57 kg) would have a minimum daily need of 28.5 g. It is customary to provide for adequacy in all situations by doubling the 0.5 g figure, thus raising the daily need in our example to 57 g—about 1 g per kg of body weight per day.

Recommended Daily Allowances for Protein

The Food and Nutrition Board of the National Academy of Sciences-National Research Council, has based its adult protein allowances on 1 g of protein per kg of body weight per day for both men and women (Table 5-1, first 6 entries in the third, sixth, and seventh columns). The Board regards this basis as a conservative one: high enough to cover individual differences and relatively easy to attain. Adults who are larger and heavier—who have a greater mass of living tissue than the "average" persons of corresponding age represented on the table—will obviously have higher daily protein allowances. Those who are smaller and lighter will have correspondingly lower daily protein allowances.

Pregnancy and lactation call for more protein. The level could reach 1½ g per

TABLE 5-1

RECOMMENDED DAILY DIETARY ALLOWANCES FOR PROTEIN [3]

	Age Years	Weight kg (lb)	Height cm (in.)	Calories	Protein g	Protein g per kg (2.2 lb)
Men	25	70 (154)	175 (69)	3200	70	1.0
	45	70 (154)	175 (69)	3000	70	1.0
	65	70 (154)	175 (69)	2550	70	1.0
Women	25	58 (128)	163 (64)	2300	58	1.0
	45	58 (128)	163 (64)	2200	58	1.0
	65	58 (128)	163 (64)	1800	58	1.0
	Pregnant (second half)			+ 300	+20	
	Lactating (850 ml daily)			+1000	+40	
Children	1–3	12 (27)	87 (34)	1300	40	3.3
	4–6	18 (40)	109 (43)	1700	50	2.8
	7–9	27 (60)	129 (51)	2100	60	2.2
	10–12	36 (79)	144 (57)	2500	70	2.0
Boys	13–15	49 (108)	163 (64)	3100	85	1.7
	16–19	63 (139)	175 (69)	3600	100	1.6
Girls	13–15	49 (108)	160 (63)	2600	80	1 6
	16–19	54 (120)	162 (64)	2400	75	1 4

kg of body weight per day during the second half of pregnancy and nearly 2 g during lactation. The greater need in the second half of pregnancy is due largely to the rapid growth of the fetus, which has now attained considerable size. At this time the daily protein allowance is 78 g, an additional 20 g daily. Even more protein is needed during lactation to provide sufficient breast milk for the baby: 40 g daily above the prepregnancy level, or a total daily protein allowance of 98 g.

► *Find your own daily protein allowance based on your body weight. (If you are 20 years of age or older, use 1 g per kg of body weight; if younger, use the allowance for boys or girls nearest your actual age, Table 5-1.) Record your protein allowance on your personal meal record.*

Compare your actual daily protein intake as shown on your personal meal record with your daily protein allowance. Account for the effect of your food choices on your total protein intake.

In this country, proteins commonly provide about 10 to 15 percent of the total calorie intake in daily meals. The specimen diet in Appendix B shows a total calorie intake of 2331, of which 276 cal (69 × 4) are derived from protein. Thus protein supplies about 12 percent of the calories (276 ÷ 2331).

► *Establish what percent of the total calories on your personal meal record was provided by protein. Does it fall within the acceptable range?*

Protein Allowances for Children [1,2]

Children need proteins not only for upkeep but also for growth. They must show a positive nitrogen balance if tissues are to grow and be nourished adequately. A child's protein requirement at any given age depends on how large he is at that time and how fast he is growing. The sixth column of Table 5-1 shows progression in protein allowances from 40 g daily for children 1–3 years of age to 100 g daily for boys 16–19 years of age. Increases in height and weight, which normally accompany increases in age, indicate a growing mass of active body tissue. A steadily increasing protein intake is needed, not only to support the growth of this tissue, but to nourish and sustain it as well. Spurts in growth, as at adolescence, call for a very high level of protein intake.

This progression in need and use of proteins by the body is reflected in the increasing amount of proteins stored in the muscles during growth (Fig. 3.5). Thus protein intake is directly related to growth in children. But protein cannot be used for growth until after its maintenance function has been fulfilled. When there is not enough protein for both maintenance and growth, growth is the loser.

Because of the growth need, children have proportionately higher protein allowances in relation to body weight than do adults. The seventh column in Table 5-1 shows that at ages 1–3 the amount of protein recommended per kg of body weight runs as high as 3.3 g. The ratio gradually decreases throughout the growth period but still remains above the adult level of 1 g of protein per kg of body weight until full adult status is reached. Total protein allowances for adults and children are thus remarkably similar. For example, a child of 7–9 years weighing 60 lbs (27 kg) has a daily protein allowance of 60 g (2.2 × 27), whereas a woman weighing more than twice as much (128 lbs or 58 kg) has an allowance of 58 g, 2 g less of protein daily than the child.

The protein needs of children are high, but they are met easily by using recommended amounts of suitable foods. The 3 food groupings shown demonstrate this point for different age groups. With only a partial listing of foods that would compose the meals, the allowances are exceeded in each case.

Importance of Quality of Protein

It is not only *quantity* of protein that counts but *quality* as well. As a matter of fact, the quality of proteins in the foods you eat determines to some degree the quantity you need. In other words, if the quality

MEETING PROTEIN ALLOWANCES FOR CHILDREN

Ages in Years	**4–6**		**10–12**		**16–19 (Boys)**	
DAILY PROTEIN ALLOWANCES	50 g		70 g		100 g	
		Protein g		**Protein g**		**Protein g**
Beef, pot roast	½ serving	12	1 serving	23	1 serving	23
Milk	3 cups	27	4 cups	36	4 cups	36
Egg	1 medium	6	1 medium	6	1 medium	6
Bread-cereals	3 servings	9	4 servings	12	5 servings	15
Fish	—	—	—	—	1 serving	17
Cheese, cheddar	—	—	—	—	1 oz	7
Total		54		77		104

is excellent, less protein suffices than if the quality of the protein is poor. And quality of protein in foods is determined by the kinds and proportions of amino acids they contain [2,4].

As you know, the basic constituents of all proteins are amino acids. They are the parts of which proteins are composed. In this form they circulate in the blood and nourish the tissues (Chap. 3). Amino acids are often referred to as the building stones of proteins or as the letters of the alphabet which, in almost endless combinations, "spell" the hundreds of "words" that represent the kinds of body protein.

There are some 22 amino acids, each of them a separate chemical entity but with certain characteristics in common with all others. Eight of these 22 are known as "essential" for adult human beings because they must be supplied ready-made in foods. The body cannot synthesize them from foods nor derive enough of them from the breakdown of tissue proteins. These are the 8 essential amino acids: tryptophan, threonine, isoleucine, leucine, lysine, methionine, phenylalanine, and valine. An additional one, histidine, is believed to be "essential" for children. Practically all of the 22 amino acids are present in most proteins in greater or lesser amounts, but it is their yield and proportion of the 8 essential amino acids that determines whether proteins are of high or of low quality.

Some progress has been made in determining human needs for the 8 essential amino acids [5,6]. Allowances have thus far been proposed for these groups: young men, young women, and infants. Moreover, a number of foods have been studied for their content of the 8 essential amino acids. It is therefore possible at the present time to examine the diets of young adults for their yields of these acids and to compare intakes of the acids with the allowances proposed. Such comparisons are interesting and they shed some light on whether the diet is satisfactory with respect to the quality of protein. But a more revealing comparison is that of the "pattern" of essential amino acids, provided by individual foods or groups of foods, with body needs as reflected by the amino acid composition of human tissue.

The amino acid "pattern" of a protein refers to the quantitative relationship—the ratios—between the essential amino acids it contains. The amino acid composition of proteins in animal foods—meats, poultry, fish, milk, cheese, and eggs—resembles the amino acid content of human tissues. Thus animal proteins can provide the amino acids in the approximate proportions needed by the body. This gives them a superior rating nutritionally, and classifies them as high quality, efficient proteins. They are referred to as "complete" proteins. The nutritive value of proteins from most plant sources—vegetables, fruits, and grains—is lower because their "patterns" of essential amino acids are less satisfactory. A poor "pattern" may be due to an incomplete assortment of essential amino acids, to their presence in too small quantities, or to unfavorable ratios between them. The proteins of soybeans and certain other legumes are more efficient than those of most vegetable sources and are nearly as useful as those in animal foods. All vegetable sources have important contributions to make to the proteins in a mixed diet.

Supplementary Value of Proteins [2,4]

Fortunately, different kinds of proteins supplement each other in behalf of good protein nutrition. This makes it possible to provide the body with plenty of high quality protein from a combination of animal and vegetable sources. When the tissues have selected from the blood the amino acids they need to form their own body protein, some leftovers remain. These are not necessarily lost. To the extent that the right amino acids are present, these "strays" team up to make other proteins that are also useful to the body.

When the day's meals provide proteins from a variety of sources, and enough of them—both animal and vegetable—good protein nutrition is practically assured. Foods that complement each other with respect to essential amino acids become partners in producing high quality proteins. Cereal grains and milk are often cited as an example of this type of union; macaroni and cheese, rice and fish are others. The idea of building essential amino acids with protein combinations is being pursued with less familiar foods in parts of the world where animal sources of protein are scarce.

Such combinations represent amino acid supplementation in the best sense. A better general appreciation of the possibilities of this type of supplementation would tend to lessen the impact of current efforts to supplement common foods with certain individual amino acids. It is the considered opinion of the Food and Nutrition Board and other professional groups that the need for supplementing the food supply of this country with synthetic amino acids has not been demonstrated [2]. Furthermore, there is some reason to believe that an excess of one amino acid may even have the unfavorable effect of creating deficiencies of other acids. This is thought possible in one of two ways: the excess of one may lessen the utilization of another amino acid, or the excess of one may increase the requirement of another [4].

Choosing Protein Foods

In choosing protein foods for meals, obviously a mixture of animal and vegetable sources is desirable. The Food and Nutrition Board's protein allowances for adults were established on the assumption of such a mixture in a diet adequate in other nutrients as well as in food energy. One-half of the total protein intake from animal sources would undoubtedly be above actual needs. However, such a proportion would not be out of line with eating practices in this country.

Experiments have also proved the wisdom of distributing animal proteins throughout the 3 meals of the day. When college women had animal protein with each meal of the day it helped distinctly to keep them in nitrogen balance. For example, nitrogen was better utilized when the students had 1 glass of milk with each of their 3 meals than when they had none at breakfast (and no other source of animal protein), 1 glass with lunch, and 2 glasses with dinner. With the exception of the variation in breakfast —with and without milk—the day's meals were identical for the comparison and were nutritionally adequate [7].

When an animal protein is eaten, the essential amino acids are available at once for tissue nourishment. When an animal protein is *absent,* the essential amino acids may not be present in the amounts and proportions to make the complete proteins that can be utilized immediately. Timing is a critical factor in the efficient use of amino acids. Apparently all essential amino acids must be available *at the same time* to make complete proteins. Those taken at one meal, as for breakfast, cannot be held over until others needed to make complete proteins are provided by later meals. Thus, in the absence of ready-made complete proteins at each meal there appears to be considerable sacrifice of amino acids, a fact that explains the difficulty in maintaining nitrogen balance under those circumstances. Recent evidence suggests that the body utilizes protein even more efficiently and completely when food is eaten in smaller more frequent meals than when eaten at the conventional breakfast, lunch, and dinner.

The specimen diet in Appendix B shows how relatively simple it is for an adult to obtain a diet adequate in total protein, nearly one-half of which is derived from animal sources. The total protein intake for the day is about 70 g, which represents a moderate margin above the allowance of 58 g. The animal sources of protein in this case are hamburger and milk with a total of 32 g (55 percent of the allowance) for the day. Examine the examples given of other food combinations, common in daily meals, which can provide as much or more protein of animal origin:

SOURCES OF ANIMAL PROTEIN

Beef	1 serving	23 g protein
Milk	2 cups	18 g protein
		—
		41 g protein
Chicken	1 serving	23 g protein
Egg	1 medium	6 g protein
Cottage cheese	¼ cup	8 g protein
		—
		37 g protein
Fish	1 serving	17 g protein
Cheese, cheddar	1 oz	7 g protein
Frankfurter	1 medium	6 g protein
		—
		30 g protein

► *What proportion of the total proteins on your personal meal record came from animal sources? Did you have a source of animal protein at each meal?*

» PROTEIN IN OUR NATIONAL DIET

You have seen that many popular foods are good sources of proteins and that it is not difficult to obtain enough high quality proteins if you have a free choice of foods. But is there sufficient protein to "go around"? Do all the foods available to the population provide enough protein for the needs of each individual? U.S. Department of Agriculture data show that the total food supply in the United States is rich in protein. On the basis of proteins available for consumption, the intake would be about 97 g per person per day if it were divided equally among all people. Of that amount, about ⅔ would be from animal sources. This proportion represents about a 16-percent increase in proteins derived from animal foods in the past 50 years; it results from an increasing supply of eggs, milk, and meat and a decreasing supply of grain products [8].

Family dietary studies point up another aspect of protein sufficiency in this country. Studies made in 1955 by the U.S. Department of Agriculture, showed that food supplies in some 6000 households provided, on the average, 103 g of protein per person per day [9]. Analysis of the family diets was made by region, by location of home—country or city—and by size of income. In the entire group, only 8 percent of the diets fell below the protein allowances of the Food and Nutrition Board. The amounts of protein consumed varied within regions (Table 6-2) and within income levels. Protein intakes of individuals in this country also vary greatly: men appear to fare better than women, boys better than girls, and young children better than older ones with respect to protein intake [10]. And even though many individuals and groups throughout the world have low protein intakes (as will be seen presently), probably the majority in this country consume more protein than their dietary allowances call for.

Evidence of high protein intakes raises the question of getting too much protein.

Is there harm in routinely eating more protein than called for by the recommended dietary allowances? Is the body subjected to undue stress resulting from the handling of excess nitrogen and discarding it via the kidneys? While the burden so imposed, is recognized, there is no evidence at present to indicate that nitrogen excesses of the magnitude common in this country are detrimental to health [2]. Lack of visible evidence, however, does not necessarily mean that it is nonexistent. Moderation in the consumption of protein would, therefore, appear to be the desirable course to pursue.

The realization that people in this country, for the most part, eat proteins unsparingly and to the point of excess, may lead you to question the validity of advertising campaigns for protein supplements such as gelatin capsules and powders. You are now equipped to examine the claims made for such supplements. You can compare the amino acids present in gelatin (printed on the container) with the list of essential amino acids given earlier in this chapter. You will find that one essential amino acid is entirely lacking in gelatin. This makes it an *incomplete* protein. If there is an actual shortage of protein in the diet and nitrogen balance is jeopardized, the addition of complete proteins in the form of everyday foods is the best guarantee of correcting the condition. If, on the other hand, no shortage of protein exists—as is usually the case—there is no justification for additions of protein in *any* form. A candid appraisal of the facts available can help you to distinguish between the sound and unsound in nutritional claims.

Diets Low in Protein

Despite the fact that protein foods are plentiful in this country, individuals and groups do not share them alike, nor in accordance with need. In other countries, similar discrepancies exist. With variations in the protein intake among nations and among the peoples of nations, including our own, it seems well to consider potential danger spots of protein malnutrition. These include:

Groups with Special Needs Protein shortages are apt to appear at periods when dietary allowances are particularly high, as in adolescence, pregnancy, and lactation. Danger of inadequate protein intake also exists during the early preschool period when children are assuming an upright position and require regular supplies of high quality protein to strengthen muscles (Chap. 3). Changes from the infancy diet at this time may be responsible for a lower protein intake than needed.

Some older people tend to eat smaller quantities of food as they increase in age. Unless they make wise choices, therefore, their protein intake may decline in both quantity and quality. In a study of women in certain western states it was found that those in the 75–79-year-old group were getting on the average 53 g of protein daily, and that this represented a gradual decline from 70 g at the 13–17-year-old level [11]. In another study, Iowa women of 70 years or older were eating less protein than those in the 30–39-year-old age range. The proportion of women in the older age group with less than 50 g of protein in their daily diets was twice as high as that in the younger age group [11].

Low Economic Levels High quality protein sources are not cheap. It is therefore logical to regard as a potential danger spot the diets of low-income groups. The U.S. Department of Agriculture household dietary studies of 1955 showed that protein in family diets tended to parallel family income in that families at lower income levels, in general, had less protein than those at higher income levels [9]. As reported, there was great variation in protein intake at all income levels, but low protein diets were found more frequently among families with low incomes. However, few family diets that failed to meet the dietary allowances for protein failed by a wide margin.

Low Calorie Diets Meals low in total amount of food (calories) in relation to need may be suspected of being low in protein. This is true whether the food supply is restricted or the individual voluntarily chooses to eat less food in order to reduce his weight. If protein intake is to be adequate under these circumstances, foods must be selected with special care. Emphasis should be placed on high-quality proteins.

Poor Food Habits People with certain fixed food habits are apt to have a low protein intake, or at least one of inferior protein quality. This is especially true if their selection of food is limited. Often the diet is composed of 2 or 3 traditional foods whose nutrients do not supplement each other adequately. People may eat such foods from long-established habit and continue to do so even when more nutritious foods are available. Groups that subsist on high-fat, high-carbohydrate diets, or on such combinations as corn pone and fat back or "tea and toast" to the exclusion of other foods, are the ones most vulnerable. Diets such as these, which are low either in total protein or in high quality protein, or both, are usually low in other nutrients as well. All too often these foods are eaten in amounts that cause excess calorie intake and undue gain in weight.

Vegetarians Obviously, strict vegetarians exclude sources of animal protein. Only by eating scientifically planned mixtures of vegetable sources, such as those described under the next topic, can they hope to obtain the essential amino acids in the amounts and proportions needed. The practical difficulties of obtaining enough protein from an all-vegetable diet are apparent in Figure 5.1. Some vegetarians, called "lacto-vegetarians," include milk in their diets and thereby receive a supply of animal protein.

► *Plan a true vegetarian diet to meet your own dietary allowances for calories and total protein. What major problems are encountered?*

Scarcity of Protein Food Sources In areas of the world where national eating habits call for low protein intake, where protein-rich foods are scarce, and where few animal proteins are available, the effects of poor protein nutrition are evident. This is true for much of Africa, for parts of the Middle East and the Far East, and for large portions of Latin America. Table 5-2 shows the daily average protein content, total and animal, and the calorie yield of food supplies of peoples in various areas of the world. There is a noticeable difference in the amount and quality of proteins consumed by different nations. It may be significant that many of the countries with low intakes of total and of high-quality proteins are also the ones with low life expectancy.

Children are the chief victims of protein-deficient diets because of their proportionately greater need for high quality protein. One condition common among young children in areas with such diets and usually seen soon after weaning is called *kwashiorkor* [12,13]. It has been reported in some 65 nations of the world (Fig. 11.1). A major cause appears to be poor quality and low total intake of protein. When weaned, children in these countries are routinely put on a cereal diet devoid of or low in animal protein and often deficient in calories. If

TABLE 5-2

PROTEIN CONTENT AND CALORIE YIELD OF FOOD SUPPLIES IN SELECTED COUNTRIES*

Average Per Capita Per Day 1957–1958

Country	Calories	Protein Grams Total	Protein Grams Animal
Argentina	2960	95	57
Australia	3200	91	60
Brazil	2520	62	18
Canada	3070	95	62
Ceylon	2110	43	6
Chile	2550	79	28
Ecuador	2130	51	13
Germany, West	2960	80	45
India	1800	47	6
Iran	1730	58	8
Israel	2750	84	33
Italy	2600	76	25
Japan	2200	68	17
Mexico	2380	64	13
Morocco	2350	72	18
New Zealand	3370	104	71
Pakistan	2010	49	8
Sweden	2890	82	53
Taiwan	2340	57	14
Turkey	2890	92	14
United Arab Republic (Egypt region)	2640	78	13
United Kingdom	3090	87	51
United States of America	3100	92	66
Uruguay	2960	96	62
Venezuela	2040	54	20

* *Yearbook of Food and Agriculture Statistics*, Rome, Italy: Food and Agriculture Organization, 1959.

this situation continues, a child becomes emaciated, his growth is stunted, his muscles are underdeveloped, the color and texture of his hair are altered, and he suffers from loss of appetite and diarrhea. Unless he receives treatment, early death may follow. When these children, at weaning, are fed dry milk or other sources of high quality protein in addition to their cereals, kwashiorkor does not usually develop. If the diet is thus improved after the onset of the disease, it can frequently be arrested or kept under control.

Organizations of the United Nations and various regional agencies concerned with the nutrition of the peoples of the world are experimenting with food mixtures of locally available, low-cost foods which will provide high quality proteins. One approach is to combine a small amount of the scarce animal-source proteins, such as fishmeal, with a larger proportion of the more abundant plant sources [12,13]. Another is to make all-plant combinations by skillfully combining the more efficient of the plant proteins [14], particularly legumes such as soybeans and peanuts, with other plant sources of lesser value that provide supplementing amino acids needed to achieve a satisfactory total protein mixture. Research on such mixtures continues. Some are designed merely as diet supplements; others may be used safely as the main or as the sole item of diet. Such mixtures, which are being tested in parts of the world where protein-deficient diets are common, hold great promise for better protein nutrition in those areas. In the meantime, efforts are also being made to increase the availability of milk for children by increasing local milk production and by importing concentrated forms of milk.

The disease *pellagra,* which is also associated with low protein intake, is discussed briefly in connection with the vitamin niacin (Chap. 7). The relation of protein to anemia is brought out in the discussion of iron (Chap. 6).

PROTEINS—A FEW HIGHLIGHTS

WHAT PROTEINS DO FOR YOU	Build and maintain all body tissues: muscles, tendons, blood, skin, bone, nails Help form glandular secretions such as hormones, digestive and other enzymes Help form antibodies to build resistance to disease Provide food energy
RECOMMENDED DAILY DIETARY ALLOWANCES	ADULT: On the average: 70 g protein (men) 58 g protein (women) (1 g per kg [2.2 lbs] of body weight per day) CHILD of school age: On the average: 50–70 g protein daily for children 4–12 years of age (2.8–2.0 g per kg [2.2 lbs] of body weight per day)
SOME OF THE BEST FOOD SOURCES	Lean meats, poultry, fish Dry legumes Cheese, milk, eggs Cereals and breads (See Fig. 5.1)
THE IMPORTANCE OF PROTEINS TO GOOD NUTRITURE	A liberal intake of proteins: a well-developed body of desirable size and muscle texture; an inadequate protein intake: an undersized, poorly developed body with poor muscle tone A diet providing a generous supply of high quality proteins: a feeling of fitness and well-being; low protein intake: lack of vigor and stamina Protein intake important in resistance to certain infections, recovery from disease, healing of wounds, and convalescence from surgery; improvement hastened if protein nutrition is adequate

REFERENCES

1. Leverton, R. M., "Proteins," *Food—The Yearbook of Agriculture.* Washington, D.C.: U.S. Department of Agriculture, 1959. p. 57.
2. Food and Nutrition Board, *Evaluation of Protein Nutrition.* Pub. 711. Washington, D.C.: National Academy of Sciences-National Research Council, 1959.
3. Food and Nutrition Board, *Recommended Dietary Allowances.* Pub. 589. Washington, D.C.: National Academy of Sciences-National Research Council, 1958.
4. Leverton, R. M., "Amino Acids," *Food—The Yearbook of Agriculture.* Washington, D.C.: U.S. Department of Agriculture, 1959. p. 64.
5. Rose, W. C., "The Amino Acid Requirements of Adult Man," *Nutrition Abstracts and Reviews,* 27 (July 1957) pp. 631–47.
6. Reynolds, M. S., "Amino Acid Requirements of Adults," *J. Am. Dietet. Assoc.,* 33 (Oct. 1957) pp. 1015–18.
7. Leverton, R. M., and Gram, M. R., "Nitrogen Excretion of Women Related to the Distribution of Animal Protein in Daily Meals," *J. Nutrition,* 39 (Sept. 1949) pp. 57–65.
8. Economic Research Service, *Consumption of Food in the United States, 1909–52.* Supplement for 1960 to Agricultural Handbook No. 62. Washington, D.C.: U.S. Department of Agriculture, August 1961.
9. LeBovit, C., and Clark, F., "Are We Well Fed?" *Food–The Yearbook of Agriculture.* Washington, D.C.: U.S. Department of Agriculture, 1959. p. 620.
10. Morgan, A. F., *Nutritional Status U.S.A.* Bull. 769. Berkeley: California Agricultural Experiment Station, University of California, Oct. 1959.
11. Phipard, E. F., "Protein and Amino Acids in Diets," *Nutrition Committee News,* May–June 1959. Washington, D.C.: U.S. Department of Agriculture.
12. Scrimshaw, N. S., "Progress in Solving World Nutrition Problems," *J. Am. Dietet. Assoc.,* 35 (May 1959) pp. 441–48.
13. Institute of Nutrition of Central America and Panama, *Am. J. Clinical Nutrition,* 9 (March–April 1961). (A series of papers on nutritional conditions in that area.)
14. "Leaf Protein as Human Food," *Nutrition Reviews,* 18 (July 1960) pp. 218–19.

READINGS

Allison, J. B., "Biological Value of Proteins," *Food and Nutrition News,* 30 (Feb. 1959) p. 1. Chicago: National Livestock and Meat Board.

Andrews, J. S., "Proteins and Nutrition," *Cereal Science Today,* 2 (Nov. 1957) pp. 242–45; 264.

Block, R. J., and Mandl, R. H., "Amino Acid Composition of Bread Proteins," *J. Am. Dietet. Assoc.,* 34 (July 1958) pp. 724–26.

Burke, B. S., Reed, R. B., van den Berg, A. S., and Stuart, H. C., "A Longitudinal Study of the Animal Protein Intake of Children from One to Eighteen Years of Age," *Am. J. Clinical Nutrition,* 9 (Sept.–Oct. 1961) pp. 616–24.

———, "Relationships between Animal Protein, Total Protein and Total Calorie Intakes in the Diets of Children from One to Eighteen Years of Age," *Am. J. Clinical Nutrition,* 9 (Nov.–Dec. 1961) pp. 729–34.

Cohn, C., Joseph, D., and Oler, A., "Feeding Frequency and Protein Metabolism," *Federation Proceedings,* 21 (March–April 1962) p. 403.

Darby, W. J., "Dietary Interrelationships," *Food and Nutrition News,* 29 (March 1958) p. 1. Chicago: National Livestock and Meat Board.

Goldsmith, G. A., "Underfed or Poorly Fed?" *Today's Health,* 36 (June 1958) pp. 36; 58–61.

Mitchell, H. H., "Our Protein Needs," *Today's Health,* 36 (Sept. 1958) pp. 56–61.

Nasset, E. S., *Your Diet, Digestion and Health.* New York: Barnes & Noble, Inc., 1962. (Chap. 5, "Utilization of Proteins.")

CHAPTER 6

Mineral elements

Certain facts about mineral elements were established in Chapter 3. You know, for example, that mineral elements, collectively, represent one of the 6 nutrient classes; that the presence of particular kinds of mineral elements is more important than the total quantity in foods; that they are not broken down in digestive processes in preparation for "nutritional service" to the body but, if soluble, are absorbed and used essentially as they occur in foods; and that, in broad terms, minerals help build the body structure and coordinate its processes.

You are now ready to consider: a) certain individual mineral elements that require particular attention in food selection, their more specific functions, and their food sources; b) how much you need of those mineral elements for which dietary allowances have been established; and c) what you can expect in terms of nutritional well-being when meals contain enough, or are deficient in, certain mineral elements. First some general considerations that will give a background for this chapter.

» ORIGIN OF MINERAL ELEMENTS

Mineral elements originate in the soil —soil fed by rocks that have disintegrated through the ages. Plants grown in the soil take up the inorganic elements they need for forming their roots, stems, and leaves. Animals eat the plants and utilize the minerals they require for their own body development and functioning. You obtain your mineral elements by eating not only plants, but also animal tissue and such products of animals as milk and eggs. Thus, indirectly, the minerals of the soil become the minerals of your body and you have another example of how the foods you eat become a part of you.

You should not draw sweeping conclusions from this fact, however. Pseudoscientists and diet quacks have associated the mineral content of soils too closely with the nutritional status of peoples living on products of those soils (Chap. 10). It is true that soils differ in mineral content, but the level of minerals in the vegetation grown on the soils may not reflect those differences. Often no relationship can be shown [1]. Iodine, and possibly fluorine, deficiencies of the soil are the only ones known to be a problem in human nutrition. And these are minimized by eating foods grown on many different soils and by other dietary practices recommended today.

In a 10-year study in which 2 groups of cows were fed through several generations on feeds grown on depleted and on well-fertilized soils, the feeds from the 2 soils showed little difference in composition [2]. And there was no significant difference in the composition and in the growth-promoting properties of the milk from the 2 groups of cows [3]. The danger of a relationship between depleted soils and human malnutrition lies in the failure of such soils to produce *enough* foods rather than in the inferior quality of the food produced.

Mineral elements may be said to be merely "on loan" from the soil to the body and to be returned to the soil unchanged. After the various minerals have been made available for body use, they are diverted to the parts of the system where needed. Here, they discharge the duties for which they are intended and then are excreted.

» MINERAL ELEMENTS USEFUL TO THE BODY

For convenience in discussing them, mineral elements may be separated roughly into 2 groups: those which occur in the body and in foods in relatively large amounts, and those called *trace elements,* which occur in foods in traces only and are needed in only minute amounts. Calcium, phosphorus, magnesium, potassium, sodium, chlorine, and sulfur belong to the first group. Iron, copper, iodine, fluorine, cobalt, molybdenum, manganese, chromium, selenium, and zinc are in the second category. They are the trace elements that are useful in nutrition. The Food and Nutrition Board has proposed daily dietary allowances for only calcium and iron [4]. It is believed that if the allowances for these and other nutrients on the recommended dietary allowance table are met, the remaining minerals will also be present in adequate amounts.

Mineral elements are identified separately, but it should be understood that they work together closely and render service in many different combinations. Therefore, while certain minerals serve special purposes in the body, they rarely act alone in achieving these purposes.

» CALCIUM AND PHOSPHORUS

A notable example of collaboration between minerals is that between calcium and phosphorus. They occur together in different parts of the body and, jointly, they meet many body needs. Both are present in relatively large amounts. The body of a man of average size contains about 2¾ lbs of calcium and about 1½ lbs of phosphorus. Both calcium and phosphorus are distributed unevenly: about 99 percent of the calcium and 80–90 percent of the phosphorus to the bones and teeth; the small remainder of each to the soft tissues and body fluids.

Your day-to-day intakes of calcium and phosphorus come from the foods you eat. How well you are nourished with respect to these two mineral elements depends on how well you choose your meals. It is of first importance, therefore, to know reliable food sources of both minerals and practical ways of applying the information to food selection.

The task is simplified by eliminating a detailed consideration of the food sources of phosphorus. This is possible because diets that supply enough protein and calcium usually "bring along" enough phosphorus. Important sources of phosphorus are lean meats, milk, cheeses, fish, dry legumes, whole-grain cereals, and eggs. Our chief concern at this point, then, is the calcium values of familiar foods, in portions commonly served.

Comparative Calcium Food Values

One way to obtain a perspective on calcium values in foods is to study the comparative calcium yields of the different foods on your own representative food list. The specimen representative list (Fig. 6.1) serves as a basis for drawing general conclusions with respect to important food sources.

It is apparent from Fig. 6.1 that calcium is present in many foods but that relatively few of them are rich sources. Of this small number, milk and cheese lead the list. Canned salmon (which includes the bones), dry legumes, and certain "greens" are next in line. All of these foods rank quantitatively as primary sources. But richness in calcium is not the sole consideration. It is also important to know how often and how much of such foods are served and whether the calcium present can be absorbed by the body. Milk is in a particularly favorable position because it lends itself to frequent use and its calcium is readily absorbed. It is also used in different forms, such as cheese and ice cream. Ice cream (not shown in Fig. 6.1) yields 75 or more mg of calcium per serving. Routine use of milk and milk-made foods in a day's meals makes it feasible to double or triple the calcium values of the individual milk items in Fig. 6.1.

In regions where collards and certain other "greens" are used daily in liberal amounts, they are also significant sources of calcium. Unfortunately, spinach contains oxalic acid (as do chard and beet greens), which probably prevents its calcium from being absorbed by the body. The calcium is said to be "unavailable." (In Appendix G it may be assumed that calcium is available in all "greens" listed unless otherwise indicated.) Several "greens" have as much or more calcium than spinach does, and in available form. Their calcium values range from 124 mg per ½ cup serving (kale) to 237 mg (collards).

Salmon and dried legumes are not usually daily items of diet in this country. Furthermore, fish, in general, are not good sources of calcium unless the bones are eaten, and this is not usually the case. Therefore, regular use of milk and milk-made foods and *carefully chosen* secondary sources of calcium give the most promise of an adequate calcium intake.

The secondary sources of calcium as shown in Fig. 6.1 are fruits (whole oranges lead the list), cottage cheese, vegetables, and eggs. The difference in values between primary and secondary sources is striking. For example, it takes 4½ servings of a high secondary source (1 medium orange, 63 mg) to equal the calcium yield of a primary source (1 cup milk, 285 mg). The calcium values listed drop off sharply, and only halfway down the list, it takes about 16 servings of a food (green peas) to equal the calcium value of 1 cup of milk.

Foods that furnish less than 20 mg of calcium per serving include all meats, all breads and cereals, and some fruits and vegetables. Meats, cereals (unless prepared with or served with milk, or fortified with calcium), and pure fats and sweets can therefore be eliminated in practical considerations of dietary calcium.

► *Arrange your own list of representative foods (sort cards) in order of their quantitative importance as sources of calcium. Analyze the list. Consider groupings representing similar calcium values and try to characterize the content of the groupings.*

Enter calcium values on your personal meal record. Total the calcium intake for the day.

Fig. 6.1 Servings of representative foods in order of their importance as sources of calcium. (Each bar represents an approximate calcium value for the series of foods listed below it.)

Food*	Weight or Approximate Measure **	Calcium Milligrams
250 mg		
Milk, fluid, skin (or buttermilk)	1 cup	298
Milk, fluid, whole	1 cup	285
Cheese, cheddar	1 1/8" cube	221
125 mg		
Salmon, canned	1/2 cup	159 (includes bones)
Beans, dry, canned	3/4 cup	129
Spinach	1/2 cup	112 (not usuable by body)
Broccoli	1/2 cup	98
50 mg		
Orange	1 medium	63
Cheese, cottage, creamed	1/4 cup	50
Sweet potato	1 medium	44
25 mg		
Cantaloup	1/2 melon	33
Egg	1 medium	27
Apricots, dried, cooked	1/2 cup	26
Squash, winter	1/2 cup	25
Beans, snap, green	1/2 cup	23
Cabbage, shredded, raw	1/2 cup	23
Grapefruit	1/2 medium	21
Prunes, dried, cooked	5 with juice	21
15 mg		
Bread, white, enriched	1 slice	19
Carrots, diced	1/2 cup	19
Pineapple juice, canned	1/2 cup (small glass)	19
Peas, green	1/2 cup	18
Strawberries, raw	1/2 cup	16
Cream, coffee	1 tbsp	15
Haddock	1 fillet	15
Oatmeal, cooked	2/3 cup	14
Orange juice, fresh	1/2 cup (small glass)	13
Peanut butter	1 tbsp	12
Lettuce leaves	2 large or 4 small	11
Rice, cooked	3/4 cup	11
Beef, pot roast	3 oz	10
Chicken	1/4 small broiler	10
8 mg		
Potato, white	1 medium	9
Tomato juice, canned	1/2 cup (Small glass)	9
Apple, raw	1 medium	8
Banana, raw	1 medium	8
Macaroni, enriched, cooked	3/4 cup	8
Pork chop	1 chop	8
4 mg		
Corn, canned	1/2 cup	5
Ham, luncheon meat	2 oz	5
Liver, beef	2 oz	5
Peaches, canned	2 halves, with juice	5
Sausage, salami	1 slice	5
Butter or fortified margine	1 tbsp	3
Corn flakes, fortified	1 1/3 cup	3
Frankfurter	1 medium	3
Bacon, crisp	2 slices	2
0 mg		
Beverage, kola type	6 oz	...
Sugar, granulated	1 tbsp	...
Oils, salad or cooking	1 tbsp	0

*Foods are in forms ready to eat. All meats and vegetables are cooked unless otherwise indicated.

**See Appendix G for further identification of these foods. On that list all foods are described more fully and both weights and measures are indicated.

Make a list of the "greens" in Appendix G with their calcium values per 1/2 cup serving. Which of them provide available sources of calcium? How much do you depend on "greens" as a source of calcium?

Make a list of the different kinds of fish in Appendix G with their calcium values per serving. Which—if any—are comparable to salmon in calcium value? What are the practical possibilities for depending on fish as a source of calcium?

Your Calcium Need

Daily needs for calcium have been assessed with balance experiments similar to those for protein. There is some dissatisfaction with the balance method as a means of determining calcium requirements, but an acceptable alternative method has not been found. The term "balance" refers to the condition of equilibrium that exists in an adult body when the daily intake of calcium in foods balances the outgo in excreta. The amount of calcium necessary to bring this about in an adult is regarded as his daily requirement. To establish the requirements for childhood, pregnancy, and lactation, essentially the same procedure is followed. The difference is that the maximum storage that can be achieved at these periods, rather than balance, is the objective.

Recommended Daily Allowances for Calcium

The Food and Nutrition Board of the National Academy of Sciences-National Research Council, proposes 800 mg as the daily calcium allowance for men and women (Table 6-1). The Board recognizes that

TABLE 6–1

RECOMMENDED DAILY DIETARY ALLOWANCES FOR CALCIUM AND IRON [4]

	Age Years	Weight (lb)	Height (in.)	Calories	Calcium mg	Iron mg
Men	25	154	69	3200	800	10
	45	154	69	3000	800	10
	65	154	69	2550	800	10
Women	25	128	64	2300	800	12
	45	128	64	2200	800	12
	65	128	64	1800	800	12
	Pregnant (second half)			+300	1500	15
	Lactating (850 ml daily)			+1000	2000	15
Infants	0–1/12					
	2/12–6/12	13	24		600	5
	7/12–12/12	20	28		800	7
Children	1 – 3	27	34	1300	1000	7
	4 – 6	40	43	1700	1000	8
	7 – 9	60	51	2100	1000	10
	10–12	79	57	2500	1200	12
Boys	13–15	108	64	3100	1400	15
	16–19	139	69	3600	1400	15
Girls	13–15	108	63	2600	1300	15
	16–19	120	64	2400	1300	15

people vary widely in individual need, but the proposed allowance is believed to be sufficiently liberal to provide for such individual differences. No specific allowance is proposed for phosphorus: an adult's desirable daily intake is believed to be about one and one-half times that for calcium.

The daily allowance for calcium during the latter half of pregnancy is nearly double that of nonpregnant women (1500 mg vs. 800 mg). Calcium and phophorus are chiefly involved in the construction of the bones and teeth of the fetus. In a full term fetus, about 65 percent of these 2 minerals are normally deposited in the last 2 months of pregnancy. The mother's diet, therefore, requires the largest amounts of calcium and phosphorus (and vitamin D) during that period. If she entered pregnancy with low calcium stores, she should increase her intake in early pregnancy and thus begin replenishing her stores before the period of greatest stress.

The mother's daily allowance for calcium during lactation is more than double that of the nonpregnant woman (2000 mg vs. 800 mg). This greatly increased allowance reflects the needs of the baby's very rapidly growing skeleton. And the mother's diet must supply the bone-building ingredients, through her breast milk, if growth is to proceed normally.

How the Average Adult Can Meet His Calcium Allowance

The specimen diet in Appendix B shows one way an adult might choose a day's meals furnishing about 800 mg of calcium. It confirms the points made earlier in discussing Figure 6.1, i.e., milk is the only rich source of calcium that is normally included in some form in almost every meal; several fruits and vegetables are good supporting sources; cereals contribute calcium when milk is used (cornflakes served with milk; bread, rolls, cake if made with milk); meat makes a negligible contribution to the day's calcium; sugar, soft drinks, and butter provide none.

The 4 food combinations in chart on page 94 show ways in which an adult may meet his calcium allowance with and without, milk and dairy foods.

No other nutrient allowance is so easily attained as that for calcium—by discriminating food selection—and none is so difficult to attain or so easily missed if the few rich sources are omitted or used in inadequate quantities. Food combinations 1, 2 and 3 given on next page show ways to reach the adult's daily calcium allowance using milk products exclusively or with other very good and good sources of calcium. Combination 4 omits dairy foods but includes other very good, good, and fair sources. This combination should not serve to minimize the nutritional importance of fruits and vegetables. Both groups make significant dietary contributions, as will be shown. Its purpose is rather to demonstrate how difficult it is to obtain enough calcium when milk and milk-made dishes are omitted from the diet. Under such circumstances, vegetables and fruits must be eaten in quantities scarcely practicable. At the same time, main-dish foods must regularly include certain selected kinds of fish, such as salmon (with bones), eggs, and dry legumes such as beans.

► *What is your own daily calcium allowance? (If you are 20 years of age or older, use 800 mg; if you are under 20 years, use the allowance nearest your age, Table 6-1). Record your calcium allowance on your personal meal record.*

How does your actual daily calcium intake as shown on your meal record compare with your daily calcium allowance? Account for the effect of your food choices

MEETING DAILY CALCIUM ALLOWANCE FOR ADULTS: 800 mg

	1	Calcium mg
Milk, skim	1 pt (2 cups)	596
Cheese, cheddar	1 oz	221
Total		817
	2	
Milk, skim	1 cup	298
Cheese, cheddar	1 oz	221
Broccoli	½ cup	98
Orange	1 medium	63
Cheese, cottage	¼ cup	50
Sweet potato	1 medium	44
Egg	1 medium	27
Total		801
	3	
Cheese, cheddar	2 oz	442
Cheese, cottage	½ cup	100
Turnip greens	½ cup	188
Orange	1 medium	63
Egg	1 medium	27
Total		820
	4	
Salmon, canned (with bones)	½ cup	159
Beans, dry, canned	¾ cup	129
Broccoli	½ cup	98
Orange	1 medium	63
Sweet potato	1 medium	44
Cantaloup	½ melon	33
Egg	1 medium	27
Apricots, stewed	½ cup	26
Squash, winter	½ cup	25
Cabbage, raw	½ cup	23
Prunes	5, with juice	21
Bread, enriched	4 slices	76
Carrots	½ cup	19
Peas, green	½ cup	18
Beets	½ cup	18
Strawberries	½ cup	16
Total		795

on your total calcium intake: whether it is high or low in relation to your allowance.

Estimate the calcium yield of the vegetarian diet you planned in Chapter 5.

How would you reply to a person who said to you: "I don't use milk but I eat lots of salads. Will they give me the calcium I need?"

Calcium Allowances for Children

Children need calcium not only for upkeep but for growth of their bones. Table 6-1 shows progression in daily calcium allowances from 600 mg during the first 6 months of life to more than twice that amount during adolescence. The increased storage and use of calcium by the growing body is shown in Figure 3.4 [5]. Because of their growth need, children have a proportionately higher allowance in relation to body weight than do adults and the actual calcium allowances for children at every age level above infancy are higher than those for adults. The full-grown man and the infant of 6 months to 1 year of age have identical daily allowances for calcium. And the adult allowance is little more than half that of the teen-ager.

The problem of meeting a child's dietary allowance for calcium is similar to that of meeting the adult's—a matter of selecting rich sources that are used regularly. The chart on page 95 shows food combinations for 3 age groups in which the allowances may be met easily.

The food combinations for children demonstrate again the wide divergence between calcium values obtained from certain important sources, eaten daily in reasonable quantities, and from less concentrated sources. In assembling the foods for the 3 combinations shown, it was assumed that milk would be a part of the diet of the

MEETING CALCIUM ALLOWANCES FOR CHILDREN

Ages in Years	**4–6**		**10–12**		**13–19 (Boys)**	
DAILY CALCIUM ALLOWANCES	1000 mg		1200 mg		1400 mg	
		Ca mg		**Ca mg**		**Ca mg**
Milk, whole	3 cups	855	4 cups	1140	4 cups	1140
Orange	1 medium	63	1 medium	63	1 medium	63
Egg	1 medium	27	—	—	—	—
Cabbage	½ cup, raw	23	—	—	—	—
Prunes	5, with juice	21	—	—	—	—
Peas green	½ cup	18	—	—	—	—
Cheese, cheddar	—	—	—	—	1 oz	221
Total		1007		1203		1424

children at each age level. Obviously other foods in the diet would add to the total calcium intake for the day. A calcium margin so provided would be "money in the bank." The teen-ager would have particular difficulty in meeting his high calorie needs if he attempted to obtain his calcium from alternate sources, chiefly from fruits and vegetables.

When Milk Is Not Available

In many parts of the world little milk is available. Some countries traditionally use cheeses made from the small amount of milk obtained from their various domesticated animals. In other countries, condensed forms of milk are imported. Even with such measures, milk and milk products still are a negligible source of calcium in parts of the Western and in much of the Eastern Hemisphere. Under these circumstances, babies are often breast fed for a prolonged period to give them the benefit of calcium from mother's milk. After weaning, the calcium content of the diet is usually very low; this deficiency results in the small bones and the short stature of the peoples on such diets. Sometimes dietary customs, such as eating tiny bones of fish and other animals, drinking the liquid after boiling such bones in vinegar (which dissolves the calcium), soaking corn in lime before making certain native dishes such as tortillas, eating very large amounts of green vegetables, are responsible for raising the calcium content of the diet. In areas where the drinking water contains calcium, it makes a small contribution to the total supply.

When milk is available, but for some reason a person cannot use it, a physician may recommend calcium and phosphorus in pure chemical forms. The body can utilize them in pills and capsules as well as in food form, but the user is deprived of the other essential nutrients in the milk and must therefore make special plans to obtain these nutrients from other foods. (See Fig. 9.2.)

How Your Body Uses Calcium and Phosphorus

During digestion, calcium and phosphorus are separated from the foods eaten and are eventually absorbed through the intestinal wall into the blood stream, which carries them to the areas of the body where they are needed. These minerals are not absorbed completely: the amounts not absorbed are excreted in the feces; those absorbed and not used are excreted in the urine.

Several factors affect the amounts of calcium absorbed from the intestinal tract [6]. Among them are:

The kinds of foods that provide the calcium. The calcium from milk is readily absorbed because of its type of sugar (lactose), its vitamin D content (vitamin D milk), and, possibly, its proteins.

The absorption of calcium from vegetables is hampered in 2 ways: by their high content of fiber, which moves them along the intestinal tract so rapidly that calcium absorption is lessened; and, in certain instances, by their oxalic acid content, which has already been mentioned. Certain "greens" and rhubarb contain oxalic acid, which combines with calcium. The oxalate that results is insoluble in the intestinal fluids. The calcium cannot be absorbed and it is thus lost in the feces.

The amount of vitamin D present. Vitamin D is necessary for the absorption of calcium from the gastrointestinal tract. (More detailed consideration of this point will be given under vitamin D, Chap. 7.)

The amount of calcium provided by the diet. The more calcium provided by food, the greater the total amount absorbed. But the body uses calcium more economically—absorbs a larger proportion of the intake—when the intake is small.

The body's need for calcium. During child growth, pregnancy, and lactation when the demands are greatest, the absorption is usually most efficient.

Control of Body Calcium The parathyroid glands, located in the neck, hold the control key to the body's use of calcium and indirectly influence its use of phosporus [6]. This key is a hormone secreted by the glands. The parathyroid hormone governs the calcium content of the blood: it keeps it at a constant low level. To maintain this level, the hormone can move calcium and phosphorus from the bones to the blood or, if the blood has an excess of these minerals, can excrete the excess via the kidneys. A reduced secretion of the parathyroid hormone causes the calcium content of the blood to drop sharply and the phosphorus content to rise, thus creating an imbalance. Any wide divergence from normal in the calcium level of the blood is a danger signal to health.

How Calcium and Phosphorus Serve You [6,7]

Calcium serves with sodium and potassium in promoting normal action of the heart muscle to maintain a steady rhythmic beat. It is essential for the clotting of the blood, for the control of the passage of fluids through cell walls, and for the action of certain enzymes. Phosphorus is an indispensable part of every cell of the body. It plays a distinctive role in maintaining the neutrality of the blood and it reacts chemically with other nutrients—proteins, fats, and carbohydrates—to provide the body with energy and material needed for growth and maintenance. Calcium and phosphorus are both necessary for normal response of nerves to stimulation and to action of all body muscles. Thus we have the first examples of the regulatory and coordinative functions of specific mineral elements. Calcium and phosphorus are equally important to body structure.

Building Functions Calcium and phosphorus are responsible for the strength and hardness of bones and teeth [8]. In chemical union, as calcium phosphates, they are carried by the blood to the bones and deposited there as tiny crystals around a framework of protein material known as the organic matrix. The crystals are provided with substances for repair by the intercellular fluid that surrounds them. A network of blood and lymph vessels and nerves runs throughout the matrix and bone crystals. Larger crystals of the same type are deposited in the teeth.

Bones change in size and character with age (Fig. 6.2). Bones of the fetus are small before birth and consist chiefly of cartilage and water. As they increase in size, calcium and phosphorus are deposited in and around the cartilage and the bones are hardened. This process is called calcification. The quantitative increase in body calcium with age is shown graphically in Figure 3.4 [5]. Normally the increase in calcium is in direct proportion to the size of the individual as he grows into an adult.

In the first few weeks of fetal life, tooth "buds" begin to form; the first teeth start to calcify by the middle of pregnancy. Certain permanent tooth buds begin to calcify at birth; most others start the process in the intervening period up to 3 years of age. Wisdom teeth often begin to calcify as late as the tenth year of age.

Bone-building requires not only calcium and phosphorus. It must have protein for building and maintaining the bone matrix and for cell content. It must have vitamins A, C, and D for specialized purposes, which are considered in Chapter 7. As would be expected, bones and teeth calcify more slowly when the diet is deficient in calcium, phosphorus, and the other nutrients needed. This fact was demonstrated in Fig. 2.4, where the retarding effect of undernutrition was shown in the poorly calcified wrist bones of a 7-year-old child.

On the other hand, a reserve supply of calcium and phosphorus can be built up in the body's bones at any age. This occurs when the diet provides enough for immediate needs, and a surplus for storage. When a surplus exists, it is deposited on the inside of the ends of the bones in needle-like crystals. This reserve supply is available for emergencies when the dietary intake does not cover day-to-day needs: it is the "money in the bank" referred to earlier. (The relationship of magnesium to bone-building should be noted here, although the

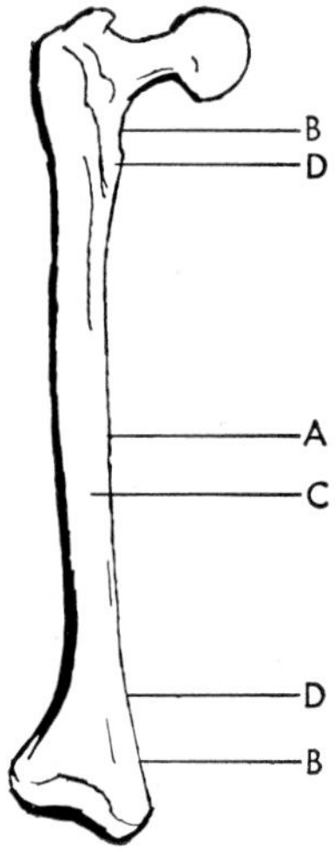

Fig. 6.2 A long bone. As a long bone grows larger, new bone material is deposited on the outside of the shaft (A), and at the two ends of the shaft (B). At the same time, the bone material on the inside of the shaft (C) and just beneath that of the ends (D) is absorbed and used by the body wherever it is needed. This "give and take" system permits the bones to increase in size without becoming "overweight." (Adapted from M. Keen, *The How and Why Wonder Book of the Human Body*. New York: Grosset & Dunlap, Inc., 1961.

discussion of this mineral is found later in this chapter. It appears possible that magnesium may substitute in a minor way for calcium stores when the intake of the latter is deficient.)

Calcium in Our National Diet

The question whether we as a nation get enough calcium may be answered in different ways, depending on the basis for the reply. One basis is the amount of calcium available per person per day from our total food supply [9]. At the present time the figure is about 1000 mg. This amount is somewhat above the 800 mg dietary allowance for adults and for very young children, but considerably below the figure for adolescence, pregnancy, and lactation (1300–2000 mg). But calcium, like other nutrients, is not distributed equally to all people, nor is it allocated on the basis of need. To determine whether we are getting enough calcium, therefore, we require information on the food habits of families and their individual members.

The comprehensive dietary study of households made by the U.S. Department of Agriculture in 1955 showed that the calcium intake of almost one-third of the families in this sample failed to measure up to their recommended dietary allowances for calcium [10]. It will be noted from Table 6-2 that calcium in family diets was lower, and more consistently low, in the different sections of the country than any other nutrient.

But family consumption data still do not pinpoint the specific groups where calcium intakes are lowest. Dietary data obtained by investigators at the State Agricultural Experiment Stations on large numbers of individuals have been analyzed by sex and age [11]. Information on average calcium intakes in relation to the recommended dietary allowances for persons 4–80 years of age is summarized in Figures 6.3 and 6.4. It will be noted that boys of almost all ages, on the average, met the calcium allowances, but that girls were low at all ages, and drastically so in the 13–20-year-age range. In the adult group the sex difference appeared again. The calcium intakes of men were, on the average, above recommended allowances; the women's intakes were low and continued to decline into old age.

A look behind the averages of groups to individual diet records does not change the picture radically. It merely sharpens the focus on the findings. It makes it possible to examine the range of diets on the scale of adequacy, i.e., to know the proportion that fell below and the proportion that rose above the allowances, and how much they varied in either direction. One piece of useful information derived from scrutiny of individual records is provided in Figure 6.5 [11]. It shows by the length of bars the

TABLE 6–2

PROPORTIONS OF FAMILY DIETS IN REGIONS OF THE UNITED STATES NOT PROVIDING RECOMMENDED AMOUNTS OF EIGHT NUTRIENTS

Nutrient	North East Percent	North Central Percent	West Percent	South Percent
Protein	7	5	5	12
Calcium	28	26	26	34
Iron	12	9	7	10
Vitamin A val.	12	13	11	26
Thiamine	22	14	16	15
Riboflavin	18	16	15	25
Niacin	7	5	6	10
Ascorbic Acid	17	19	23	37

Food, The Yearbook of Agriculture, 1959, Washington, D. C.: U. S. Department of Agriculture. p. 623.

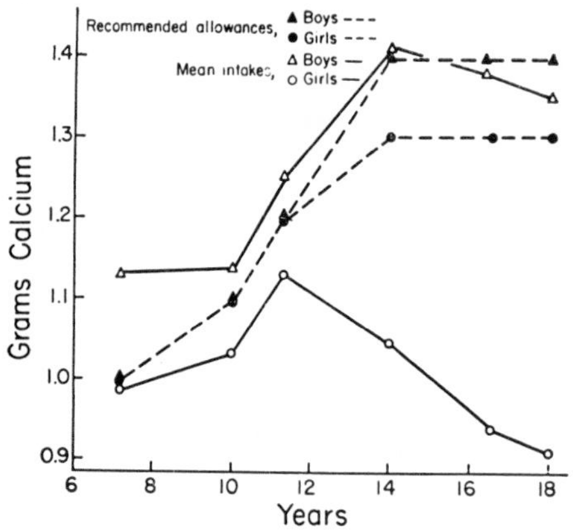

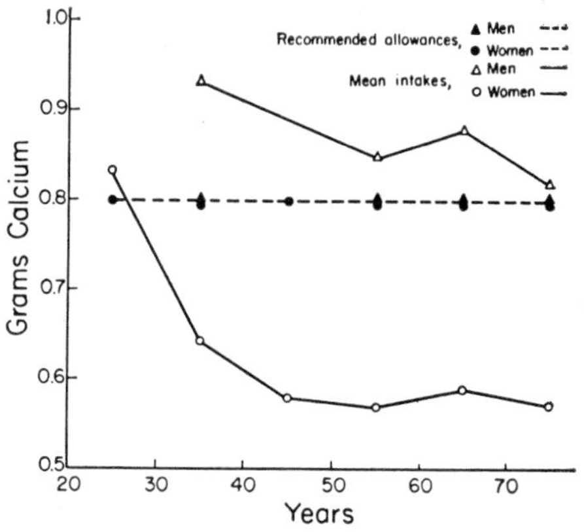

Figs. 6.3 and 6.4 Calcium intake in relation to daily dietary allowances. (*left*) Average daily calcium intake of boys and girls 4–20 years of age. (*right*) Average daily calcium intake of men and women from 20 to more than 80 years of age. (A. F. Morgan [Ed.], *Nutritional Status U.S.A.* Bull. 769. Berkeley, Calif.: University of California, Division of Agricultural Sciences, Agricultural Experiment Station, p. 33.)

percentage of adolescent boys and girls whose daily intakes of several nutrients fell below two-thirds of the recommended allowances for those nutrients. The twin bars at the top on either side of the figure pertain to calcium. They serve to accent the findings from group averages: a larger percentage of girls than of boys had low intakes of calcium, and there were more girls with low intakes at the 15–18-year-old level than at the 12–14-year-old level. But Figure 6.5 tells us still more: nearly one-half of the older girls had daily intakes that failed to meet even two-thirds of the recommended allowances for calcium; one-third of both boys and girls 12–14 years of age fell below two-thirds of the calcium allowance for that age period.

Because calcium is so closely identified with milk, consumption data on calcium usually reflect the status of milk consumption. At the present time, milk and milk products, other than butter, provide more than three-fourths of all the calcium available to consumers in the United States [9].

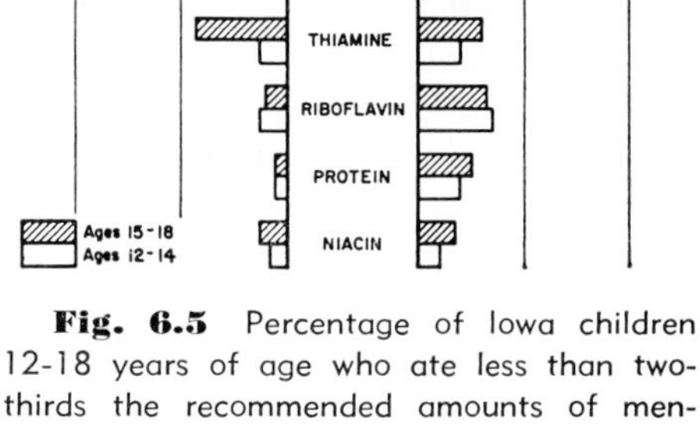

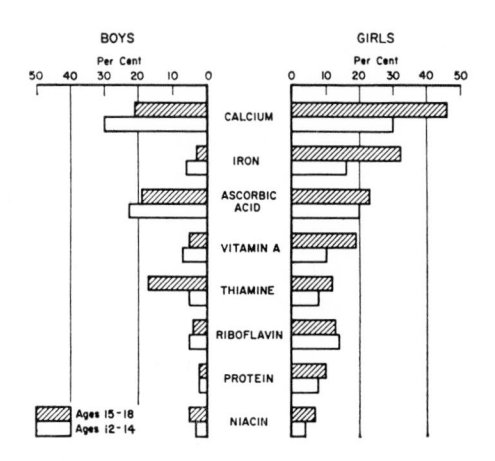

Fig. 6.5 Percentage of Iowa children 12-18 years of age who ate less than two-thirds the recommended amounts of mentioned nutrients. (A. F. Morgan [Ed.], *Nutritional Status U. S. A.* Bull. 769. Berkeley, Calif.: University of California, Division of Agricultural Sciences, Agricultural Experiment Station, p. 43.)

Next in line are fruits and vegetables, which, as a group, yield about one-tenth the total amount. The calcium content of the food supply in this country has increased by about one-fourth in the period during which records were kept—from 1909 to the present. Family dietary studies likewise show an increased intake of calcium as well as an increased consumption of milk during the latter half of the same period. Although this trend is favorable, comparisons of actual with desirable intakes of calcium, as shown in Figures 6.3–6.5 indicate the need for continued increases, particularly among certain age groups. Adolescents—especially girls—and women of all ages appear to be those in greatest need of higher milk consumption.

Calcium intakes should be sufficiently liberal to allow for special needs. Several investigators have found that emotional stress—sorrow, anxiety, joy—among subjects has greatly decreased their ability to retain calcium [12]. It is apparent that calcium consumption must be ample to tide one over such situations when the body's utilization capacity is at low ebb. Studies made at the University of Illinois on teen-age boys sought to establish calcium intakes that would assure positive calcium balance and good calcium nutrition in these years of extremely rapid growth [13]. The boys had been well fed throughout life and had consumed milk regularly. In general, they were considered well nourished. Nevertheless, it proved impossible in most cases to establish practical calcium intakes that would assure maximum retentions. This emphasizes the need for building body stores with liberal intakes of calcium in the preadolescent years. The increase in height of our population above that of certain other peoples may well imply a higher calcium requirement to provide for growth and maintenance of the larger skeleton.

Results of Good and Poor Calcium Nutriture

A reserve of calcium and allied minerals, with adequate replenishment from daily food, serves the body in the many ways that have been discussed. The result to be expected is a well-functioning body with good bone growth and development and a high level of health and vigor. When the diet is deficient in calcium and phosphorus, these minerals are taken from reserves in the bone structure itself. If this situation continues, the bones become deficient in calcium content, fail to grow properly, and eventually become thin and weak.

Difference in Growth Growth imposes heavy demands for calcium, as has been suggested by the high dietary allowances recommended during childhood [4]. Studies with young experimental animals indicate that planned low calcium intakes result in smaller, poorer bones. Because comparable experiments with children are not feasible, such a direct cause-and-effect relationship has not been demonstrated in human beings. Moreover, the mixed heritage of human beings clouds the picture of growth possibilities. Nevertheless, the sizes of peoples in various parts of the world suggest a calcium-growth relationship. For example, populations of parts of South and Central America who have lived for generations on low calcium intakes are of notably small frame and short stature. Children 5–10 years of age in these areas may be as much as 3 years behind in skeletal growth compared with the children of countries on larger intakes [14]. Japanese children reared in Japan, where rich sources of calcium are not plentiful, have already been shown to be smaller, age for age, than Japanese children reared in this country (Chap. 2). In populations deficient in calcium, there are usually shortages of other nutrients that undoubtedly also contribute to their impeded growth. However, in the areas mentioned, lack of calcium appears to be a major deficiency, common to all.

Difference in Quality of Bone It is logical that a poorly calcified, weakened bone would break easily and heal slowly when broken. Research and observations on animals shows this to be the case [16]. However, clear-cut experimental evidence on human beings has not been available. When a child or adult has bone-healing difficulties, many factors frequently complicate the picture. More and more, however, it seems evident that diet, and notably a prolonged calcium deficiency, is an important factor. Repeated cases of slow bone healing in patients with a history of allergy to milk since birth, for example, have strengthened the conviction that there is a relationship between bone with low calcium reserve and its ability to mend promptly. Middle-aged and older persons who have routinely consumed calcium-poor diets may be expected to have brittle, demineralized bones, which are susceptible of breakage and offer problems in healing [6]. There is also evidence to show that the size and formation of teeth is affected by nutritional conditions during the period of tooth development, and that poorly formed teeth, with pits and fissures, are more caries-susceptible than are well-formed teeth.

Abnormalities in Bones [15,16] Several abnormal conditions in bones are related directly or indirectly to diet. *Rickets* in children results when calcium and phosphorus are not deposited properly in the bones. The bones become weakened and eventually bend easily. An imbalance of calcium, phosphorus, and vitamin D in the body is chiefly responsible for rickets. The period of greatest susceptibility is from prebirth through the preschool age. The condition was common in this country until the discovery of vitamin D and recognition of its function in bone formation. Now that vitamin D has become part of the routine diet during pregnancy and early childhood —in the form of cod liver oil, vitamin D concentrates, and vitamin D milk—rickets is seldom seen here.

Osteomalacia, "adult rickets," is also caused in main by an imbalance of calcium, phosphorus, and vitamin D. It is well known in the Far East. Women there are particularly susceptible because of their heightened needs for calcium in pregnancy and lactation in the face of a supply often insufficient even for maintenance. Vitamin D shortage is attributed to insufficient exposure to direct sunshine.

Osteoporosis is a condition that exists when bones become porous and fragile because calcium is being withdrawn faster than it is being deposited. It usually occurs in older people, especially women, and frequently when they have had a generally poor diet over many years. The precise cause of this type of faulty bone formation is not known. It appears to be a disorder of metabolism, notably a failure of the organic matrix to function properly. This condition may be aggravated by deficiencies of bone-building nutrients and/or poor use of them by the body [16]. Treatment usually includes a diet high in calcium and vitamin D.

Strontium-90 has become well known as a product of atomic explosions. It settles on soils and plants and enters the body, in and on foods. It is radioactive and therefore an accumulation of it in the bones could be a health hazard. High concentrations have been known to cause bone cancers. At the present time, the amount found in human beings is small in relation to the amount considered dangerous to health. Calcium in the diet appears to have a protective function with respect to strontium-90 [6,12]. Apparently the bones accept and deposit calcium in preference to strontium when the former is present in abundance.

Some concern has been expressed recently that people in this country may get too much rather than too little calcium. Those defending this position cite cases of the calcification of soft tissues of the body and particularly the formation of kidney stones. In refutation, it has been pointed out that high calcium intakes and calcified soft tissues do not consistently parallel each other [16]. Also, repeat stone formers and large-stone formers have been reported to be low calcium consumers. And children whose milk (calcium) consumption is relatively high are practically free from stone formation. Some authorities in the field of calcium metabolism are convinced that our dietary allowances for calcium are conservative rather than high; that actual intakes are low rather than high; and that clinical evidence suggests deficiency rather than excessive use of calcium in this country.

» MAGNESIUM, POTASSIUM, SODIUM, CHLORINE, AND SULFUR

Other minerals that occur in the body in relatively large amounts also play important roles in nutrition [17]. Most of them are widely distributed in plant and animal foods. None of this group, which includes magnesium, potassium, sodium, chlorine, and sulfur, appears on the table of recommended daily dietary allowances. Exact information with respect to need is lacking in most cases, but presumably dietary shortages are not common. In several cases the Food and Nutrition Board has suggested desirable daily intakes; in others, it has indicated use of certain foods to cover probable needs.

Magnesium

Magnesium is present in the body in both bones and soft tissues—70 percent in the bones and 30 percent in the soft tissues and blood. It acts in the utilization of calcium and phosphorus. It also serves in many complex relationships with other nutrients, is important in several enzymatic reactions, and helps in the building of proteins. This much is clear, but the full significance of magnesium in animal nutrition is not yet completely understood. Deficiency of magnesium in human beings results in disturbances of calcium metabolism; excesses of magnesium are believed to cause deposition of calcium in the soft tissues.

It has been estimated that 250–300 mg magnesium per day will satisfy an adult's need, and that a child requires about 6 mg magnesium daily for each pound of body weight. There seems no danger that a person will be deficient in magnesium, and slight danger that he will get too much from an ordinary mixed diet. Magnesium is quite well distributed in both animal and vegetable foods.

Potassium, Sodium, and Chlorine

The 3 mineral elements—potassium, sodium, and chlorine—are discussed together because of their overlapping functions. They are found in relative abundance in the body, next in line quantitatively to calcium and phosphorus. Sodium and chlorine, well known because they occur together in common salt, are found chiefly in the fluids that circulate *outside* body cells; potassium is present mostly in fluids *inside* the cells. All 3 are important in the function of osmosis, by which substances pass back and forth between the cells and the surrounding fluids. They also are necessary in keeping a normal balance of water between fluids and cells. An increase or decrease in one of these minerals may create an imbalance. Nerve response to stimulation, travel of nerve impulses to the muscles, and muscle contraction (including the beat of the heart [Chap. 3]) are all dependent on the presence of sodium and potassium. And, together with chlorine, they help to keep a balance between the amount of acid and alkali in the blood.

There is usually no deficiency of these minerals unless there are sudden large losses from the body. Extreme heat that causes heavy perspiration can result in large losses of sodium. This can be replaced by adding sodium chloride to the diet. Pellets of common salt are used. Sodium in excess of needs can be handled well under ordinary circumstances. The body does this by excreting what is not needed. When the body's mechanism fails to rid itself of excess sodium—as in certain types of heart and kidney diseases—the sodium is retained and the patient suffers from edema, a condition in which the tissues retain water.

Table salt is our most concentrated source of sodium (43 percent). Most other foods contain some sodium naturally and many have sodium or salt added to them in such preparation processes as curing meats, brining fish and vegetables. With liberal use of table salt, many people eat far in excess of their need for sodium. Foods of animal origin are the richest natural sources. Vegetables and fruits are low in sodium, except when sodium products are added in preserving them. Cereal grains are low in sodium unless it is used in processing them. Waters vary greatly in sodium content. A *moderate* use of table salt is regarded as the simplest way to avoid excessive intake of sodium.

Potassium and chlorine are distributed widely in common foods, and chlorine is present in salt. There is no indication at present that the average person need be concerned with his potassium or chlorine intake. No daily allowance has been proposed for sodium, potassium, or chlorine.

Sulfur

Sulfur is closely identified with protein. It is an integral part of sulfur-containing amino acids and is found in every cell of the body. Proteins vary in yield of sulfur as they vary in content of these amino acids. No dietary allowance has been proposed for sulfur. It seems safe to assume that the sulfur needs of the body will be met if the protein intake is adequate.

» TRACE MINERAL ELEMENTS

"It is important to remember," says the Yearbook of Agriculture, "that life is a delicate balance of a seemingly infinite number of competing chemical and physiological processes. The trace elements are obviously of great importance to those processes and to that balance" [18]. Our knowledge is still incomplete with respect to the exact functions and nutritional requirements of most of the trace elements. It is known, however, that certain of them have important work in building body substance and regulating body processes. They are indispensable parts of catalytic systems that speed up nutritive activities in the cells. Natural body catalysts are called enzymes. Some enzymes contain one or more of the trace elements. A large part of the vital processes of life is dependent upon activities of enzyme systems.

» IRON

The body of an adult man contains about one-seventh of an ounce of iron—about one three-hundredth that of calcium. The greater part of the iron is in the blood; the remainder is in the muscle cells, in other body cells, and in respiratory enzymes. Iron is closely related in function with other nutrients. The indispensability of copper to iron is discussed later in this chapter. Iron is found in various combinations and associations with proteins.

Iron is best known for its partnership with hemoglobin, a protein of the red blood cells. When iron is absorbed through the walls of the small intestine, a large part of it is carried to the bone marrow. Here the red blood cells are manufactured and the iron becomes a part of hemoglobin. The hemoglobin, which supplies the red coloring matter to the blood, carries oxygen from the lungs to all the cells of the body and carries back to the lungs carbon dioxide which is exhaled.

Comparative Iron Values in Foods

A regular and adequate supply of iron from daily meals is important for carrying on body functions. It is thus important to know how to select foods that provide the needed iron. The comparative iron yields of the items on your representative food list will indicate the range of values among common foods. The specimen representative list (Fig. 6.6) serves here as a basis for discussion of comparative iron sources. Average servings of the foods are arranged in order of their quantitative importance, from rich sources to those with little or no iron.

The importance of protein foods as concentrated sources of iron is apparent from Figure 6.6. Organ meats such as liver, lean muscle meats of all kinds, and dry legumes, head the list; 2 oz of cooked beef liver stands out as nearly twice as rich as 3 oz of cooked lean beef. The livers of different animals and some other organ meats are likewise higher in iron than similar amounts of lean muscle meats (Appendix G).

Dark green leafy vegetables (represented by spinach on the list), dried fruits (represented by prunes and apricots), eggs (yolk), whole grain, restored, and enriched cereals and breads are all good sources of iron.

Those foods which supply only ½ mg of iron or less per serving (the entire lower half of the list), and are thus negligible sources, include fresh fruits, many vegetables of high water content other than the green leafy varieties, unenriched, highly milled cereals, fat meats such as bacon, milk, and cheeses. These foods can be counted on to provide some iron in the diet, but unless the greater part of the allowance is met by the richer sources, these lesser sources will not yield the necessary amount. It will be noted that milk and meat have practically reversed their positions on the calcium and iron lists, respectively (Figs. 6.1 and 6.6).

The pure fats, sugar, and soft drinks provide no iron. Molasses is an exception in the sugar group. Some iron is retained at the molasses stage but is refined out by the time it becomes sugar. (See Chap. 10 for comparative iron values.) However, molasses cannot be considered an important source of iron in the U.S. food supply because of the relatively insignificant amount used. Sugars and syrups, as a group, provide little more than 3 percent of the country's total iron supply.

The foods in Figure 6.6 lend themselves to a system for *estimating* iron values. The values are low and easy to count; the foods can be grouped conveniently. In general, livers can be assigned a value of 5 mg,

Fig. 6.6 Servings of representative foods in order of their importance as sources of iron. (Each bar represents an approximate iron value for the series of foods listed below it.)

Food *	Weight or Approximate Measure **	Iron Milligrams
5 mg		
Liver, beef	2 oz	4.4
3 mg		
Beans, dry, canned	3/4 cup	3.3
Beef, pot roast	3 oz	2.9
Pork chops	1 chop	2.2
2 mg		
Spinach	1/2 cup	1.8
Apricots, dried, cooked	1/2 cup	1.5
Ham, luncheon meat	2 oz	1.5
Peas, green	1/2 cup	1.5
Prunes, dried, cooked	5 with juice	1.5
Chicken	1/4 small broiler	1.4
1 mg		
Egg	1 medium	1.1
Oatmeal, cooked	2/3 cup	1.1
Sausage, salami	1 slice	1.1
Broccoli	1/2 cup	1.0
Macaroni, enriched, cooked	3/4 cup	1.0
Sweet potato	1 medium	1.0
Cantaloup	1/2 melon	0.8
Frankfurter	1 medium	0.8
Squash, winter	1/2 cup	0.8
Strawberries, raw	1/2 cup	0.8
0.5 mg		
Banana, raw	1 medium	0.7
Corn, canned	1/2 cup	0.7
Potato, white	1 medium	0.7
Salmon, canned	1/2 cup	0.7
Bread, white, enriched	1 slice	0.6
Pineapple juice, canned	1/2 cup (small glass)	0.6
Bacon, crisp	2 slices	0.5
Beans, snap, green	1/2 cup	0.5
Carrots, diced	1/2 cup	0.5
Cornflakes, fortified	1 1/3 cup	0.5
Grapefruit	1/2 medium	0.5
Haddock	1 fillet	0.5
Tomato juice, canned	1/2 cup (small glass)	0.5
Apple, raw	1 medium	0.4
Peaches, canned	2 halves with juice	0.4
Peanut butter	1 tbsp	0.4
Rice, cooked	3/4 cup	0.4
0.3 mg		
Cabbage, shredded, raw	1/2 cup	0.3
Cheese, cheddar	1 1/8" cube	0.3
Orange	1 medium	0.3
Orange juice, fresh	1/2 cup (small glass)	0.3
Cheese, cottage, creamed	1/4 cup	0.2
Lettuce leaves	2 large or 4 small	0.2
Milk, fluid, skim (or buttermilk)	1 cup	0.1
Milk, fluid, whole	1 cup	0.1
0 mg		
Butter or fortified margarine	1 tbsp	trace
Beverage, kola type	6 oz	...
Sugar, granulated	1 tbsp	...
Cream, coffee	1 tbsp	0
Oil, salad or cooking	1 tbsp	0

*Foods are in forms ready to eat. All meats and vegetables are cooked unless otherwise indicated.

**See Appendix G for further identification of these foods. On that list all foods are described more fully and both weights and measures are indicated.

lean muscle meats and beans, 3 mg, green leafy vegetables, dried fruits, ham, and chicken, about 2 mg. Eggs, whole-grain and enriched cereals, and several vegetables and fruits yield about 1 mg per serving.

U.S. Department of Agriculture data show that nearly one-third of the iron available to consumers in this country comes from meat, poultry, and fish; about one-fourth from flour and cereal products, many of them enriched; one-tenth from dry legumes and nuts; the remainder divided in smaller amounts among other food groups [9]. This distribution is in sharp contrast to the concentration of calcium (76 percent) in one food group—milk and dairy foods, excluding butter. It is apparent that we must "shop around" for iron and that a knowledge of the types of foods where it is most apt to be found is important to good iron nutrition.

Whole grain, restored and enriched cereals and breads are important for iron, not only because they are relatively good sources but because cereals, in some form, are eaten at practically every meal. Whole-grain cereals are those which retain all or a large part of the germ and outer coats of the grain, and the nutrients therein, after light milling. Restored cereals are those to which certain nutrients are "restored" to high natural levels after they have been lost in the milling process. Enriched cereals and breads are made from highly milled grains and flours to which specified amounts of iron and certain vitamins are added to a given amount of the cereal product [19].

The practice of *enrichment* emerged from World War II. By the beginning of the war, nutritionists were aware that the diet in this country was declining in content of iron and those vitamins affected by lessened use of potatoes and whole-grain cereals. In 1940 the Food and Nutrition Board developed suggested levels of enrichment for white flour and baker's bread. In 1943, War Food Order No. 1 was issued, requiring nation-wide enrichment of white bread and rolls with iron, thiamine, riboflavin, and niacin, with calcium and vitamin D as optional ingredients. By the end of the war when the order was revoked (1946), 19 states had made enrichment compulsory. By 1958, 27 states, Hawaii, and Puerto Rico had passed legislation requiring enrichment. At the present time, nearly all bread and flour is also enriched in the states *not* having legislation, and it is estimated that, in this country as a whole, 80–90 percent of all white bread and family flour is now enriched [19].

Progress has also been made in the enrichment of cornmeal and rice. Federal standards have been established. In several southern states, all degerminated cornmeal and grits sold are required by law to be enriched to the same levels as flour. Table 6-3 shows present federal enrichment standards for flour, bread, corn, and rice.

Enrichment of bread and flour has been a specific factor in raising the content of iron in the food supply despite the continued decline of cereal consumption. Within 2 years after the issuance of War Food Order No. 1, the amount of iron available in the food supply increased about 12 percent per capita, per day [9]. This increase was undoubtedly due in large part to the enrichment of bread and flour and the greater use of these products in wartime when certain other foods were scarce. Probably some of the rise could be attributed to the greater use of leafy green vegetables from wartime gardens. An examination of family diets in 1948 showed that households on low incomes were getting, on the average, 14 percent more iron from their diets than would have been possible without enrichment. This is regarded as a significant change and in many cases would make the difference between adequacy and inadequacy in intake of iron and the other

TABLE 6–3

ENRICHMENT STANDARDS FOR FLOUR, BREAD, CORN MEAL AND GRITS, AND RICE [19]
(Milligrams per Pound unless Otherwise Stated)

	Flour		Bread		Corn		Rice	
	Minimum	Maximum	Minimum	Maximum	Minimum	Maximum	Minimum	Maximum
Thiamine	2.0	2.5	1.1	1.8	2.0	3.0	2.0	4.0
Riboflavin	1.2	1.5	0.7	1.6	1.2	1.8	1.2‡	2.4‡
Niacin	16.0	20.0	10.0	15.0	16.0	24.0	16.0	32.0
Iron	13.0	16.5	8.0	12.5	13.0	26.0	13.0	26.0
Calcium*	500.0	625.0	300.0	800.0	500.0	750.0	500.0	750.0
Vitamin D† (USP units)	250.0	1000.0	150.0	750.0	250.0	1000.0	250.0	1000.0
Wheat germ†	In flour and bread to extent of not more than 5 percent by weight of finished product.							
Dried yeast†	In corn meal and grits to extent of not more than 1.5 percent by weight of finished product.							

* Required in self-rising flour: minimum: 500 mg; maximum: 1500 mg per lb.
† Optional.
‡ The requirement for riboflavin has been stayed. A public hearing will be held on the issue of whether the standard of identity shall include riboflavin as a required ingredient of enriched rice.

nutrients involved in enrichment. Further aspects of enrichment will be considered in connection with the B vitamins, the other enrichment factors.

► *Arrange your own list of representative foods in order of importance as sources of iron. Analyze the list. Suggest groupings representing similar iron values. Characterize the foods in each grouping.*

Enter iron values on your personal meal record. Total the iron intake for the day.

Make a list of the organ meats in Appendix G with their iron values per serving. How much do you depend upon organ meats as sources of iron?

Compare servings of "greens" in Appendix G with spinach as sources of iron.

Your Iron Needs

The daily needs for iron have been assessed with iron balance experiments. Originally, the traditional chemical balance method was used exclusively. In recent years, a radioactive balance method has been introduced in which the difference between the radioactivity of tagged iron ingested and that excreted in the feces is determined.

Recommended Daily Allowances for Iron The Food and Nutrition Board, on the basis of available evidence from balance experiments, has proposed allowances of 10 mg for men of all ages and 12 mg daily for women (Table 6-1)[4]. Iron is the only trace element for which allowances have been established. The human body is remarkably thrifty with its iron. It uses it over and over again. When red blood cells are destroyed, the iron is salvaged and re-utilized. Actually, men can get along with daily intakes of less than 10 mg of iron if there is no loss of blood. The 10 mg give a margin of safety. The additional 2 mg daily for women are proposed to meet their special needs, as will be shown.

The daily allowance for iron during the latter half of pregnancy and for lactation is 15 mg—a 25 percent increase over the nonpregnancy allowance. This high figure for pregnancy is needed to cover the requirements of the developing fetus and to provide for its storage of iron. The lactation allowance, which does not increase above that for pregnancy, is believed to be sufficient to provide for the small amount of iron in the breast milk.

How the Average Adult Can Meet His Iron Needs The specimen diet in Appendix B shows one way an adult might choose a day's meals furnishing more than 12 mg of iron. Representatives of good sources of iron (Fig. 6.6) are easily found in the diet: hamburger, baked beans, enriched cereals (in toast, rolls, and gingerbread). The yield of iron from the gingerbread may be a surprise until you realize that eggs and molasses are among the ingredients and that it is made with enriched flour. The foods on the diet that yield the least iron, or none—as would be expected from a study of Figure 6.6—are cole slaw, celery, milk, butter, jelly, cake, and the soft drink.

The following 4 food combinations show ways in which a woman can meet her daily iron allowance.

MEETING DAILY IRON ALLOWANCE FOR WOMEN: 12 mg

	1	Iron mg
Liver, beef	2 oz	4.4
Beans, dry, canned	¾ cup	3.3
Spinach	½ cup	1.8
Prunes	5, with juice	1.5
Egg	1 medium	1.1
Total		12.1

	2	Iron mg
Beef, pot roast	3 oz	2.9
Beans, dry, canned	¾ cup	3.3
Egg	1 medium	1.1
Bread, enriched	1 slice	0.6
Spinach	½ cup	1.8
Peas, green	½ cup	1.5
Prunes	5, with juice	1.5
Total		12.7

	3	
Beef, pot roast	3 oz	2.9
Egg	1 medium	1.1
Oatmeal	⅔ cup	1.1
Bread, enriched	3 slices	1.8
Macaroni, enriched	¾ cup	1.0
Peas, green	½ cup	1.5
Squash, winter	½ cup	0.8
Corn	½ cup	0.7
Apricots, stewed	½ cup	1.5
Total		12.4

	4	
Frankfurter	1 medium	0.8
Egg	1 medium	1.1
Salmon, canned	½ cup	0.7
Bread, enriched	3 slices	1.8
Oatmeal	⅔ cup	1.1
Potato	1 medium	0.7
Cauliflower	½ cup	0.7
Banana	1 medium	0.7
Beets	½ cup	0.6
Carrots	½ cup	0.5
Grapefruit	½ medium	0.5
Bacon	2 slices	0.5
Cornflakes	1⅓ cup	0.5
Tomato juice	½ cup	0.5
Peaches, canned	½ cup	0.4
Peanut butter	1 tbsp	0.4
Cheese, cheddar	1 oz	0.3
Cheese, cottage	¼ cup	0.2
Milk, whole	1 cup	0.1
Total		12.1

It is obvious that unless the richest sources of iron are chosen, larger or more frequent servings of the lesser sources are required. Combination 1 shows how simply the iron allowance can be met with 1 serving each of liver, baked beans, spinach, prunes, and egg. Such a combination is not a practical solution. At least the first 2 items are rarely daily food items in this country. Combination 2 substitutes beef roast—a muscle meat—for liver, and retains the beans. It takes additional good food sources to make up the difference in iron content between the muscle meat and the liver. Combination 3 retains the beef, omits the beans, and adds several foods, some of them of lesser iron value than those in Combination 2. The serving of bread is tripled. Combination 4 shows the result of including no major source of iron—although the first 3 items belong to the meat group and might be assumed to be high in iron, as are many other protein foods. A much larger number of items is required in Combination 4 to meet the allowance than in Combination 3. The triple servings of bread proved to be the single richest source of iron in combination 4.

The importance of knowing and choosing, daily, one or more concentrated sources of iron is apparent from the above combinations and accompanying discussion. It is doubtful whether most individuals who fail to take this precaution choose the variety and number of lesser sources required to meet the allowances for iron.

► *What is your iron allowance? (Obtain this from Table 6-1 on basis of age, as you did your calcium allowance.)*

How does your iron intake as shown on your meal record compare with your daily iron allowance? Whether your intake is above or below your allowance, account for the situation in terms of your food selection.

Estimate the iron yield of the vegetarian diet you planned earlier. Was the diet adequate in iron content? If not, how could you make it adequate without changing its vegetarian character?

Iron Allowances for Children As is true of practically every other nutrient, recommended allowances for iron increase with the age of children (Table 6-1). In the teen years the allowances remain the same but they are twice those of the preschool years. This progression is due to the factors of growth: increasing blood supply, and the growing number of iron-bearing muscle cells and respiratory enzymes.

The problem of meeting a child's dietary allowances for iron is similar to that of meeting the adult's—a matter of selecting certain concentrated sources for each day's meals and "filling in" with lesser sources. The food groupings in chart on page 110 for 3 age periods show ways in which the recommended daily allowances may be met with essentially the same foods.

The first combination, for the preschool child, shows a grouping of foods good in iron and commonly eaten by children of this age, which easily meets the relatively low allowance of 8 mg. These same foods serve as the nucleus for the second grouping. Here the beef is increased from a half to a whole serving, an extra slice of enriched bread is included, and a banana and a serving of ham are added to meet the 12-mg allowance of the elementary school child. These foods, in turn, form the nucleus for the third grouping, with beef increased to 1½ servings, the number of eggs doubled, and an apple included. Thus we see that children of different ages can meet their varying iron needs at the family table, chiefly by adjusting the size of servings of certain foods in line with their total energy needs.

MEETING IRON ALLOWANCES FOR CHILDREN

Ages in Years	4–6		10–12		13–19	
DAILY IRON ALLOWANCES	8 mg		12 mg		15 mg	
		Iron mg		Iron mg		Iron mg
Beef, pot roast	1½ oz	1.5	3 oz	2.9	4½ oz	4.3
Peas, green	½ cup	1.5	½ cup	1.5	½ cup	1.5
Prunes	5, with juice	1.5	5, with juice	1.5	5, with juice	1.5
Egg	1 medium	1.1	1 medium	1.1	2 medium	2.2
Oatmeal	⅔ cup	1.1	⅔ cup	1.1	⅔ cup	1.1
Bread	3 slices	1.8	4 slices	2.4	4 slices	2.4
Ham	—	—	2 oz.	1.5	2 oz	1.5
Banana	—	—	1 medium	0.7	1 medium	0.7
Apple	—	—	—	—	1 medium	0.4
Total		8.5		12.7		15.6

Iron in Our National Diet

On the basis of the amount of iron available per person per day from our total food supply, the question whether we as a nation are getting enough iron may be answered in the affirmative. About 16.5 mg of iron are thus available. This figure is greater than the daily allowance for any age or condition and should serve to reassure us. However, it is to be understood that the 16.5 mg of iron represents the iron from the foods in their entirety, including kitchen and plate wastes, whereas the allowances represent quantities for actual consumption. Also, it presupposes that the total amount of iron available is divided evenly among the entire population. This, of course, is not the case. Studies of iron intakes by families and by individuals compared with dietary allowances, therefore, present a different picture.

Family diets studied by the U.S. Department of Agriculture in 1955 did not, on the average, provide fully the recommended amounts of iron in any of the 4 geographical regions studied [10]. Table 6-2 shows that the extent of the deficit varies in the 4 regions from 7 to 12 percent. These are not large deviations, particularly in comparison with those for calcium, represented on the same table.

Experiment Station investigators have studied their subjects by sex and age groups, and have compared average intakes with recommended allowances for iron [11]. Figures 6.7 and 6.8 summarize this information for persons ranging in age from 4 to 80 years. It will be noted that children up to about 12 years of age have satisfactory iron intakes (Fig. 6.7). During adolescence, the average intakes of boys more than meet the allowances, but those for adolescent girls fail to do so to a marked degree. In the adult group, the men's averages range well above the allowance level; most of the women's averages fall below it (Fig. 6.8). After 55 years of age there is a sharp decline in women's iron intake. Figures 6.7 and 6.8 resemble their counterparts for calcium (Figs. 6.3 and 6.4) in revealing that adolescents are less well nourished with respect to iron than younger children, that girls are less well nourished than boys, and women less well nourished than men.

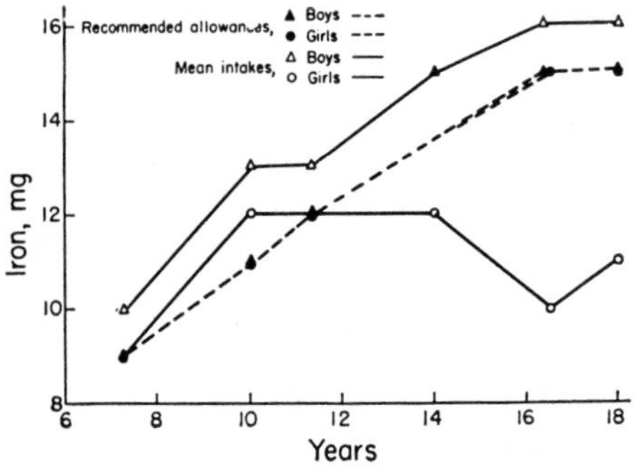

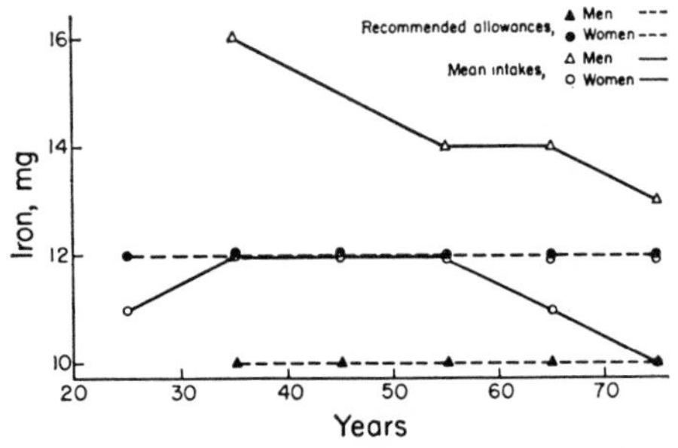

Figs. 6.7 and 6.8 Iron intake in relation to daily dietary allowances. *(left)* Average daily iron intake of boys and girls 4–20 years of age. (*right*) Average daily iron intake of men and women from 20 to more than 80 years of age. (A. F. Morgan [Ed.], *Nutritional Status U.S.A.* Bull. 769. Berkeley, Calif.: University of California, Division of Agricultural Sciences, Agricultural Experiment Station, pp. 33 and 35, respectively.)

The findings of the Iowa study (Fig. 6.5), pinpoint the iron deficiencies for adolescents, as they do the calcium deficiencies. Again, the picture is far more favorable for boys than for girls. Here the standard has been lowered to two-thirds of the recommended iron allowance [11].

How Your Body Uses Iron [7]

Iron is released from the intestine, for the body's use, only when it is needed. Iron that has been absorbed into the blood stream usually is disposed of in 3 ways: some is used immediately, some is stored, and a little is excreted. As indicated earlier, a large share goes into the making of hemoglobin. Iron is stored chiefly in the liver, bone marrow, and spleen. Stored iron exists with protein in combinations that can be mobilized by the body for hemoglobin synthesis when iron is needed for that purpose. The body excretes some iron daily despite its remarkable ability to conserve its iron content. Some iron is lost through the feces. In addition, there is a small loss from the urine and from the many cells that are discharged from the body in a variety of ways. All cells contain some iron; therefore, even secretions of the skin carry away small amounts of iron.

Special Stresses For women and children, there are special needs for iron that make more difficult the attainment of iron balance [20,21].

Menstrual Flow It is estimated that women from adolescence to the menopause lose from 35 to 70 cc of blood every 28 days. This loss amounts, on the average, to 0.5 mg–1 mg of iron daily, with a median value of 0.75 mg. Excessive menstrual flow, which may not be uncommon, can more than double the loss. If a woman's intake of iron is 12 mg daily (Fig. 6.8) and she absorbs 10 percent of it (both may be optimistic assumptions), she has theoretically a slight positive iron balance (1.2 − 0.75 − excretion loss).

Child Bearing The additional 3 mg of iron daily during pregnancy called for by the recommended allowances is met in part by conserving the iron from menstrual losses. Even with this saving, however, a negative iron balance for the mother is a strong possibility unless iron intake is increased up to or beyond the daily allowance of 15 mg. Only when the iron supply in the mother's body is adequate does the fetus have enough for its own development and an accumulation in the liver to carry it satisfactorily through early infancy. Data on women's diets indicate that they are poor in iron at ages when stresses are greatest (Fig. 6.8). Unless steps are taken to prevent iron deficiency, frequent pregnancies may deprive the mother, the fetus, and eventually the infant of adequate amounts of iron [22].

Childhood The factor of growth constitutes a stress during childhood. The body of an infant contains about 0.5 g of iron; the adult body, 3–5 g. There must therefore be a steady gain in body content of iron over the period from infancy to adulthood. The total gain would be 2.5–4.5 g, with a net increase of about 0.3–0.6 mg per day over the entire period. Assuming that a 10-year-old child meets his daily iron allowance of 12 mg and absorbs 10 percent of it (1.2 mg), he may store 0.5 mg and have a surplus of 0.7 mg. How much of this represents a positive balance depends on how much iron is excreted—a subject about which there is almost nothing known for the childhood years. There is certain to be some excretion, however. This being the case, a normal child who meets his iron allowance perhaps has only a slight positive iron balance. And such a balance can be wiped out easily by a diet poor in iron, or by poor absorption of iron, or by even a mild infection.

Blood Donations Donations of blood for transfusions result in considerable loss of iron and therefore constitute a type of stress. When a pint of blood is given, the donor may lose as much as 250 mg of iron. Spread over a year, this means a loss of about 0.68 mg per day. An adult man, the most frequent donor, is in the best position to lose this amount if his diet meets the recommended allowances in all nutrients—particularly in protein and iron—and if he absorbs the iron efficiently. However, if he makes more than one annual blood donation, physicians often recommend a supplement of iron salts to such a diet.

Results of Poor Iron Nutriture

The foregoing section has suggested the circumstances that help to create iron deficiencies. What difference do such deficiencies make in nutrition and health when they do occur? How are they identified? A shortage of iron in the diet, poor absorption, and/or certain stresses that increase the need for iron may lead to iron-deficiency anemia, called *hypochromic anemia* [21]. One is said to be "anemic" when the hemoglobin content of the blood is below normal. "Normal" is not a hard and fast standard, nor is it the same for everyone. It is higher for men than for women, higher for boys than for girls. Neither is there entire agreement on ranges that may be considered satisfactory. However, men and women in a good state of iron nutrition usually have about 14–18 and 12–16 g of hemoglobin per 100 ml of blood, respectively. Older boys test about the same as men; older girls, slightly less than women. Children in the age range of 8–12 years normally have hemoglobins of about 11–15 g. The degree of deviation below "normal" that may be called anemia is likewise not regarded as the same for all. Twenty-five percent below "normal" usually places a person in the danger zone. A physician should decide the level to be regarded as anemia in any individual case.

Lowered hemoglobin results in decreased ability to carry oxygen to the cells and to return carbon dioxide to the lungs for exhalation. With less oxygen and more carbon dioxide in the cells, body processes become sluggish and efficiency is lowered. A person in this condition is usually listless and dispirited. He is pale in appearance because the color-bearing (red) hemoglobin of his blood is reduced in amount.

There is no way of knowing the exact extent of iron-deficiency anemia. After discussing the hazards of maintaining iron balance, one authority points out that "Iron deficiency anemia is one of the most common nutritional deficiencies and one of the most prevalent anemias," and concludes, "Healthy persons probably maintain a positive iron balance by a narrower margin than was formerly believed" [20].

It should be pointed out that there are several types of anemia other than the one caused by iron deficiency. Also, that dietary faults other than inadequate iron may contribute to low hemoglobin. The essential role of dietary protein in the formation of hemoglobin is increasingly recognized, and the parts played by certain vitamins and by other minerals are more and more appreciated. These factors are discussed at appropriate points in the text. A generally excellent diet, including all of these nutrients, is the best way to prevent low hemoglobin or to return it to normal if it is low. Proof that one suffers from a true iron-deficiency anemia exists only if the hemoglobin increases when iron alone is administered.

» TRACE MINERAL ELEMENTS—COPPER, IODINE, AND FLUORINE

Copper

Copper bears an interesting relationship to iron. It appears to be necessary for the absorption of iron from the alimentary tract, for its incorporation into certain iron-containing enzymes and into hemoglobin. Copper is thus needed in the making of hemoglobin, even though hemoglobin contains no copper [21]. Normal use of iron in the body is therefore dependent on adequate intake and utilization of copper.

Deficiency of copper in human beings has been seen only in young children. First proof of the existence of the deficiency was furnished when an anemic condition was relieved by the administration of a copper salt. Apparently, adults are resistant to copper deficiency even on grossly inadequate diets. The Food and Nutrition Board has proposed an allowance of about 2 mg daily for an adult; 0.05 mg per kg (2.2 lb) of body weight during growth [4]. Copper is contained in a variety of foods and is often present as a contaminant. If a diet even approaches the tentative allowance, it will usually provide all the copper needed. Copper occurs in many of the same foods as iron. Meats, particularly liver, are excellent sources.

Iodine

Iodine is an essential constituent of the hormone thyroxine, produced by the thyroid gland. As discussed in Chapter 4, thyroxine is a vital factor in controlling basal energy metabolism. Thyroxine is also necessary for growth and development in the young; for successful pregnancy and lactation in the adult. When there is a deficiency in the secretion of thyroxine, children fail to develop physically. And with prolonged, severe deficiency, they suffer from cretinism, which involves both physical and mental retardation.

Simple goiter—an enlargement of the thyroid gland—is due to a deficiency of iodine. The thyroxine level of the blood declines and the gland is enlarged in its effort to increase its production of the hormone. Goiter occurs chiefly in regions of the world where the soil is poor in iodine [18]. In this country, the strongly goitrous regions are around the Great Lakes and in the Pacific Northwest.

Goiter has been known for centuries, but its cause and specific treatment were discovered only in the last 50 years. The importance of iodine as a preventive measure was demonstrated in Akron, Ohio, in a study started in 1917. Two grams of sodium iodide were fed semiannually for 2½ years to more than 2000 young girls. About the same number of girls served as controls, with no iodine added to their diets. Of the group receiving iodine, only 5 developed goiter; of those receiving no iodine, about 500 developed goiter.

As the result of this and other studies, a movement was launched in 1922 to provide and sell iodized salt as a means of supplying iodine to goitrous regions. Follow-up studies have shown that the incidence of goiter has dropped since that time from nearly 50 percent to less than 5 percent among children in Great Lakes regions. This drop is attributed largely to the increased use of iodized salt. Despite the fact that less than half the salt in the United States is iodized and is manufactured and distributed on a voluntary basis, recent dietary studies show that about three-fourths of families use it regularly. A contributing factor to the decline in simple goiter is the present system of marketing foods far from their points of origin, thus increasing the possibility that goitrous regions will receive some of their foods from areas where the soil is iodine-rich.

The daily requirement for iodine is not known with certainty because satisfactory methods of determining need have not been found. The Food and Nutrition Board has therefore not suggested a daily dietary allowance [4]. The need for iodine is known to increase during the periods of most rapid growth and during pregnancy. As a result, girls and women are particularly susceptible to simple goiter.

There is only a minute quantity of iodine in the body. It is also present in foods in very small amounts. The same kind of food may vary widely in iodine content from sample to sample, depending on the iodine content of the soil on which it is grown. Salt-water fish and fish that live a part of their lives in salt water are the best food sources of iodine. Foods grown on iodine-rich soils are good secondary sources. Iodized salt is the most dependable source if used routinely. The habit of using it is strongly recommended by professional groups, particularly for goitrous regions.

Fluorine

The chief known function of fluorine is to help prevent dental caries. Its relation to dental caries was discovered through observations of the effects on teeth of excessive fluorine in the drinking water in certain regions of the United States. It was noted that although great excesses of fluorine caused a mottled, unsightly condition in teeth, particularly in children who used the water regularly, these teeth did not decay readily. And when the water naturally contained a definite but small amount of fluorine, the teeth were *not* mottled and they still resisted decay. This finding led in 1945 to the first experiments in which fluorine was added in minute amounts to drinking water naturally low in fluorine content to observe effects in checking dental caries [21].

Such studies were carried on in 2 cities on a control basis: the drinking water in 1 city was fortified with fluorine; that in a comparable second city, not fortified. Samples from the child population in both cities were given annual dental and medical examinations, in some cases for as long as 10 years. The findings were startling. For example, at the end of the 10-year period, in Newburgh, New York, where the community water supply was fortified to a level of 1 part per million of fluoride, children had an average of 60 percent fewer decayed teeth than children in Kingston, New York, with whom they were being compared. Kingston, 30 miles distant, had no fluoridation. The greatest benefits in Newburgh were observed in children who had used the fluoridated water since birth. No unfavorable effects from the fluoridation were found in the medical examinations. When this type of experiment was repeated in other localities, the outcomes were essentially the same [21].

Such results led to campaigns in many cities for the fluoridation of community water supplies naturally low in fluorine content. At the present time, it is estimated, nearly 2000 communities have added to the fluorine content of their drinking water in an effort to control dental caries. The practice is spreading to other countries. Fluoridation has been endorsed by the American Dental Association, the American Public Health Association, and leading medical groups as desirable from the standpoint of dental health and as harmless to general health. Some strides have been made in developing a method of applying a dilute solution of fluorine directly to the teeth. Such a plan could be helpful in areas where people do not have a public water supply and where the well water is below the desirable level for fluorine content.

Fluorine is not widely distributed in common foods. Milk, meat, fruits, and vegetables contain little. Fish and dry legumes are fairly good sources.

Other Trace Mineral Elements

Other trace elements are being studied for their possible significance in nutrition. Of these, cobalt, molybdenum, manganese, and zinc appear to be factors in animal nutrition. Thus far there are few clues to their relationship to human nutrition. Obviously no dietary allowances have been established, and knowledge is incomplete with respect to the occurrence of these mineral elements in common foods. A fully adequate diet, including enough calcium and iron to meet the established allowances, would undoubtedly cover human needs. The brief comments that follow on the four elements mentioned serve chiefly to indicate alignments of these trace elements with other nutrients—which may be the key to an eventual understanding of their nutritional importance to human beings.

Cobalt is a component of the vitamin B_{12} molecule [4]. Cattle and sheep eat only plant foods and these provide little or no vitamin B_{12}. If the diet of these ruminants contains sufficient cobalt, they can make their own B_{12}. Vitamin B_{12}, in turn, functions in the formation of red blood cells (Chap. 7). Where pastures and soils are poor in cobalt, animals suffer from a cobalt deficiency.

Molybdenum, like cobalt, functions indirectly in animal nutrition. It is necessary for the nourishment of bacteria in the rumen of sheep, which must break down cellulose to a form of carbohydrate that sheep can use. Directly, molybdenum functions in the rat and dog in the formation of certain intestinal enzymes. Animals apparently are subject to an excess rather than to a deficiency of molybdenum [21].

Manganese deficiency in certain laboratory animals leads to problems with reproduction and lactation. Others are affected by impaired leg bone formation. Toxicity due to excesses of manganese in laboratory animals has appeared in the form of retarded growth and gastric disturbances. In man, manganese toxicity has manifested itself in persons exposed to the mining and loading of the ore in the following ways: crippling of the legs, tremor of the hands, and blurring of the speech [21].

Zinc is attached to two important enzymes in the animal body and is a part of the chemical structure of the hormone insulin [4]. On a zinc-deficient diet, rats and mice fail to grow normally and lose hair around their necks and shoulders. There is some evidence that excessive zinc creates problems in the utilization of copper.

MINERAL ELEMENTS—A FEW HIGHLIGHTS

	Calcium	**Iron**	**Copper**	**Iodide**
WHAT MINERALS DO FOR YOU	Helps build bones and teeth; keeps them rigid and strong Helps blood to clot Helps control muscular action, including beat of the heart	Is essential part: of every blood and tissue cell; of hemoglobin of the red blood cells, which carries oxygen to every body cell	Acts with iron in formation of hemoglobin	As essential constituent of thyroxine, is necessary to normal functioning of thyroid gland Controlling factor in basal energy metabolism
RECOMMENDED DAILY DIETARY ALLOWANCES	ADULTS: 800 mg 1500 mg preg. 2000 mg lact. CHILDREN (above infancy): 1000–1400 mg	10 mg men 12 mg women 15 mg preg., lactation 7–15 mg	2 mg, proposed .05 mg per kg body weight	No iodine allowance proposed Use of iodized salt will supply adequate amount
SOME OF THE BEST FOOD SOURCES	Milk Cheeses, hard "Greens" except spinach, beet, chard Dry legumes Citrus fruits Eggs	Organ meats Lean muscle meats Dry legumes Dark green leafy veg. Dried fruits Eggs Cereals, whole-grain and enriched	Essentially the same foods that provide iron	Iodized salt Salt-water fish Foods grown on iodine-rich soil Water in nongoitrous regions

REFERENCES

1. Gray, L. F., "Factors Which Affect the Nutrients in Plants," *Food—The Yearbook of Agriculture*. Washington, D.C.: U.S. Department of Agriculture, 1959. p. 389.
2. Duncan, C. W., *Effects of Fertilizer Practices on Plant Composition*. East Lansing, Mich.: Michigan State University Centennial Symposium (Nutrition of Plants, Animals, Man), Feb. 1955.
3. Cederquist, D. C., and Ohlson, M. A., *Nutritive Value of Milk Produced by Cows Fed Rations from Low and High Fertility Soils*. East Lansing, Mich.: Michigan State University Centennial Symposium (Nutrition of Plants, Animals, Man), Feb. 1955.
4. Food and Nutrition Board, *Recommended Dietary Allowances*. Pub. 589. Washington, D.C.: National Academy of Sciences-National Research Council, 1958.
5. Leitch, I., and Aitken, F. C., "The Estimation of Calcium Requirement: A Re-examination," *Nutrition Abstracts and Reviews,* 29 (April 1959) pp. 393–407.
6. Hathaway, M. L., and Leverton, R. M., "Calcium and Phosphorus," *Food—The Yearbook of Agriculture*. Washington, D.C.: U.S. Department of Agriculture, 1959. p. 112.
7. *The Heinz Handbook of Nutrition*. New York: McGraw-Hill Book Company, Inc., 1959. (Chap. 12.)
8. "Incorporation of Dietary Calcium into Growing Bone," *Nutrition Reviews,* 17 (Jan. 1959) pp. 14–15.
9. Economic Research Service, *Consumption of Food in the United States, 1909–1952*. Supplement for 1960 to Agricultural Handbook No. 62. Washington, D.C.: U.S. Department of Agriculture, August 1961.
10. Le Bovit, C., and Clark, F., "Are We Well Fed?" *Food—The Yearbook of Agriculture*. Washington, D.C.: U.S. Department of Agriculture, 1959. p. 620.
11. Morgan, A. F., *Nutritional Status, U.S.A.* Bull. 769. Berkeley: California Agricultural Experiment Station, University of California, Oct. 1959.
12. Hunscher, H. A., "Pertinent Factors in Interpreting Metabolic Data," *J. Am. Dietet. Assoc.,* 39 (Sept. 1961) pp. 209–19.
13. Smith, J., "Calcium Needs of Teen-age Boys," *Nutrition News,* 10 (April 1947) p. 13. Chicago: National Dairy Council.
14. Shank, R. E., *Findings from Calcium Research Conference* (Proceedings of Summer Conference). Chicago: National Dairy Council, 1958.
15. Ohlson, M. A., and Stearns, G., *Calcium Intake of Children and Adults* (Symposium on Effects of High Calcium Intakes). *Federation Proceedings,* 18 (Dec. 1959) pp. 1076–1085.
16. Whedon, G. D., *Effects of High Calcium Intakes on Bones, Blood and Soft Tissue; Relationship of Calcium Intake to Balance in Osteoporosis* (Symposium on Effects of High Calcium Intakes). *Federation Proceedings,* 18 (Dec. 1959) pp. 1112–18.
17. Leverton, R. M., "Sodium, Potassium and Magnesium," *Food—The Yearbook of Agriculture*. Washington, D.C.: U.S. Department of Agriculture, 1959. p. 119.

18. Monty, K. J., and McElroy, W. D., "The Trace Elements," *Food—The Yearbook of Agriculture.* Washington, D.C.: U.S. Department of Agriculture, 1959. p. 122.
19. Food and Nutrition Board, *Cereal Enrichment in Perspective, 1958.* Washington, D.C.: National Academy of Sciences-National Research Council, 1958.
20. Moore, C. V., and Dubach, R., "Metabolism and Requirements of Iron in the Human," *J. Am. Med. Assoc.*, 162 (Sept. 15, 1956) pp. 197–204.
21. Wohl, M. G., Goodhart, R. S. (Eds.), *Modern Nutrition in Health and Disease.* 2nd ed. Philadelphia: Lea & Febiger, 1960. (Chap. 10, "Iron and Essential Trace Elements.")
22. Sisson, T. R. C., and Lund, C. J., "The Influence of Maternal Iron Deficiency on the New Born," *Am. J. Clinical Nutrition,* 6 (July–Aug. 1958) pp. 376–85.

READINGS

Better Teeth for Life . . . Fluoridation. Public Health Service Pub. 636. Washington, D.C.: U.S. Department of Health, Education and Welfare, Division of Dental Health.

Burke, B. S., Reed, R. B., van den Berg, A. S., and Stuart, H. C., "A Longitudinal Study of the Calcium Intake of Children from One to Eighteen Years of Age," *Am. J. Clinical Nutrition,* 10 (Jan. 1962) pp. 79–88.

"Calcium Metabolism in Osteoporosis," *Nutrition Reviews,* 19 (Sept. 1961) pp. 269–72.

Council on Foods and Nutrition, *Nutrition in Tooth Formation and Dental Caries.* Symposium 8. Chicago: American Medical Association, 1961.

Darby, W. J., *Interrelationship of Quality of Soil and Human Nutrition.* East Lansing, Mich.: Michigan State University Centennial Symposium (Nutrition of Plants, Animals, Man), Feb. 1955.

Mann, G. V., "Sulphur Metabolism," *Food and Nutrition News,* 34 (Dec. 1960) p. 1. Chicago: National Livestock and Meat Board.

Massler, M., "Calcification Pattern of Human Teeth," *Nutrition News,* 25 (Feb. 1962) p. 1. Chicago: National Dairy Council.

Whedon, G. D., "Calcium Needs of Adults and Older People," *Nutrition News,* 23 (April 1960) p. 5. Chicago: National Dairy Council.

Wonderful Human Machine. Chicago: American Medical Association. Adapted from *Today's Health,* 1961. (Part I. "The Skeleton.")

CHAPTER 7

Vitamins

In earlier chapters, certain facts about vitamins were established: that vitamins, as a group, represent one of the 6 nutrient classes; that their importance in nutrition is out of all proportion to the small quantities of them that are found in foods and are required by the body; that vitamins in foods are not broken down in the digestive processes in preparation for "nutritional service" to the body, but are absorbed essentially as they occur; that vitamins, in broad terms, contribute to the building of the body structure and help regulate its processes.

You are now prepared to consider: a) some of the individual vitamins in relation to nutrition and health; b) how much you need of those vitamins for which daily dietary allowances have been established; c) how you obtain the vitamins to which attention must be given in food selection; and d) the outcomes in nutritional status when there is enough, or a deficiency, of certain vitamins. First some general considerations that will give a background for this chapter.

» VITAMINS AS A GROUP

Vitamins make up the newest nutrient group. The first of the vitamins was discovered as recently as 1913, although their presence was suspected before that. Scientists had realized for some time that natural foods contained "accessory factors" necessary to the life and health of experimental animals and that such factors were not present in pure proteins, fats, carbohydrates, and mineral elements, heretofore believed to be the sole components of an adequate diet. As vitamins were discovered, they were identified by letters of the alphabet. The first part of the word vitamin stems from the Latin word *vita,* meaning life; the second part of the word is without significance at the present time. The discovery of vitamins introduced what came to be known as the newer knowledge of nutrition.

Originally it was thought that the various vitamins were chemically related. But as each of the major vitamins was identified, it became apparent that they differed in chemical nature and in body functions and had little in common except the group title, "vitamin" [1]. Most of the vitamins have now been given scientific names that suggest their individual character.

A dozen or more vitamins occur naturally in foods and have been shown to contribute to human nutrition [2]. Vitamins are "essential" in the sense that they must be present in daily foods—they cannot be synthesized in the body in sufficient quantities to satisfy body needs. They do not furnish a measurable amount of energy even though they are organic substances. Six vitamins are included by the Food and Nutrition Board on its daily dietary allowance table (Appendix C)[3]. It is to these 6 we need give special attention in selecting meals. If they and other nutrients listed on the table are supplied in amounts to meet the allowances, other vitamins required by the human body probably also will be provided adequately by those same meals. Tentative allowances have been suggested for several of these other vitamins.

The term "coordinator" is often applied to vitamins because of their ability to work with each other and with other nutrients in coordinating body functions. This action is chiefly catalytic. Beyond that, their exact functions differ so greatly it is impossible to generalize. Each vitamin has essential duties to perform. A severe shortage of any one of the vitamins leads eventually to a characteristic nutritional disorder. Such disorders had been known for centuries, in some cases, and frequently food "cures" had been applied successfully (such as lemons for scurvy) long before vitamins were discovered. However, it was not until a deficiency of each major vitamin was linked by research to a specific nutritional disorder in people that the cause-and-effect relationships were fully established. Such relationships are pointed out in the discussions of individual vitamins.

Much present-day information on vitamins originated with studies on animals. Some of the basic research on the performance of vitamins in metabolism could be done only with animals. Suitable methods of working with human subjects are constantly being developed. All research has been strengthened as pure vitamins have been made available. Pure vitamins have made it possible to determine more precisely the characteristic responses of animals to specific vitamins. When comparable effects are identified in human beings, the functions of individual vitamins in human nutrition are clarified.

The occurrence of vitamins in foods is varied in quantity and source. The 6 vitamins on the dietary allowance table and certain others are discussed here individually. Emphasis is placed on the positive contributions to nutritional well-being of including adequate amounts of vitamins in daily foods rather than on the conditions created by serious vitamin deficiencies.

All vitamins fall into 2 classes with respect to their solubility: some are soluble in water; some are soluble in fat and in the solvents of fat, such as ether. They are considered here in these 2 categories.

» FAT-SOLUBLE VITAMINS

Vitamins A, D, E, and K belong to the group soluble in fats [4]. Solubility offers a practical basis for a discussion of vitamins because of its relation to the retention of vitamin values in foods. In the main, fat-soluble vitamins are more stable to ordinary handling and cooking processes than are water-soluble vitamins. All fat-soluble vitamins are stored in the body in some degree. This fact has a bearing on the distribution of fat-soluble vitamins in the animal foods people eat and on the ability of people to build up a reserve of these vitamins in their own bodies. Vitamins A and D were among the first to be discovered. Considerable is known about their functions, food sources, and the body's need for them under different conditions.

Vitamin A

Vitamin A activity is vested in several related compounds. They will be considered here under two representative headings: *vitamin A,* as such, and the plant pigment *carotene.* Both occur in the body and in foods. Some of the carotene provided by foods is converted into vitamin A, mainly in the intestinal wall during digestion, and serves the body in the vitamin form. Because of its ability to make this transfer, carotene is called *pro*vitamin A. Vitamin A, as such, present in foods, is called *pre*formed vitamin A. Carotene is present in both animal and vegetable foods; vitamin A is present only in animal foods. The total vitamin A activity of a food is referred to as its *vitamin A value.* In the average diet in this country, about two-thirds of the vitamin A value is derived from carotene and one-third from preformed vitamin A [3].

Vitamin A and Resistance to Infection [2,4] Vitamin A is needed for the maintenance and functioning of the mucous membranes of the body: the outer skin covering and the linings of various body passages and cavities such as the eyelids and eyes, nose and mouth, and respiratory, genitourinary, and digestive tracts. When the diet provides sufficient vitamin A, the membranes are moist, pliable, and intact; they provide a protective covering to the organs and resist bacterial invasion. When the diet is deficient in vitamin A, the membranes are thin, dry, porous, and flaky. They are unable to perform their protective functions and bacteria have ready access. A shortage of vitamin A may, therefore, be said to lower barriers to certain infections.

Vitamin A and Vision Vitamin A is needed for vision. Vitamin A deficiency results in a condition known as *night blindness.* In this condition, one is unable to see well in dim light, particularly after exposure to a bright light. The "blindness" is explained by the fact that vitamin A is united to a protein in the retina of the eye to form a pigment, called visual purple, which is bleached in strong light. The vitamin A is lost in this process. If the body has sufficient vitamin A to draw upon, regeneration of the visual purple is rapid, the eyes adapt quickly in subdued light, and one can see almost at once. When there is a vitamin A deficiency, the regeneration of visual purple is slow and night blindness is the consequence. You may experience some degree of night blindness when you step from a brightly lighted lobby or from brilliant sunshine into a partially darkened theatre, or when you face a dark road at night after being confronted with the glare of oncoming automobile headlights. Since night blindness is sometimes due to a physical defect in the eye, or other causes, the vitamin-A-deficient condition is referred to as *functional* night blindness.

Night blindness may be prevalent in this country. There is no sure way of knowing how much there is and to what degree it exists. It is well known to people who are subjected routinely to strong light for long periods and then plunged into darkness. This is the situation of fishermen when they face the glare of sun on water for hours, and then try to make their way home in darkness. There are many tragic stories of the fishermen of Newfoundland and Labrador, in earlier days, who were lost at sea under these circumstances. Their basic diets were almost devoid of vitamin A value and they did not realize that one of the richest sources was within their reach, i.e., the livers of the fish with which they had filled their boats.

Vitamin A and Eye Disease In cases of extreme shortage of vitamin A value over a long period of time, an infectious eye disease, *xerophthalmia,* may develop. Unless vitamin A is introduced in some form, the condition worsens and blindness develops eventually. Xerophthalmia grows out of a change in the epithelial tissue of the eye. Failure of tear glands to function results in a dry eye and severe damage to the cornea.

Xerophthalmia is almost never seen in this country. It is known in areas of the Far East where diets are low in fats that carry vitamin A, and in vegetables and fruits rich in carotene. A now-famous outbreak of the disease occurred in children of Denmark during World War I. Butterfat, the country's chief source of vitamin A, was being exported to England in the form of butter. The Danish children, on skim milk, developed xerophthalmia. Many lost their eyesight. The physicians of Denmark associated the condition with that of experimental animals, reported from laboratories in the United States. The eye condition had been created in the laboratories by feeding a purified diet and was cured by adding butterfat or egg yolk fat to the diet. As a result of this work, vitamin A had been discovered only a few months earlier. The children of Denmark likewise responded to the addition of butterfat to their diets. When exports of Danish butter were curtailed and the children were returned to whole milk, the eye disease was brought under control. Thus the condition was recognized as a deficiency of vitamin A.

Other functions of vitamin A have been suggested chiefly by findings of research on laboratory animals. They have shown that adequate amounts of vitamin A are required for desirable body growth, including size of skeleton, for development of teeth and enamel formation, and for health, vigor, stamina, successful reproduction, and lactation.

Food Sources of Vitamin A and Carotene Color is a distinguishing feature of vitamin A value in foods. Vitamin A itself is a very pale yellow. Carotene, so called because it was first found in carrots, is a deep yellow-orange. Since carotene is present in both animal and vegetable foods, it can be readily identified in the pale yellow color of egg yolk, butter, fish-liver oils and in the yellow cast of liver itself, as well as in the orange color of carrots, sweet potatoes, and cantaloup. In addition, there is the characteristic color of carotene in green vegetables, although it is obscured by the green chlorophyll in these plants. Identifying colors are evident in Figure 7.1.

The specimen list of representative foods in Figure 7.1 is arranged in descending order of vitamin A values. It will be noted that the values are expressed in International Units (IU) rather than in grams or milligrams. One IU of vitamin A activity is that provided by 0.3 μg (microgram) of pure vitamin A or by 0.6 μg of carotene.

A 2-oz serving of cooked beef liver stands at the top of Figure 7.1. It provides about 3 times as much vitamin A value as does 1 serving each of the next 3 sources: sweet potatoes, leafy green vegetables, and carrots. Liver is the chief storage organ for vitamin A in the animal body. The striking contrast between liver and muscle as storage points for vitamin A in the animal body is demonstrated in the contrast between beef liver and beef roast as sources of vitamin A value: 30,330 IU vs. 30 I.U. Livers of different animals vary in vitamin A value but they are all concentrated sources.

In general, the yellow-orange color diminishes in intensity as the vitamin A values of foods decrease. Cantaloup, for

Fig. 7.1 Servings of representative foods in order of their importance as sources of vitamin A value. (Each bar represents an approximate vitamin A value for the series of foods listed below it.)

Food *	Weight or ** Approximate Measure	Vitamin A Value International Units
30,000 IU		
Liver, beef	2 oz	30,330
10,000 IU		
Spinach	1/2 cup	10,600
Carrots, diced	1/2 cup	9,065
Sweet potato	1 medium	8,970
6,000 IU		
Cantaloup	1/2 melon	6,590 (deep orange varieties)
Squash, winter	1/2 cup	6,345
2,000 IU		
Broccoli	1/2 cup	2,550
Apricots, dried, cooked	1/2 cup	2,287
Tomato juice, canned	1/2 cup (small glass)	1,270
500 IU		
Prunes, dried, cooked	5 with juice	733
Egg	1 medium	590
Peas, green	1/2 cup	575
Peaches, canned	2 halves with juice	500 (yellow varieties)
Butter or fortified margarine	1 tbsp	460
350 IU		
Beans, snap, green	1/2 cup	415
Milk, fluid, whole	1 cup	390
Cheese, cheddar	1 1/8" cube	380
Orange	1 medium	290
250 IU		
Lettuce leaves	2 large or 4 small	270
Chicken	1/4 small broiler	260 broiler
Corn, canned	1/2 cup	260 (yellow corn)
Orange juice, fresh	1/2 cup (small glass)	250
150 IU		
Banana, raw	1 medium	190
Cream, coffee	1 tbsp	130
Beans, dry, canned	3/4 cup	105
Cheese, cottage, creamed	1/4 cup	100
Pineapple juice, canned	1/2 cup (small glass)	100
60 or less IU		
Salmon, canned	1/2 cup	60
Apple, raw	1 medium	50
Haddock	1 fillet	50
Strawberries, raw	1/2 cup	45
Cabbage, shredded, raw	1/2 cup	40
Beef, pot roast	3 oz	30
Grapefruit	1/2 medium	10 (white fruit)
Milk, fluid, skim (or buttermilk)	1 cup	10
0 IU		
Bread, white, enriched	1 slice	trace
Potato, white	1 medium	trace
Beverage, kola type	6 oz	...
Cornflakes, fortified	1 1/3 cup	...
Frankfurter	1 medium	...
Oil, salad or cooking	1 tbsp	...
Bacon, crisp	2 slices	0
Ham, luncheon meat	2 oz	0
Macaroni, enriched, cooked	3/4 cup	0
Oatmeal, cooked	2/3 cup	0
Peanut butter	1 tbsp	0
Rice, cooked	3/4 cup	0
Oil, salad or cooking	1 tbsp	0
Sausage, salami	1 slice	0
Sugar, granulated	1 tbsp	0

*Foods are in forms ready to eat. All meats and vegetables are cooked unless otherwise indicated.

**See Appendix G for further identification of these foods. On that list all foods are described more fully and both weights and measures are indicated.

example, is about 3 times as rich as apricots per serving; apricots about 4 times as rich as peaches; peaches about 3 times as rich as bananas. But depth of color is not the sole gauge of vitamin A value in egg yolks and butterfat (whole milk, cream, butter), which contain both carotene and preformed vitamin A. Different breeds of animals differ in their ability to convert carotene to vitamin A in their bodies. Therefore, egg yolks or butterfat of deep yellow color do not necessarily contain more vitamin A value than those of paler color. The deeper color may merely mean the presence of more unconverted carotene. Also, nature has not been entirely consistent in associating the orange color with provitamin A. In rutabagas, for example, she has produced an orange-colored food, but the chief pigment is not carotene. Thus, one-half cup of cooked rutabagas yields 270 IU of vitamin A value, the same amount of carrots provides 9,065 IU vitamin A value.

The association of vitamin A value with certain fats is shown in Figure 7.1 in the difference between the value for 1 cup of whole milk (390 IU) and for the same amount of skim milk (10 IU). In recognition of the preference of many adults for skim milk to lower the fat content of their diets, the Food and Nutrition Board has approved the restoration of vitamin A to skim milk to "the average year-round level present in the whole milk supply." In many areas, therefore, skim milk has the same vitamin A value as whole milk. Federal specifications for fortified margarine require a minimum of 15,000 IU of vitamin A per pound, the approximate amount provided by butter.

Nearly one-half of the foods in Figure 7.1 furnish only 50 IU or less of vitamin A value per serving. This group includes all of the muscle meats, all of the fish except salmon, all of the cereals and breads, the cooking fats and salad oils, sugar, and a few fruits and vegetables. These are obviously negligible sources.

Vitamin A Content of the National Food Supply The U.S. Department of Agriculture reports that vegetables and fruits provide about 60 percent of all the available vitamin A value in the food supply of this country [5]. And about one-half of this amount comes from leafy green and yellow vegetables. The remaining 40 percent of vitamin A value comes chiefly from 4 sources: 14 percent from dairy products, excluding butter; 8 percent each from fats and eggs; 10 percent from meats. Clearly, vegetables are quantitatively a more important source of vitamin A value than are animal foods. The 10 percent of vitamin A value supplied by meats appears low in view of the fact that liver, an organ meat, is richer per serving than any other food. Since muscle meats are a negligible source of vitamin A, this low yield from meats would seem to reflect the negative attitude of the public toward the use of liver, reported in Chapter 1. It also emphasizes the point made in foregoing pages that the importance of a food as a source of any nutrient depends more on the frequency with which it is eaten than on the concentration of the nutrient in the food.

Stability of Vitamin A and Carotene Vitamin A and carotene are insoluble in water and resistant to ordinary cooking temperatures [6]. They are not lost or destroyed in boiling vegetables, for example, nor in freezing and canning processes. Vegetables, fruits, and eggs, dried in air, may lose much of their vitamin A value; those dried in a vacuum retain much of their vitamin A value. Fats exposed to air at warm temperatures become rancid. Rancidity destroys vitamin A and carotene.

► *Arrange your own list of representative foods (sort cards) in order of their quantitative importance as sources of vitamin A value. Study the list with a view to associating kinds of foods with their vitamin A values.*

Enter vitamin A values on your personal meal record. Total the vitamin A values for the day.

Familiarize yourself with the relative vitamin A values within the 3 sources—yellow vegetables, yellow fruits, and vegetable "greens"—from Appendix G. Also note the wide difference in vitamin A values between green vegetables, such as green beans, and the dark green leafy vegetables, such as kale.

Meeting Vitamin A Needs An important consideration in establishing and meeting the nutritional need for vitamin A is the proportion of carotene to vitamin A in the daily diet. Experiments have shown that carotene is used less efficiently by the body than is the preformed vitamin. This situation poses a problem since the two are associated in some foods and their values are expressed jointly as International Units of vitamin A. In arriving at the vitamin A activity of foods, carotene is given half the value of the preformed vitamin [3]. But this ratio may be even less favorable to carotene in some cases because of the wide range in the availability of carotene to the body under different conditions. The amount of absorption of carotene and the efficiency of its conversion to vitamin A varies with individuals and depends on such factors as the kinds of foods (vegetables) that provide the carotene, how they are prepared, and the presence of certain other nutrients. Thus a high vitamin A intake, if obtained largely from vegetable sources, could present an overly optimistic picture of vitamin A nutrition. A practical solution for meeting vitamin A needs with assurance would seem to be to choose some foods daily that supply the preformed vitamin and to make allowances for possible losses of carotene by using in abundance foods rich in this provitamin.

Other kinds of losses may prevent an individual from meeting vitamin A needs. A common one is that resulting from the indiscriminate use of mineral oil as a laxative. Vitamin A, as well as carotene, may be dissolved in the oil in the digestive tract. Since the oil is not absorbed, the vitamin may be discarded from the body along with the oil. This problem can be minimized by taking the oil several hours after eating a meal [4].

Recommended Daily Allowances for Vitamin A On the basis of available data, the Food and Nutrition Board has proposed allowances of 5000 IU daily for men and women of various ages (Table 7-1). An addition of 20 percent is made for the second half of pregnancy (6000 IU) and of 60 percent for lactation (8000 IU). The allowances are double the minimal amounts required to protect against vitamin A deficiency, and requirements are proportional to body weight. The allowances assume a diet whose vitamin A composition is two-thirds the provitamin, carotene, and one-third preformed vitamin A. Thus the Board has applied roughly the 60–40 ratio of carotene to preformed vitamin A available in the national food supply. Minimal values were doubled because of evidence that intakes above actual need are beneficial to health. Also, storage of vitamin A in the human liver makes it possible to draw upon this reserve supply for a considerable period of time without apparent harm to the body, if the current diet should provide little or none.

How the Average Adult Can Meet His Vitamin A Allowance The specimen diet in Appendix B shows how an adult

TABLE 7-1

RECOMMENDED DAILY DIETARY ALLOWANCES FOR VITAMINS A AND D [3]

	Age Years	Weight lb.)	Height (in.)	Calories	Vitamin A IU	Vitamin D IU
Men	25	154	69	3200	5000	
	45	154	69	3000	5000	
	65	154	69	2550	5000	
Women	25	128	64	2300	5000	
	45	128	64	2200	5000	
	65	128	64	1800	5000	
	Pregnant (second half)			+300	6000	400
	Lactating (850 ml daily)			+1000	8000	400
Infants	0–1/12					
	2/12–6/12	13	24		1500	400
	7/12–12/12	20	28		1500	400
Children	1– 3	27	34	1300	2000	400
	4– 6	40	43	1700	2500	400
	7– 9	60	51	2100	3500	400
	10–12	79	57	2500	4500	400
Boys	13–15	108	64	3100	5000	400
	16–19	139	69	3600	5000	400
Girls	13–15	108	63	2600	5000	400
	16–19	120	64	2400	5000	400

may choose a diet which *appears* fairly satisfactory but which provides only about 2300 IU of vitamin A value—less than one-half the allowance of 5000 IU per day. The butter and whole milk in the meals furnish 1255 IU of the vitamin A value of the diet, or about half of that available from all of the foods.

Examination of the items on the specimen diet shows that no rich source of vitamin A value was chosen from the vegetable-fruit group. The addition of half a serving of any one of the deep yellow or deep green leafy vegetables would have more than completed the daily allowance. In terms of meal planning, this would amount to a full serving of one rich source every other day. Thus the problem of obtaining a diet adequate in vitamin A value lies not in scarcity of the vitamin in common foods, but in knowing and using, at suitable intervals, the excellent sources available.

The 4 food listings given show ways in which an adult can meet his daily vitamin A allowance (page 127).

The first listing suggests the usefulness of liver as a source of vitamin A value on a weekly basis, especially if concentrated vegetable sources are used sparingly. The second suggests how a rich vegetable source can serve on an every-other-day basis. The third listing shows how an excellent source can be supplemented with a lesser source, such as green peas, and thus attain the daily allowance. The fourth suggests a possible combination when excellent sources are

MEETING DAILY VITAMIN A ALLOWANCE FOR ADULTS: 5000 IU

		A IU Vitamin
	1	
Liver, beef	2 oz	30,330
	2	
Spinach	½ cup	10,600
	3	
Carrots	¼ cup (½ serving)	4,533
Peas, green	½ cup	575
Total		5,108
	4	
Apricots, stewed	½ cup	2,287
Tomatoes, canned	½ cup	1,270
Egg	1 medium	590
Milk, whole	1 cup	390
Orange	1 medium	290
Lettuce	2 leaves	270
Total		5,097

omitted. The specimen diet already considered illustrates the possibilities for failure in attaining the allowance that can result when no important sources of vitamin A value are included. Reluctance to use vegetables, particularly the kinds highest in vitamin A value, may be traced to the dislike for vegetables on the part of both adults and children, as discussed in Chapter 1.

► *What is your daily dietary allowance for vitamin A value? (Find on Table 7-1, on the basis of your age.)*

How does your intake, as shown on your meal record, compare with your daily allowance for vitamin A value? In terms of food selection, explain why it falls below the allowance or exceeds the allowance. If it falls below, how could you correct it without changing your food habits drastically?

Vitamin A Allowances for Children Since vitamin A needs are based on body weight, it is logical that the dietary allowances for vitamin A value should increase from infancy to adolescence. However, once the adolescent has reached the 5000 IU level considered liberally adequate for the adult, the allowance is not further increased throughout the teens (Table 7–1).

The problem of meeting a child's allowances for vitamin A value is not unlike that of meeting the adult's—a matter of making sure that certain excellent sources are included at suitable intervals to provide for an adequate daily average intake of the vitamin. The 3 combinations, page 128, show how children at different ages may meet their vitamin A allowances when their meals include recommended amounts of whole milk and one egg daily and are supplemented with vegetables, which are excellent sources of vitamin A value.

Milk represents about one-third of the vitamin A allowance in each of the columns. The amounts of milk used are the same as those included on the corresponding calcium lists in Chapter 6. The egg in each column makes a moderate but significant contribution. The portion of vegetable in each case merely suggests the frequency with which a concentrated source could be served to complete the allowance. In combination 1, for example, a vegetable as rich in vitamin A value as winter squash could be used every 5 or 6 days to complete the preschool child's allowance; in combination 2, a vegetable as concentrated as spinach could be served every 3 or 4 days to meet the school-age child's allowance; and in combination 3, a vegetable as rich as carrots could be served every 2 or 3 days to meet the vitamin A needs of adolescence. These vegetables are obviously among the richest sources of carotene. Different vegetables have been used in the 3 combinations to illustrate the possibilities for variety. The use of minimum amounts is not to suggest curtailment of vegetable eating. Quite the

MEETING VITAMIN A ALLOWANCES FOR CHILDREN

Ages in Years	**4-6**		**10-12**		**13-19**	
DAILY VITAMIN A ALLOWANCES		2500 IU		4500 IU		5000 IU
		Vit. A IU		**Vit. A IU**		**Vit. A IU**
Milk, whole	3 cups	1170	4 cups	1560	4 cups	1560
Egg	1 medium	590	1 medium	590	1 medium	590
Squash, winter	1/6 serving*	1060	—	—	—	—
Spinach	—	—	¼ serving*	2650	—	—
Carrots	—	—	—	—	⅓ serving*	3022
Total		2820		4800		5172

* 1 serving: ½ cup.

reverse. Such rich sources may be used daily with profit. As has been pointed out, a surplus of carotene may be needed to make up for that which is not absorbed. However, rich sources may, with safety, be alternated with less concentrated vegetable sources and still provide the body with a desirable surplus of vitamin A value.

Excesses of Vitamin A Despite the fact that amounts of vitamin A value greater than the allowances are believed to be beneficial to health, there is increasing evidence that large excesses are toxic [7]. Such excesses do not result from eating rich food sources, but from highly potent concentrates taken in liquid or capsule form. The Council on Foods and Nutrition of the American Medical Association has sounded a warning that there is definite possibility of harm from taking in excess of 50,000 IU of vitamin A daily over a prolonged period. Children are more susceptible than adults. Many symptoms of toxicity from such excesses have been reported, including loss of appetite, irritability, and bone and joint pains.

Vitamin A Value in Our National Diet On the basis of the vitamin A value available from our total food supply, there is potentially enough for each individual to have more than 7000 IU daily [5]. This amount is considerably greater than the daily allowance for any age or condition. However, it does not represent actual intake by families or by individuals.

Family diets analyzed by the U.S. Department of Agriculture in 1955 did not provide fully the recommended amounts of vitamin A value in any of the 4 geographical regions studied. Table 6-2 shows that the percentage deviations below allowance levels varied in different regions of the United States: 12, 13, 11 and 26 percent in the North East, the North Central, the West and the South respectively [8]. These data do not reveal the amount of deviation below the allowances, but it may be suspected that some of the diets were low enough to be hazardous to good vitamin A nutrition.

State Experiment Station studies give a picture of vitamin A consumption by age groups and by sex [9]. Figures 7.2 and 7.3 summarize the information for persons of both sexes, ranging in age from 4 to 80 years. At all ages—adults and children—average intakes exceeded allowance values. The men and boys had considerably larger average intakes than the women and girls. Even in so favorable a situation as this, however, many individual diets may fail to meet allowances. This proved to be the case

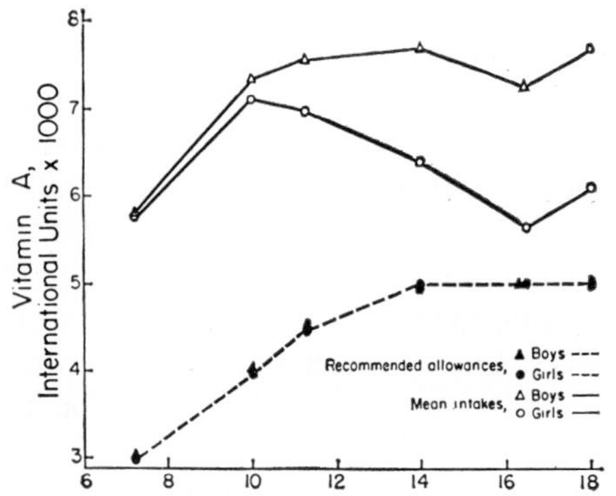

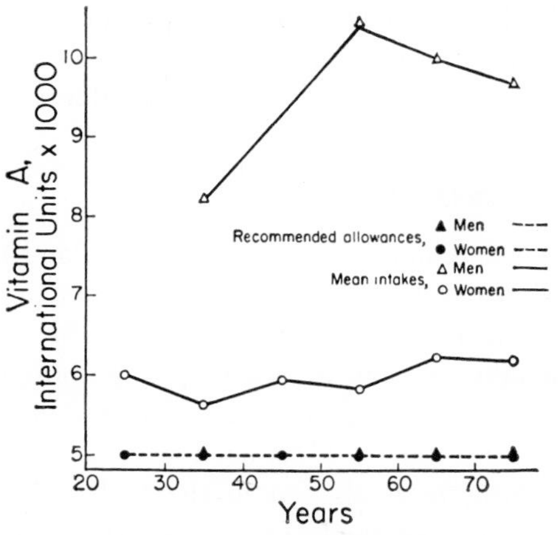

Figs. 7.2 and 7.3 Vitamin A intake in relation to daily dietary allowances. *(left)* Average daily vitamin A intake of boys and girls 4-20 years of age. *(right)* Average daily vitamin A intake of men and women from 20 to more than 80 years of age. (A. F. Morgan [Ed.], *Nutritional Status U.S.A.* Bull. 769. Berkeley, Calif.: University of California, Division of Agricultural Sciences, Agricultural Experiment Station, p. 35.)

at least in one locality [9]. When diets of adolescents were examined (Fig. 6.5) about 20 percent of the girls 15–18 years of age failed to attain even two-thirds of their dietary allowance for vitamin A value. The diets of about 10 percent of the girls 12–14 years were similarly deficient. The boys had a better record. Less than 10 percent of the boys at the 2 age levels fell below two-thirds of their dietary allowances for vitamin A value.

How To Assess Vitamin A Nutriture Average vitamin A value intakes for families and for different age groups appear reassuring. Also, the national food supply is rich in the vitamin. But we cannot overlook the fact that individuals vary widely in their intake of vitamin A and some may be seriously deficient. Just what difference such variations make in terms of human health has been the subject of many studies on children and adults. These have been made by measuring levels of vitamin A and of carotene in the blood, and by examining individuals for outward signs of vitamin A deficiencies, especially skin and eye conditions. These findings have then been compared with diet records in an attempt to discern diet-health relationships.

In general, diets poor in vitamin A and carotene were found to be associated with low blood levels of vitamin A, or of carotene, or both. And such signs as roughness of skin and inflammation of the mucous membranes of the eyes, related to vitamin A deficiency, were found more frequently in those persons with low blood levels than in those with satisfactory blood levels [9]. But there were many exceptions to this occurrence—exceptions due largely perhaps to the problem inherent in the double nature of vitamin A value itself. Low levels of carotene in the blood suggest a current dietary deficiency of carotene; high levels indicate adequate current intake. On the other hand, satisfactory levels of vitamin A in the blood may merely mean a stored supply of vitamin A resulting from previous high intakes of vitamin A and/or carotene. Low vitamin A blood levels indicate a low dietary intake and reduced stores. Finally, adequate blood levels of both vitamin A and carotene would seem to indicate satisfactory nutrition with respect to total vitamin A value.

Vitamin D

Vitamin D occurs in the body and in foods in 2 forms: as the preformed vitamin D, and in provitamin forms [2,4]. The provitamin, present in animals, is a form of cholesterol; in plants it is called *ergosterol.* The provitamin is changed to vitamin D, as such, in foods and in the body (skin) when it is exposed to ultraviolet rays of the sun or of an ultraviolet lamp.

Functions of Vitamin D Vitamin D is needed primarily for the most efficient utilization of calcium and phosphorus in the normal nourishment of bones and teeth. This need is particularly critical in childhood, pregnancy, and lactation but it continues to some extent throughout adult life.

There must be a satisfactory balance of calcium and phosphorus in the body if bones are to grow properly and become rigid and strong. Vitamin D assists in the absorption of calcium and phosphorus from the intestinal tract into the blood stream, in maintaining a proper calcium-phosphorus level in the blood, and in depositing these minerals properly in the bones and teeth [4]. If there is a shortage of calcium, phosphorus, or vitamin D, bones and teeth do not develop normally. The bones bend easily and, in extreme conditions, malformations such as bowed legs are extensive. This condition is known as *rickets.* During periods of rapid growth—before birth and during the first two years—children are most susceptible to rickets. Teeth are also poorly formed, erupt late, and are prone to early decay. *Osteoporosis,* and *osteomalacia,* bone diseases in adults are discussed under calcium in Chapter 6.

Rickets has been known as a bone disease of infants for centuries. The usefulness of cod-liver oil in controlling rickets was recognized in some countries in the nineteenth century, but vitamin D, the curative property in the oil, was not identified for another 100 years. Since the discovery of vitamin D in 1922, its use in various forms as a supplement to a child's diet has increased rapidly. Pediatricians now prescribe it routinely from the first few days of life. As a result, rickets, at least in exaggerated form, has largely disappeared in this country.

Sources of Vitamin D Vitamin D, as such, occurs in common foods in very small amounts. The comparative vitamin values on page 131 illustrate this and other points with respect to sources of vitamin D. Liver, butterfat and egg yolk contain some vitamin D. Most salt-water fish are relatively good sources: the vitamin is concentrated in the liver oil, but is also present in the body oil. Fish-liver oils are the richest natural sources of vitamin D. (They are also good sources of vitamin A.) The most concentrated source of vitamin D is produced by irradiating the provitamin, ergosterol, from yeast. The product is then dissolved in oil and marketed in this form. Viosterol is a well-known name for such a product. It is so potent a source of vitamin D that the dosage is prescribed in drops. Vitamin D is measured in terms of International Units (IU). Each unit is based on the activity of 0.025 μg (microgram) of pure crystalline vitamin D.

Several strong contrasts may be noted from the same listing: corn oil is a negligible source of vitamin D in comparison with the oils from animal sources; there is a wide range in vitamin D values between liver oils of different species of fish; and there is a considerable variation in the liver oils of

COMPARATIVE VITAMIN D VALUES OF A FEW SELECTED SOURCES

Food	Measure	Weight, oz	Weight, g	Vitamin D, IU
Butter	2 tbsp	1.0	28.0	22
Egg yolk	1 yolk	0.6	17.0	26
Liver, beef		3.0	85.0	29
Milk, vitamin D fortified	1 qt	34.4	976.0	400
Salmon, canned	½ cup	3.0	85.0	267*
Sardines, canned	8 halves	3.0	85.0	1173*
Corn oil	1 tsp	0.17	4.6	0.42
Cod-liver oil	1 tsp	0.17	4.6	467–4,296†
Halibut-liver oil	1 tsp	0.17	4.6	5,604–10,741†
Concentrates of fish-liver oils and Irradiated products of pure provitamins	available in different strengths; may be as much as 250 times richer in vitamin D than cod-liver oil*			

* See reference No. 2 at end of chapter.
† See reference No. 10 at end of chapter.

different members of the same species. When sold, all products are standardized and labelled for potency. The dosage should always be prescribed by a physician. Vitamin-D-fortified milk falls between natural food sources and the fish-liver oils quantitatively as a source of vitamin D. Its value lies in part in the fact that it supplies the vitamin automatically, in significant amounts, in routine daily meals.

Fortification of Food Sources When it was realized that foods supply little vitamin D, a movement was started to bring about the fortification of one staple food with this vitamin. Professional groups agreed upon milk as the most logical food for fortification because of the universality of its use and its calcium and phosphorus content. Fresh, evaporated, and some dried milks are fortified with vitamin D by adding a known amount of a vitamin D concentrate to a specified quantity of milk. The final product provides on the average 400 IU vitamin D per quart, as fresh or reconstituted milk. Homogenization distributes the vitamin evenly throughout the product. The 400 IU yield of vitamin D milk per quart was planned to correspond with the daily dietary allowances for the vitamin.

Recommended Daily Allowances for Vitamin D The Food and Nutrition Board's daily dietary allowances for vitamin D are identical for all ages covered—400 IU (Table 7-1). No values are assigned to the adult except for pregnancy and lactation. There is evidence that vitamin D is needed throughout the growth period, but the exact requirement at the different age levels has not been determined specifically. It has been demonstrated that 400 IU of vitamin D is sufficient for good calcium nutrition in children if the calcium and phosphorus intakes are also sufficient.

Meeting Vitamin D Needs The required intake of vitamin D at any age depends on the basic amount normally created in the body by exposure to sunlight. There is no way of measuring this source of vitamin D precisely, but it is known to vary widely with the potency of the ultraviolet rays that reach the skin. In the tropics, for example, where clothing is scanty, people live out of doors, and the sun's rays are direct, rickets is little known. In zones where the days are shorter, the ultraviolet rays are less direct, where people spend much time indoors, and where heavy clothing covers the body, rickets has been a serious problem. The condition of the atmosphere in any climate is an important factor. A clear atmosphere, free of clouds, dust, fog, and smoke permits the maximum vitamin D activity from the sun [4].

During the second half of pregnancy and in lactation the requirements for calcium and phosphorus are greatly increased to satisfy the needs of the baby's developing skeleton. Vitamin D is also required then to play its usual role of helping to utilize these 2 minerals to the fullest. Probably other adults do not need a supplementary source of vitamin D unless they are routinely deprived of sunlight, either by occupation, as night workers, or by clothing, as in the case of some religious orders. Older people may benefit by small amounts of extra vitamin D if they are closely housed. When adults have a low calcium intake, increased vitamin D does not compensate for the lack of this mineral.

Storage of Vitamin D Vitamin D is stored in the body to some extent. After it is absorbed from the intestine or formed in the body, it goes to the liver. Here most of the excess is kept until it is needed. Body reserves of the vitamin undoubtedly help to prevent some vitamin D deficiencies.

Stability of Vitamin D Vitamin D is stable to ordinary cooking temperatures, as well as to aging and storage. Heated vitamin D milk does not lose its vitamin D content; fish-liver oils retain their vitamin D value after holding.

Excesses of Vitamin D Amounts of vitamin D beyond need do not increase calcium retention or improve rates of growth or dentition. An excess of vitamin D is toxic [7]. Early signs of toxicity may be loss of appetite, nausea, and diarrhea, followed by more serious symptoms if the excess continues. Toxic effects are seen most often in infants from unintentional overdosage of highly concentrated sources of vitamin D and in adults using excessive amounts as therapy. The quantity of vitamin D that constitutes overdosage varies with individuals and depends on such factors as the amount of their exposure to ultraviolet light and their intake of calcium and phosphorus. Vitamin D intakes should be under the supervision of a physician, except in the case of vitamin D milk.

Vitamin E [11]

Vitamin E was discovered in 1922. Its functions for several animal species have been well defined, but only recently has there been assurance of its essentiality for man. Vitamin E is an antioxidant. Its importance to the human body appears to lie in this property—in its ability to unite with oxygen and thus protect red blood cells from such blood-destroying agents as hydrogen peroxide [4]. By combining with oxygen, vitamin E also prevents the destruction of vitamin A and carotene by oxidation in the body (in the gastro-intestinal tract) and in foods. Fats exposed to air (oxygen) become rancid; rancidity destroys vitamin A and carotene. Vitamin E acts by uniting with oxygen, prevents rancidity, and thus prevents destruction of the other fat-soluble vitamin.

Such signs of vitamin E deficiency in animals as reproductive failure, degeneration of skeletal muscles, and paralysis of hind quarters do not appear to be applicable to human beings. Their occurrence in animals, however, has led to misunderstandings on the part of the public with respect to such applications. Efforts to treat human cases of muscular dystrophy and spontaneous abortion with large doses of vitamin E have not proved successful.

Vitamin E is stored in the body, chiefly in the muscles and fat deposits; it is thus possible to maintain a reserve supply. The vitamin is not sensitive to usual cooking temperatures. And, because it is fat-soluble, vitamin E is not dissolved in cooking water and discarded. A shortage of vitamin E is highly unlikely because it is widely distributed in common foods. Wheat germ and wheat-germ oil are concentrated sources. It is also present in leafy vegetables, legumes, whole grains, vegetables, oils, liver, butter, milk, and eggs. No daily requirement for vitamin E has been established and no dietary allowance has yet been recommended.

Vitamin K

Vitamin K is essential to the normal clotting of the blood and to normal functioning of the liver. Its relation to blood clotting is not fully understood, but it is believed that this vitamin enables the liver to form prothrombin, a protein required for clot formation. When clots fail to form, there is danger of bleeding to death. A small amount of vitamin K is stored in the liver. When there is injury to the liver and vitamin K cannot be stored, there is a reduction of prothrombin in the blood [2,4].

For some time it has been routine practice to administer vitamin K to mothers during the last month of pregnancy, or to the infant during the first few days of life. This has been done to prevent hemorrhage in newborn babies. The procedure is now being questioned on several grounds including the difficulty of proving that low levels of prothrombin cause hemorrhage or that routine administration of vitamin K lowers the incidence of hemorrhage. There is also question as to the possible effects on the health of the infants of altering the normal coagulation process. It now appears that infants normally have low levels of prothrombin and other coagulation factors at birth; that these levels decrease further during the first weeks of life; and that they then rise naturally to normal concentrations [3].

The human requirement for vitamin K has not been determined, nor have dietary allowances been recommended. There are 2 chief natural sources of vitamin K: common foods, and the vitamin K synthesized by the bacteria of the intestinal tract. The prevalence of vitamin K in a wide variety of green leafy vegetables, in egg yolk, and in organ meats makes a dietary shortage quite improbable. There seems to be no reason to supplement diets in this country with vitamin K unless there is liver injury or some other condition for which a physician prescribes additional amounts of the vitamin [3].

» WATER-SOLUBLE VITAMINS

The water-soluble vitamins make up a large group. All but one belong to the B complex. The remaining water-soluble vitamin is ascorbic acid or vitamin C. For the most part, water-soluble vitamins are not stored in the body. Excesses are largely excreted, thus eliminating the possibilities for toxicity that exist with overdosage of fat-soluble vitamins.

At least 11 vitamins compose the B complex. Seven of them are essential in human nutrition and must be provided in daily meals; 3 of these are included on the allowance table of the Food and Nutrition Board [12]. These 3 are thiamine (vitamin B_1), riboflavin (vitamin B_2), and niacin. They were once thought to be one substance. Gradually, their separate identities were established. Certain overlapping characteristics and functions delayed the process of separation. For example, the fact that each is soluble in water led to difficulties in recognition. And all are concerned together in the task of providing the body with energy. Their function basically is converting sources of energy in the body, especially carbohydrate, into "living" energy. In effect, they make it possible for carbohydrate to "burn" at body temperature. In addition, each has its own characteristic contributions to make in nourishing the body. All 3 occur in very small amounts in every body cell.

Thiamine

Functions of Thiamine (Vitamin B_1) Thiamine teams up with an enzyme in the body to form what is known as a *coenzyme*. The latter acts as a catalyst in the oxidation process, which prepares glucose in the body to supply energy [12]. Thus thiamine helps carbohydrate metabolism through its intermediary stages. If there is enough thiamine, the process proceeds normally. If there is not enough, there is an accumulation in the blood of one of the intermediary products of carbohydrate metabolism, *pyruvic acid*. This condition may lead to poor functioning of the gastrointestinal tract and may be related to loss of appetite, which follows thiamine deficiency. Because of its association with the desire to eat, thiamine is sometimes referred to as the *appetite* vitamin. Fatigue, nausea, and general apathy are often accompaniments of appetite failure.

Adequate intake of thiamine is also necessary to a functionally normal nervous system. A moderately low thiamine intake over a period of time can lead to specific symptoms: mental depression, moodiness, irritability [12].

Thiamine Deficiency Disease A very low intake of thiamine leads eventually to *beriberi*—a dietary deficiency disease. Beriberi is characterized by degeneration of nerve tissue, especially in the arms and legs, by muscle weakness, heart disease, edema, and eventually paralysis. Beriberi has been known for centuries. It was, and still is, rampant in parts of the world that subsist almost exclusively on white rice. Beriberi plagued the Japanese Navy for generations. Sailors on ships' rations, mainly rice, usually became ill and many did not survive long sea voyages. Meats or legumes added to the diet prevented or cured the disease. This favorable effect was mistakenly attributed to protein.

In the late nineteenth century it was discovered by accident that a diet of white rice could produce a beriberi-like disease in chickens, and that polishings of the rice would cure it. A concentrate from the rice polishings brought about dramatic recovery when administered to people with beriberi. The curative property in the polishings was isolated about 40 years later and was named vitamin B. In another 10 years the chemical structure of the vitamin was determined, and it was synthesized. Its official name then became *thiamine* [1].

Food Sources of Thiamine Thiamine is widely distributed naturally in plant and animal foods, but with the exception of a few highly concentrated sources, the amounts are relatively small. Furthermore, whole grains, which naturally carry significant amounts of thiamine in their outer coats and germs, are used today in small quantities in comparison with the more acceptable highly milled flours and breakfast foods. Recognition of these facts on the part of nutritionists led to the enrichment of flour and bread with thiamine and certain other nutrients. (See Chapter 6 for a statement of the history of enrichment, the enrichment standards established, and the present status of enrichment in this country.)

Enrichment of bread and flour has been a specific factor in raising the content of thiamine in the food supply, even in the face of declining cereal consumption. Figure 7.4 shows graphically the extent to which enrichment has been responsible for the increased thiamine. In 1941, 2 years before enrichment was required by War Food Order No. 1, 1.68 mg of thiamine was available per person per day in foods in this country. By 1945, 2 years after the issuance of the order, the thiamine content had risen to 2.08 mg per person. Measuring the increase in another way: In the period 1935–1939, 19 percent of the thiamine in the food supply came from cereal grains; in the period 1942–1945, during which time the enrichment order went into effect, the percent of thiamine from cereal grains had risen to 33.5 percent [5]. It should be pointed out that, whereas consumption of grain products as a whole has decreased in the past 50 years, the consumption of flour in the form of bread and other baked products has increased. It may be assumed that many of these products are made from enriched flour [13].

The percentage of thiamine available in the nation's food supply from cereal grains remains today about the same as in 1945—32 percent or nearly one-third of the total; about one-fourth (25 percent) of the thiamine is from meat, poultry, and fish; about one-eighth (11 percent) from dairy products, excluding butter; and lesser amounts are from different categories of vegetables and fruits and from eggs. With some reservations the comparative thiamine yields on the specimen representative food list (Fig. 7.5) bear out the general picture of thiamine availability. Average servings of the foods are arranged in descending order of their quantitative importance as sources of thiamine.

It is apparent from Figure 7.5 that lean pork, fresh or cured, is a very rich source of thiamine per serving, and that several other meats, including liver, rank above enriched bread as sources of thiamine. The point made repeatedly that regular use is the chief consideration in making any food an important source of a nutrient is borne out again. Breads, breakfast foods, and other grain products, which are on every menu, tend to overshadow the richer sources of thiamine, eaten less often. Milk is another case in point. It also may contribute a significant amount of thiamine if taken daily in recommended amounts.

As with iron, we have the problem of "shopping around" for thiamine. Aside from the foods mentioned, the very small amounts in most vegetables and fruits and the total, or almost total, lack in fats, oils, and sugars, makes it important to know where to "shop." Thiamine is unusual in that it takes several servings of even the richest food sources to attain the adult dietary allowances.

Fig. 7.4 The effect of enrichment on the thiamine content of the diet.

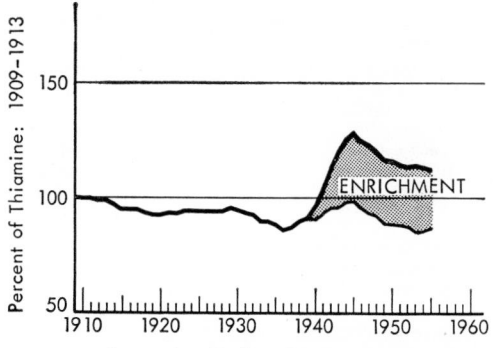

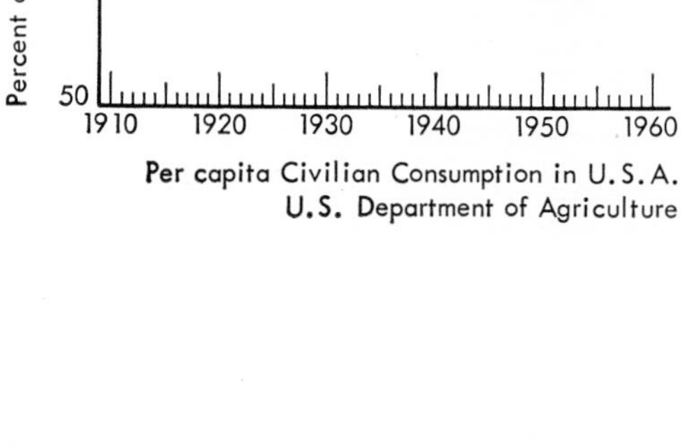

Fig. 7.5 Servings of representative foods in order of their importance as sources of thiamine. (Each bar represents an approximate thiamine value for the series of foods listed below it.)

Food *	Weight or ** Approximate Measure	Thiamine Milligrams
0.6 mg		
Pork chop	1 chop	0.63
Ham, luncheon meat	2 oz	0.57
0.15 mg		
Peas, green	1/2 cup	0.20
Sausage, salami	1 slice	0.16
Liver, beef	2 oz	0.15
Oatmeal, cooked	2/3 cup	0.15
Macaroni, enriched, cooked	3/4 cup	0.14
Cornflakes, fortified	1 1/3 cup	0.12
Orange	1 medium	0.12
0.10 mg		
Orange juice, fresh	1/2 cup (small glass)	0.11
Beans, dry, canned	3/4 cup	0.10
Milk, fluid, skim (or buttermilk)	1 cup	0.10
Potato, white	1 medium	0.10
Sweet potato	1 medium	0.10
Cantaloup	1/2 melon	0.09
Bacon, crisp	2 slices	0.08
Milk, fluid, whole	1 cup	0.08
Rice, cooked	3/4 cup	0.08
Frankfurter	1 medium	0.08
0.06 mg		
Pineapple juice, canned	1/2 cup (small glass)	0.07
Spinach	1/2 cup	0.07
Bread, white, enriched	1 slice	0.06
Tomato juice	1/2 cup (small glass)	0.06
Banana, raw	1 medium	0.05
Beans, green, snap	1/2 cup	0.05
Broccoli	1/2 cup	0.05
Egg	1 medium	0.05
Grapefruit	1/2 medium	0.05
Squash, winter	1/2 cup	0.05
0.03 mg		
Apple, raw	1 medium	0.04
Beef, pot roast	3 oz	0.04
Carrots, diced	1/2 cup	0.04
Chicken	1/4 small broiler	0.04
Corn, canned	1/2 cup	0.04
Cabbage, shredded, raw	1/2 cup	0.03
Haddock	1 fillet	0.03
Prunes, dried, cooked	5 with juice	0.03
Salmon, canned	1/2 cup	0.03
Cheese, cottage, creamed	1/4 cup	0.02
Lettuce leaves	2 large or 4 small	0.02
Peanut butter	1 tbsp	0.02
Strawberries, raw	1/2 cup	0.02
0.01 mg or less		
Cheese, cheddar	1 1/8" cube	0.01
Peaches, canned	2 halves with juice	0.01
Apricots, dried, cooked	1/2 cup	trace
Beverage, kola type	6 oz	...
Butter or fortified margarine	1 tbsp	...
Cream, coffee	1 tbsp	0
Oil, salad or cooking	1 tbsp	0
Sugar, granulated	1 tbsp	0

*Foods are in forms ready to eat. All meats and vegetables are cooked unless otherwise indicated.

**See Appendix G for further identification of these foods. On that list allfoods are described more fully and both weights and measures are indicated.

Stability of Thiamine An additional problem in obtaining enough thiamine is that the vitamin is unstable to heat [14]. Some losses in cooking are therefore unavoidable. Cereals, which are cooked slowly at low temperatures and the water utilized, lose little thiamine. Baked products lose about 15–30 percent. Meat losses may be about one-third. In addition to destruction by heat, some of this water-soluble vitamin may be drained off or carried into drippings to be discarded. Any foods that are soaked and drained may lose large portions of thiamine. Thiamine values for foods in Appendix G and those used in this chapter take into consideration what appear to be normal losses from cooking processes. With careless handling, foods may lose much more thiamine.

► *Arrange your own list of representative foods (sort cards) in order of their importance as sources of thiamine.*

Enter thiamine values on your meal record. Total the thiamine values for the day.

What are the main sources of thiamine on the specimen diet for an adult in Appendix B? How do they differ from the sources on your own meal record?

Compare the thiamine value of one slice of white enriched bread with the same amount of whole-wheat bread and white unenriched bread.

TABLE 7–2

RECOMMENDED DAILY DIETARY ALLOWANCES FOR THIAMINE, RIBOFLAVIN, NIACIN, ASCORBIC ACID [3]

	Age Years	Weight (lb.)	Height (in.)	Calories	Thiam. mg.	Ribo. mg	Niacin mg equiv.	Asc. Acid mg
Men	25	154	69	3200	1.6	1.8	21	75
	45	154	69	3000	1.5	1.8	20	75
	65	154	69	2550	1.3	1.8	18	75
Women	25	128	64	2300	1.2	1.5	17	70
	45	128	64	2200	1.1	1.5	17	70
	65	128	64	1800	1.0	1.5	17	70
	Pregnant (second half)			+300	1.3	2.0	+3	100
	Lactating (850 ml daily)			+1000	1.7	2.5	+2	150
Infants	0–1/12							
	2/12–6/12	13	24		0.4	0.5	6	30
	7/12–12/12	20	28		0.5	0.8	7	30
Children	1 – 3	27	34	1300	0.7	1.0	8	35
	4 – 6	40	43	1700	0.9	1.3	11	50
	7 – 9	60	51	2100	1.1	1.5	14	60
	10–12	79	57	2500	1.3	1.8	17	75
Boys	13–15	108	64	3100	1.6	2.1	21	90
	16–19	139	69	3600	1.8	2.5	25	100
Girls	13–15	108	63	2600	1.3	2.0	17	80
	16–19	120	64	2400	1.2	1.9	16	80

Recommended Daily Allowances for Thiamine The Food and Nutrition Board's daily dietary allowances for thiamine are related to total calorie need because of thiamine's function in energy metabolism. The minimal requirement of adults is considered to be approximately 0.23 mg of thiamine for each 1000 calories. The allowance figure was set at about twice that amount (0.5 mg per 1000 cal) because of large individual variations in need, and the inability of the body to store quantities of thiamine. With adult calorie intakes below 2000 cal, the thiamine intake should not fall below 1.0 mg per day. The recommended daily dietary allowance (Table 7-2) shows how thiamine allowances are related to calorie allowances. Men 25 years of age, for example, with a daily calorie allowance of 3200, have a 1.6 mg thiamine allowance. (3.2 × 0.5)[3]. Thiamine allowances are calculated throughout on this basis, including those for infancy, pregnancy, and lactation.

How the Average Adult Can Meet His Thiamine Allowance The specimen diet for an adult in Appendix B shows how, even with a varied selection of foods, the allowance for thiamine may not be met. The margin of failure is narrow and cannot be considered a real shortage in view of the fact that the allowances represent desirable intakes, not requirements. Cereals in all forms provide about 40 percent of the thiamine in this diet. Pork does not appear on the menu in any form; it therefore contains no excellent source of thiamine. If pork were substituted for the hamburger or for the baked beans, it would assure a comfortable surplus of thiamine. The small contributions made by a large number of the foods on the specimen diet illustrate the point made earlier: thiamine is widely distributed in common foods but is concentrated in only a few.

The following 4 food combinations show ways in which a man about 25 years of age can meet his daily thiamine allowance.

MEETING DAILY THIAMINE ALLOWANCE FOR YOUNG MEN: 1.6 mg (3200 cal)

	1	Thiamine mg
Pork	2 chops	1.26
Oatmeal	⅔ cup	0.15
Bread, enriched	4 slices	0.24
Total		1.65
	2	
Ham	4 oz	1.14
Potatoes	2	0.20
Milk, skim	1 pt	0.20
Beans, dry, canned	¾ cup	0.10
Total		1.64
	3	
Lamb	6 oz	0.26
Potatoes	2	0.20
Peas, green	½ cup	0.20
Oatmeal	⅔ cup	0.15
Macaroni, enriched	¾ cup	0.14
Bread, enriched	6 slices	0.36
Orange	1 medium	0.12
Milk, skim	1 cup	0.10
Eggs	2 medium	0.10
Total		1.63
	4	
Lamb	3 oz	0.13
Potatoes	2	0.20
Cornflakes	1⅓ cup	0.12
Milk, skim	1 cup	0.10
Beans, dry, canned	¾ cup	0.10
Frankfurters	2	0.16
Bread, enriched	6 slices	0.36
Eggs	2 medium	0.10
Vegetables	4 servings	0.20
Fruits	2 servings	0.10
Total		1.57

Combinations 1 and 2 show the ease with which the allowance can be met by using forms of pork. The man has a calorie allowance of 3200, which means that his total intake of food is large and that multiple portions of meat, potatoes, and cereal foods can be assumed. Combinations 3 and 4 show the need for taking account of lesser thiamine sources when other meats are substituted for pork—in combination 3, when double servings of the meat are used; in combination 4, when a single serving is used. As with corresponding lists for other nutrients, the fewer the excellent sources used, the greater the dependence on a larger number of less concentrated sources. Combinations 1, 3, and 4 show how the use of enriched bread, in quantity, adds to the total thiamine intake.

► *What is your daily allowance for thiamine? Obtain this from Table 7-2 on the basis of your age. How does the value on the table differ from a calculated value, based on your actual calorie intake?*

How does the thiamine intake as shown on your meal record compare with your daily allowance for thiamine? In terms of food selection, explain why it falls below the allowance or exceeds the allowance. If it fell below the allowance, could you correct it easily? How?

Thiamine Allowances for Children

Thiamine allowances for children increase with calorie intake as do those of adults. Boys in the 16–19-year-old group have the highest thiamine allowance for any age or condition—1.8 mg—which corresponds with the highest calorie allowance, 3600 (Table 7–2). As is demonstrated next, children of different ages may meet their thiamine allowances by eating different amounts of the same foods. This is the practical way of meeting the problem when children in the family eat at the same table. As a child grows older, his calorie and thiamine needs increase simultaneously.

The amounts of milk proposed in the 3 combinations are those used in corresponding lists for nutrients previously discussed. Although milk is not listed among the concentrated sources of thiamine, it supplies a significant amount when taken in the quantities indicated. It seems likely that in many cases milk would make the difference between adequacy and inadequacy in thiamine intake. Other foods are given in graduated quantities to suggest the manner in which

MEETING THIAMINE ALLOWANCES FOR CHILDREN

Ages in Years		**4-6**		**10-12**		**16-19 (Boys)**
DAILY THIAMINE ALLOWANCES		0.9 mg		1.3 mg		1.8 mg
DAILY CALORIE ALLOWANCES		1700 cal		2500 cal		3600 cal
		Thiamine mg		**Thiamine mg**		**Thiamine mg**
Milk, whole	3 cups	0.24	4 cups	0.32	4 cups	0.32
Egg	1 medium	0.05	1 medium	0.05	2 medium	0.10
Oatmeal	⅓ cup	0.08	⅔ cup	0.15	1 cup	0.23
Lamb	1½ oz	0.07	3 oz	0.13	6 oz	0.26
Potato, white	1 medium	0.10	1 medium	0.10	2 medium	0.20
Bread, enriched	3 slices	0.18	6 slices	0.36	8 slices	0.48
Orange	1 medium	0.12	1 medium	0.12	1 medium	0.12
Vegetables	2 servings*	0.10	2 servings*	0.10	4 servings*	0.20
Total		0.94		1.33		1.91

* 1 serving vegetable: ½ cup.

servings could be increased as needs for calories and thiamine become greater with age.

Thiamine in Our Daily National Diet The U.S. Department of Agriculture reports that there would be 1.8 mg of thiamine available daily from the nation's food supply for each person in this country if it were all usable and were divided equally among all persons [5]. This amount is considerably above the allowances for young children but it is only slightly above those for various periods of adult life. It is identical with the allowance for boys in the late teens (Table 7-2). Experience in analyzing other nutrients suggests that many individual and family diets, which represent actual food intakes, would be expected to fall below daily allowances for thiamine intake. Family diets studied by the U.S. Department of Agriculture in 1955 in 4 geographic regions in this country showed this to be the case [8]. Table 6-2 shows the deviations below the allowances for thiamine to be 22, 14, 16, and 15 percent, respectively, for the North East, the North Central, the West and the South. In the country as a whole, farm families came nearer to meeting the allowances than did city families in the same areas, possibly due to greater use of cereal and pork products on farms.

Studies made by the State Experiment Stations have brought out information with respect to habits by age groups and by sex [9]. Information was assembled on boys and girls, men and women, from the ages 4 to 80 years (Figs. 7.6 and 7.7). Children up to about 12 years of age have thiamine intakes which, on the average, meet or exceed allowances. During the teens, the diets of boys and girls barely meet or fall below; the girls' diets are more consistently below than the boys' (Fig. 7.6). From 20 years of age through adult life, men's thiamine intakes run below the allowances; women's intakes run little, if at all, below (Fig. 7.7).

Teen-age diets appear to offer problems in meeting thiamine allowances. A study made of Iowa young people 12–18 years of age (Chap. 6), gives some insight into the particular ages most vulnerable and the extent of deviation below the allowances (Fig. 6.5). About 15 percent of the girls in the 15–18-year-old group had intakes of thiamine that were less than two-thirds of their daily allowances (considered borderline); almost 10 percent of the 12–14-year-old girls were in this category. Nearly 20 percent of the boys in the 15–18-year-old group had intakes of less than two-thirds of their daily allowance for thiamine; and about 5 percent of the 12–14-year-old boys were similarly low [9].

How To Assess Thiamine Nutriture It appears from the above that many individuals may have intakes of thiamine below desirable levels despite the fact that the total food supply in this country probably provides enough for all. What, if any, evidence do we have that the nutritional status of individuals is affected by such shortages? Is it possible to relate dietary information to signs of thiamine deficiency in human beings? Chemical methods of studying thiamine values in blood and urine have not been perfected to the point where the thiamine nutrition of population groups can be assessed accurately. And, as suggested earlier, physical signs of moderate thiamine deficiency are not easily identified. Recognizable symptoms are often those which may originate from deficiencies of other vitamins. Many indefinite symptoms related to digestion and associated with chronic fatigue may result from less than desirable amounts of thiamine.

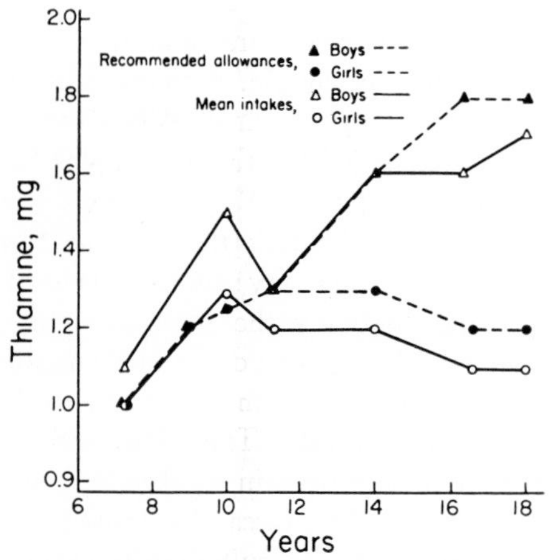

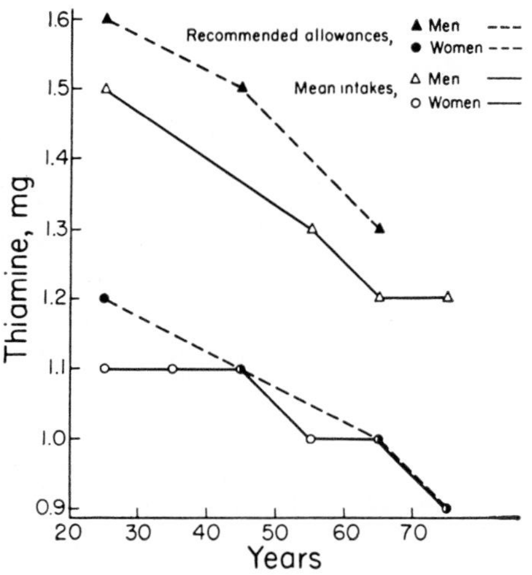

Figs. 7.6 and 7.7 Thiamine intake in relation to daily dietary allowances. *(left)* Average daily thiamine intake of boys and girls 4-20 years of age. *(right)* Average daily thiamine intake of men and women from 20 to more than 80 years of age. (A. F. Morgan [Ed.], *Nutritional Status U.S.A.* Bull. 769. Berkeley, Calif.: University of California, Division of Agricultural Sciences, Agricultural Experiment Station, p. 35.)

Beriberi, as such, is little known in the United States. Undoubtedly there are many persons on diets moderately low in thiamine who have various undiagnosed symptoms, described earlier. In rice-eating areas of the Far East, beriberi remains a major problem wherever native diets remain limited and efforts to introduce enriched rice have failed [15].

Excesses of Thiamine If adequate amounts of thiamine are beneficial, are added quantities better? One worker undertook to answer this question with studies on orphanage children of school age. In one series that extended over a period of 6 weeks, she fed each child a 2-mg thiamine tablet daily. A control group received only the thiamine naturally occurring in the orphanage diet, about 0.9 mg daily. All children were tested with 18 tasks, including measures of mental functions, motor skills, and strength. The group receiving the added thiamine showed superior scores as early as 1 week after the start of the supplementation, and continued to lead throughout the period. A repetition of the experiment with certain refinements, after the findings were challenged, proved inconclusive [16]. Similar studies by other research workers showed no significant differences between the accomplishments of children receiving a moderate amount of thiamine in daily meals and those given an additional 2 mg in tablet form. (It has already been established that there is almost no storage of water-soluble vitamins; and that amounts above need are eliminated.) It seems likely that the children in the original study who received the extra thiamine improved in nutritional status and general physical well-being, at least up to the point where their daily needs for the vitamin were satisfied. Undoubtedly more physical endurance resulted, and perhaps greater ability to concentrate. There is no proof that mental capacity, as such, is altered by changing nutritional status (Chap. 2).

Riboflavin

Functions of Riboflavin (Vitamin B_2) Riboflavin, like thiamine, unites with enzymes to help cells use oxygen—an essential step in the process of converting sources of energy in the body into energy itself [12]. When there is a shortage of riboflavin in the body, certain characteristic physical signs appear. Some are concentrated in the area of the mouth, lips, tongue, and nose. The mouth becomes sore and the tongue smooth and purplish in color; the lips are inflamed, with cracking at the corners of the mouth; and the skin is rough and scaly, particularly at the folds of the nose.

Other signs of riboflavin deficiency pertain to the eyes. The eyelids become rough; there may be a blurring of vision, and often there is sensitivity to light. Similar eye and mouth symptoms may arise from other causes, including deficiencies of other vitamins. Thus a cause-and-effect relationship with riboflavin cannot always be established unless the conditions clear up as a result of administering pure riboflavin. Experiments with laboratory animals show that liberal intakes of riboflavin result in long productive life, an extended period of adult efficiency, and vigorous health. On the contrary, animals on low riboflavin intakes are retarded in growth and development; their lives are shortened; they suffer from digestive disturbances; they display nervous symptoms and other signs, including early onset of aging and the eye and dermatitis symptoms discussed above [2].

Riboflavin Deficiency Disease A dietary deficiency disease, called *ariboflavinosis,* results from a long-continued drastic dietary shortage of riboflavin. The disease does not have a long history like that of beriberi, with gradual identification of symptoms, eventual association with a specific food as the cure, and finally the discovery of the vitamin. Actually, the vitamin became known first. When it was finally separated from the B complex and was synthesized (1935) its functions were identified. Withholding the vitamin from the diets of laboratory animals gave the first clues. Studying the physical signs of individuals living on diets low in riboflavin gave more information as to its importance for health. The skin and eye symptoms are present in marked degree in ariboflavinosis. The disease is usually seen in persons who are suffering from other vitamin deficiencies, particularly those of the B complex.

Food Sources of Riboflavin Riboflavin is widely distributed in plant and animal foods, but its major sources are from 3 food groups—milk, meats and grains. Eighty percent of the riboflavin in the United States food supply is concentrated in these 3: dairy products, excluding butter (48 percent); meat, poultry, and fish (18 percent); flour and cereal products (14 percent). Riboflavin is one of the nutrients of enrichment in flour and breads (Table 6-3). Since the enrichment program began, the proportion of riboflavin available from cereal-grain products has doubled from 7 to 14 percent. In 1941, 2 years before enrichment was required by War Food Order No. 1, the amount of riboflavin available daily per capita was 1.99 mg. In 1945, 2 years after enrichment started, the amount had risen to 2.52 mg. Today it is only slightly less than this high value.

Figure 7.8 presents the riboflavin values for the foods on the specimen representative food list. Average servings of the foods are arranged in descending order with respect to the vitamin values. Liver is by far the

Fig. 7.8 Servings of representative foods in order of their importance as sources of riboflavin. (Each bar represents an approximate riboflavin value for the series of foods listed below it.)

Food *	Weight or ** Approximate Measure	Riboflavin Milligrams
2.00 mg		
Liver, beef	2oz	2.25
0.50 mg		
Milk, fluid, skim (or buttermilk)	1 cup	0.44
Milk, fluid, whole	1 cup	0.42
0.17 mg		
Beef, pot roast	3 oz	0.18
Pork chop	1 chop	0.18
Spinach	1/2 cup	0.18
Cheese, cottage, creamed	1/4 cup	0.16
Salmon, canned	1/2 cup	0.16
Squash, winter	1/2 cup	0.16
Cheese, cheddar	1 1/8" cube	0.15
Chicken	1/4 broiler	0.15
Egg	1 medium	0.15
Ham, luncheon meat	2 oz	0.15
Sausage, salami	1 slice	0.15
0.10 mg		
Broccoli	1/2 cup	0.11
Peas, green	1/2 cup	0.11
Frankfurter	1 medium	0.10
Beans, dry, canned	3/4 cup	0.08
Haddock	1 fillet	0.08
Macaroni, enriched, cooked	3/4 cup	0.08
0.06 mg		
Cantaloup	1/2 melon	0.07
Corn, canned	1/2 cup	0.07
Sweet potato	1 medium	0.07
Banana, raw	1 medium	0.06
Beans, snap, green	1/2 cup	0.06
Prunes, dried, cooked	5 with juice	0.06
Bacon, crisp	2 slices	0.05
Bread, white, enriched	1 slice	0.05
Strawberries, raw	1/2 cup	0.05
0.03 mg		
Apricots, dried, cooked	1/2 cup	0.04
Carrots, diced	1/2 cup	0.04
Lettuce leaves	2 large or 4 small	0.04
Potato, white	1 medium	0.04
Tomato juice, canned	1/2 cup (small glass)	0.04
Cabbage, shredded, raw	1/2 cup	0.03
Cornflakes, fortified	1 1/3 cup	0.03
Oatmeal, cooked	2/3 cup	0.03
Orange	1 medium	0.03
Orange juice, fresh	1/2 cup (small glass)	0.03
Peaches, canned	2 halves with juice	0.03
Apple, raw	1 medium	0.02
Cream, coffee	1 tbsp	0.02
Grapefruit	1/2 medium	0.02
Peanut butter	1 tbsp	0.02
Pineapple juice, canned	1/2 cup (small glass)	0.02
Rice, cooked	3/4 cup	0.02
0 mg		
Beverage, kola type	6 oz	...
Butter or fortified margarine	1 tbsp	...
Oil, salad or cooking	1 tbsp	0
Sugar, granulated	1 tbsp	0

*Foods are in forms ready to eat. All meats and vegetables are cooked unless otherwise indicated.

**See Appendix G for further identification of these foods. On that list all foods are described more fully and both weights and measures are indicated.

richest source shown. Liver yields five times as much riboflavin per serving as 1 cup of milk and would, at first glance, appear to challenge milk's place as the nation's first source of riboflavin. However, regularity of use and multiple servings in a day explain the rank of milk foods. For the same reasons, whole-grain and enriched cereal products are important sources of riboflavin.

It is evident that obtaining enough riboflavin is largely a matter of knowing and choosing a few concentrated sources, as in the cases of calcium and vitamin A, rather than picking "bits" here and there, as in the cases of thiamine and iron. Some of the less excellent sources, such as eggs and green vegetables, used regularly, may add important amounts of riboflavin to individual diets even though they do not provide significant proportions of the riboflavin supply in the total American diet. Many vegetables, most fruits, fats, and sweets are negligible sources of riboflavin (Fig. 7.8).

Stability of Riboflavin [14] Riboflavin is stable to the heat of ordinary cooking temperatures but, because it is water-soluble, some of the vitamin is lost in discarded cooking water and in meat drippings. It is important to cook vegetables quickly in a small amount of water. Soaking vegetables or simmering them may mean heavy losses of the vitamin. Riboflavin is unstable when exposed to direct sunlight, daylight, or artificial light. Nearly half of the riboflavin in milk may be lost in 2 hours if the milk is exposed to direct sunshine in clear glass bottles. Brown glass bottles and paper containers afford protection from the light.

► *Arrange your own list of representative foods (sort cards) in order of their importance as sources of riboflavin.*

Enter riboflavin values on your meal record. Total the riboflavin values for the day.

Compare the riboflavin value of 1 slice of white enriched bread with that of the same amount of whole wheat bread and white unenriched bread.

Recommended Daily Allowances for Riboflavin The daily dietary allowances proposed by the Food and Nutrition Board are computed from the protein allowances, although a direct relationship between riboflavin and protein has not been established. This plan takes advantage of the similar conditions that increase the need for riboflavin and for protein: growth, increase in body weight, pregnancy, and lactation. The allowances for riboflavin (Table 7-2) were obtained by multiplying the protein allowances in each case by the factor, 0.025. A man of 25 years, for example, with a protein allowance of 70 g has a riboflavin allowance of 1.8 mg, (70 × .025). Riboflavin allowances are calculated throughout on this basis, including those for pregnancy and lactation. And, since protein allowances are based on body weight, men have higher riboflavin allowances than women (except in pregnancy and lactation); older boys and girls have higher allowances than younger children.

How the Average Adult Can Meet His Riboflavin Allowance The specimen diet for an adult in Appendix B provides 1.21 mg of riboflavin. Thus it fails by about 20 percent to meet the daily allowance value of 1.5 mg for a woman. This cannot be considered a significant deficit. About 44 percent of the riboflavin is provided by the 1¼ cup of milk at breakfast and lunch; nearly one third is furnished by the cereals in the form of breakfast food, bread, and other baked products. In these meals the 2 servings from the meat group—hamburger and baked beans—contributed less than 10 percent of the day's riboflavin; the vegetables and fruits provided a total of about 15 percent. The allowances could be met easily with another cup of milk or another serving of meat, such as lamb. Liver, on a once-a-week basis, would help to maintain a high average level of riboflavin intake. Regular use of leafy green vegetables would assure maximum contribution of riboflavin from the vegetable group.

The listings given show 4 ways of selecting sources of riboflavin, each of which would assure an adequate daily intake for a man.

The first 2 listings show that a man can meet his riboflavin allowance by

MEETING DAILY RIBOFLAVIN ALLOWANCE FOR MEN: 1.8 mg (3200 cal)

		Riboflavin mg
	1	
Liver, beef	2 oz	2.25
	2	
Milk, skim	4 cups	1.76
	3	
Milk, skim	2 cups	0.88
Lamb	3 oz	0.23
Beef, pot roast	3 oz	0.18
Bread, enriched	6 slices	0.30
Bread–cereals	2 servings	0.16
Broccoli	½ cup	0.11
Total		1.86
	4	
Cheese, cheddar	2 oz.	0.30
Chicken	3 oz	0.15
Frankfurters	2 medium	0.20
Eggs	2 medium	0.30
Bread, enriched	6 slices	0.30
Bread-cereals	3 servings	0.24
Potatoes	2 medium	0.08
Corn	1 cup	0.14
Beans, green	½ cup	0.06
Orange	1 medium	0.03
Apple	1 medium	0.02
Total		1.82

eating reasonable amounts of a single food. It is not suggested that liver be a daily item of diet, but its concentration recommends its regular inclusion in meals. Nor is it necessary for an adult to drink a quart of milk daily. As shown in combination 3, a pint of milk still makes the best contribution among other good sources. Cheddar cheese (combination 4) and other kinds of cheese, including cottage cheese, may be used in place of milk to provide riboflavin if sufficient amounts of other sources of the vitamin are added to make up the difference. As less concentrated sources of riboflavin are used, more servings of these sources must be added to attain the allowance.

► *What is your daily allowance for riboflavin? Obtain it from Table 7-2 on the basis of your age. Does this value differ from the one based on your calculated protein allowance?*

How does your riboflavin intake as shown on your meal record compare with your daily allowance for riboflavin? In terms of food selection, explain why your intake falls below the allowance or exceeds the allowance. If it falls below, can you correct it by making certain changes compatible with present food habits? How?

Can a strict vegetarian obtain a diet adequate in riboflavin? Explore the problem with rough estimates of riboflavin values in relation to total daily allowance.

Riboflavin Allowances for Children The increasing riboflavin allowances throughout childhood reach their peak in the teen periods for boys and girls, the time of fastest growth and greatest body weight (Table 7-2). Boys in the 16–19-year-old group have the highest daily allowance—2.5 mg—for any age or condition, except lactation, which has the same high value. Although high, allowances can be met easily at all ages, as shown in the next groupings

MEETING RIBOFLAVIN ALLOWANCES FOR CHILDREN

Ages in Years		**4-6**		**10-12**		**16-19 (Boys)**
DAILY RIBOFLAVIN ALLOWANCES		1.3 mg		1.8 mg		2.5 mg
		Riboflavin mg		**Riboflavin mg**		**Riboflavin mg**
Milk, whole	3 cups	1.26	4 cups	1.68	4 cups	1.68
Egg	1 medium	0.15	1 medium	0.15	2 medium	0.30
Beef, pot roast	—	—	—	—	3 oz	0.18
Bread, enriched	—	—	—	—	8 slices	0.40
Total		1.41		1.83		2.56

of foods. The foods in combinations 1 and 2 are identical with the first 2 items on the corresponding table for thiamine. A comparison of the thiamine and riboflavin tables shows that 2 foods—milk and eggs—alone supply all or a large share of the riboflavin allowance for the different ages of childhood. In contrast, milk and eggs require the addition of substantial amounts of several foods if the combination is to attain the corresponding thiamine allowances.

Riboflavin in Our Daily National Diet The nation's food supply has enough riboflavin to provide an average of 2.33 mg for each member of the population in this country [5]. This amount is greater than the daily allowance for any age or condition except lactation and the late teens, 16–19 years of age, for boys. Considering that nutrients are not divided evenly among people and are not divided according to need, it could be expected that actual intakes in relation to allowances would vary greatly among individuals, families, and age groups.

Family diets studied by the U.S. Department of Agriculture in 1955 showed considerable deviation below the allowances for riboflavin in 4 geographic regions of our country: 18, 16, 15, and 25 percent respectively in the North East, the North Central, the West, and the South (Table 6-2)[8]. Age groups studied by Experiment Station investigators presented a mixed picture [9]. Boys, on the average, had high intakes in relation to the allowances up to 20 years of age; girls were above only until 14 years of age and then fell somewhat below (Fig. 7.9). Men maintained a riboflavin intake well above their allowances; women were well below except for a short period from 20 to 35 years of age (Fig. 7.10). It would appear that men and boys are generally in a better state of riboflavin nutrition than women and girls, and that the latter are most vulnerable to riboflavin deficiency in the late teens and in the period past middle life.

In the diets of the Iowa boys and girls, 12–18 years of age (Fig. 6.5), more girls than boys failed to attain two-thirds of their dietary allowances, and almost as many in the lower as in the upper teens were thus deficient [9]. This information is significant in that two-thirds of the allowance for any nutrient may approximate actual need in contrast to the full allowance, which represents desirable intake.

How To Assess Riboflavin Nutriture The foregoing facts suggest that many people in this country may have intakes of riboflavin below need, and certainly below amounts that foster the best riboflavin nutrition. Is there supporting evidence for these dietary data? Are there physical manifestations of riboflavin deficiency that correspond

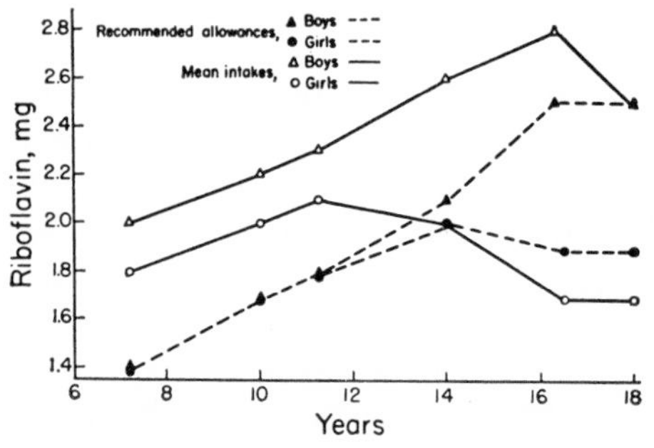

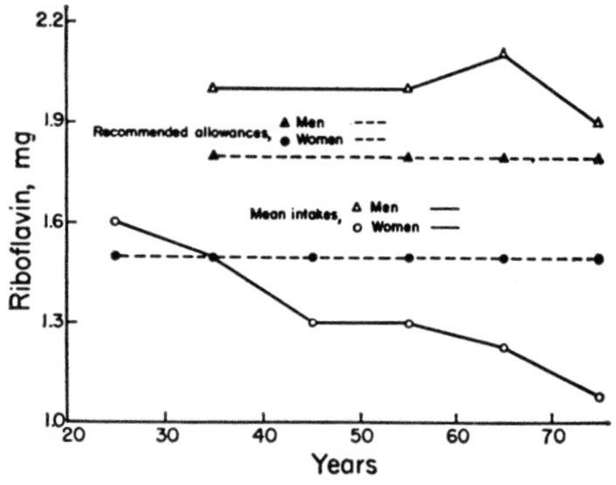

Figs. 7.9 and 7.10 Riboflavin intake in relation to daily dietary allowances. *(left)* Average daily riboflavin intake of boys and girls 4-20 of age. *(right)* Average daily riboflavin intake of men and women from 20 to more than 80 years of age. (A. F. Morgan [Ed.], *Nutritional Status U.S.A.* Bull. 769. Berkeley, Calif.: University of California, Division of Agricultural Sciences, Agricultural Experiment Station, p. 37.)

with low intakes? In the Experiment Station studies, physical signs were noted in relation to the dietary content of riboflavin. Comparisons of findings were made between certain states and between sections of the country. For example, of 4 states where the average intakes of riboflavin (and of vitamin A) were the same for all, 2 states had a greater incidence of skin and eye symptoms than did the other two. A closer look at the dietary findings revealed the significant fact that the 2 states with more physical symptoms also had more than twice as many children who received less than two-thirds of the recommended allowances for these two vitamins.

A few Experiment Stations reported special studies relating blood levels of riboflavin to intake of the vitamin. In one state, adults lived for specified periods on diets adequate in all nutrients except riboflavin: in one period, they received from one-half to two-thirds of the allowance for riboflavin; in another period, they were given 35–40 percent of their allowance. Blood levels of riboflavin fell off proportionately with lowered intake. The conclusion was reached that blood levels soon reflect inadequacy of riboflavin in daily meals [9].

There is no way of knowing at present how much riboflavin deficiency exists. Cases of outright ariboflavinosis are probably seldom seen in this country. When they do occur, they are usually complicated with multiple vitamin deficiencies. No comprehensive blood studies have been made that could indicate the extent of moderate deficits of riboflavin. The fact that the various skin, eye, and mouth symptoms are not always specific for riboflavin deficiency makes diagnosis difficult. It is possible that some of them are attributable to long-continued low intakes of riboflavin. Nutrition and medical organizations of the United Nations report ariboflavinosis as one of the frequently recorded indications of clinical malnutrition in parts of the world where diets are deficient in other B-complex vitamins and in good quality proteins.

Niacin

Functions of Niacin Niacin, along with thiamine and riboflavin, is concerned with vital processes of translating sources of energy into energy in expendable form. This is its most important positive contribution to good nutrition [12].

A prolonged deficiency of niacin leads to the disease *pellagra.* Pellagra has been called the disease of the three D's: dermatitis, diarrhea, and dementia. Rough and irritated skin is characterized by identical lesions appearing on opposite sides of the body; for example, on both elbows or on both hands. Symptoms are aggravated when the skin is exposed to the sun. Chronic digestive disturbances, with alternating constipation and diarrhea, are common accompaniments. The mucous membranes of the gastrointestinal tract become irritated; the tongue is inflamed and swollen. If the disease continues without treatment, dementia ensues and eventually death follows.

Pellagra—A Dietary Deficiency Disease Pellagra was known in southern Europe in the eighteenth century. Its cause was commonly associated with poor diet. When pellagra became known in this country, in the nineteenth century, there were various theories as to its cause. Pellagra was seen most often in persons who lived on limited diets that included large amounts of corn meal. From this observation evolved a theory, widely accepted at the time: that the disease was due to an infection caused by eating spoiled corn. In 1915 this theory was disproved and the diet theory upheld. Researchers from the U.S. Public Health Service were able to produce pellagra in healthy male subjects (prisoner volunteers) with an experimental diet of the type commonly eaten by pellagra sufferers—corn meal, fat pork, and syrup, with no milk and only a few vegetables. Attendants who lived in the identical environment but ate a different diet did not develop pellagra. From then on, pellagra was acknowledged as a dietary deficiency disease, but the specific factor involved still remained a mystery. Ten years later the same investigators announced their discovery of a new vitamin, which they called the pellagra-preventive factor [1].

Discovery of Niacin In an effort to identify the substance more specifically, research workers learned to produce pellagra in dogs (called "black tongue")[12]. This accomplished, they were in a position to test various substances for their effect on the disease in these animals. Finally, in the late 1930's, nicotinic acid, isolated from liver, proved to be the important factor. It was promptly tested on human beings also. When administered to pellagra patients it was effective in clearing up most of the symptoms of the disease. To avoid confusion with the nicotine of tobacco, with which nicotinic acid has no connection, the vitamin was called *niacin,* evolved from contractions of the original name.

As soon as the niacin values of foods became known, a puzzling problem arose: Why did many people fail to develop pellagra when their diets were low in niacin? Specifically, persons on diets that contained only moderate amounts of milk and were known to be low in niacin failed to develop pellagra, while those receiving more niacin, but no milk, developed pellagra symptoms. The answer lay in the essential amino acid, *tryptophan,* present in milk and in a variety of other foods. Tryptophan was found to be a precursor of niacin in the body. In effect, foods providing tryptophan were basically sources of niacin as well [3].

Niacin, therefore, is available in foods and in the body in 2 forms: niacin itself, and its proniacin form, tryptophan. The sum of the 2 is known as "niacin equivalent." In order to arrive at niacin equivalent values, it was necessary to find out how much tryptophan it takes to provide a given amount of niacin. The answer was obtained from experiments on human beings. It was found that the human body can make 1 mg of niacin from 50–60 mg of tryptophan. The accepted conversion factor is 60; tryptophan values can be converted to niacin values by simple division (mg of tryptophan ÷ 60 = mg of niacin).

Recommended Daily Allowances for Niacin The Food and Nutrition Board, in its 1958 table of revised allowances, has expressed niacin allowances as niacin equivalents (Table 7-2). Needs are related both to calorie intake and to body weight. To arrive at the allowances, preliminary calculations were made on both bases, using a suitable factor for each. The higher figure was chosen in each case and the amount increased by 50 percent to represent the daily dietary allowance at each of the age levels. Research on men and women was carried out to establish the minimal requirement of niacin to prevent pellagra. This requirement served as the base line for the calculated allowances.

How To Meet Your Niacin Equivalent Allowance At the present time there is no precise, generally applicable way for determining the niacin equivalent value of a diet. The niacin values for many foods —raw, cooked, and in prepared mixtures— are known and are often included with other nutrients in food composition tables. However, knowing the content of one's diet in niacin alone presents only a partial picture of intake. It is necessary to know the tryptophan content as well, and to translate its contribution in terms of niacin.

The tryptophan content of a large number of foods is known, but there are still many gaps in data, particularly for processed and prepared foods. Until such time as tables provide niacin equivalent values for many common foods in their various forms and in household measures, it is not practicable to consider sources in great detail [17]. In view of the problems as outlined, niacin has not been included in Appendix G. Nor are niacin values given for the specimen representative foods or the specimen diet for an adult. This does not mean that one has nothing to govern his niacin equivalent intake. In choosing foods he may follow 2 leads: those foods rich in niacin, as such, and foods that are important sources of tryptophan. The combined list offers a guide for choosing a diet adequate in niacin equivalent.

Sources of Niacin Nearly one-half of the niacin in the food supply of the United States is provided by meat, poultry, and fish, and about one-fourth is furnished by flour and cereal products. (Niacin is one of the nutrients of enrichment given in Table 6-3.) Lesser but important amounts are available from legumes and nuts; peanuts are a particularly good source.

Sources of Tryptophan Milk and eggs are among the better sources of tryptophan. Meats, legumes, and nuts are good sources of tryptophan, as well as of niacin. The U.S. Department of Agriculture reports that the average diet in the United States, which contains a liberal amount of protein, provides enough tryptophan to increase the niacin value by about one-third.

Sources of Niacin Equivalent By choosing a variety of foods with emphasis on the 2 groupings just cited, there should be no danger of a dietary shortage for either adults or children. The combined list to choose from should include these foods: lean meats, poultry, fish, milk, eggs, legumes, whole-grain and enriched cereals.

Stability of Niacin Niacin is relatively stable to heat, particularly in a dry medium. However, the fact that it is water-soluble makes it important to use the same care in cooking as for other water-soluble vitamins [14]. In addition, meat drippings and waters in which vegetables are cooked should be used when feasible.

Some Unresolved Problems of Niacin and Pellagra How is tryptophan used in the body in its dual capacity—as an amino acid and as a provitamin? In carrying through its function as a building stone of protein, tryptophan enters into the building and repairing of body tissue. If this is its first responsibility, how can we tell how much will be left to be diverted to the making of niacin? While this basic question remains unanswered, it will be impossible to tell how much of the dietary tryptophan we can depend upon to bolster the total niacin equivalent [17].

Other problems relate to pellagra and to the unanswered questions involved in its cause and treatment. Niacin is known to be the central factor in curing the disease, but riboflavin is often required to remove mouth and tongue symptoms, and thiamine is needed to clear up the neural signs completely. Certain unresolved problems respecting corn continue to puzzle the investigators. They know that pellagra is more common among corn-eaters than among non-corn-eaters. It is not clear, however, whether this is solely because corn is low in both niacin and tryptophan. It is known that some of the niacin of corn may not be readily available, and there may be other interfering factors as well. Although much is known about pellagra, some of its complicated story is yet to be learned.

Niacin in Our Daily National Diet At present, it is impossible to determine the adequacy of niacin equivalent in the foods eaten in the United States. In all dietary studies, niacin alone has been assessed. The fact that the dietary allowances are in terms of niacin equivalent makes it impossible to make exact comparisons. Two criteria serve as rough measures of adequacy: the favorable composition of our diet with respect to sources of niacin and tryptophan; and the lack of widespread physical symptoms related to niacin deficiency.

People in this country have a high per capita consumption of animal foods—meat, poultry, fish, milk, eggs—and intakes of these foods have been on the increase over recent years. These foods are excellent sources of niacin or tryptophan or both, as has been pointed out. Furthermore, enriched flour and bread, of which niacin is an added nutrient, is now estimated to make up 80–90 percent of all the white bread and white family flour produced in this country.

Pellagra has been a waning problem in the United States since the discovery of niacin. In the early 1900's it was a leading cause of death in southern areas of this country. It is rarely seen now, except among people whose meals are routinely limited in variety and fail to contain some of the good sources of niacin or tryptophan. Subclinical forms, which may exist particularly among low economic groups and persons who are allergic to certain proteins, are difficult to identify with certainty.

Pellagra Elsewhere in the World The medical and nutrition organizations of the United Nations report pellagra in many tropical areas of the world. Since 1940 the disease has been reported from the majority of countries of Latin America, Puerto Rico, Portugal, Spain, India, Italy, Egypt, and Southern Rhodesia. It usually accompanies a gross restriction of variety in foods and a predominance of corn [15]. Pellagra is practically unknown, even where diets are relatively poor, when an appreciable quantity of legumes or of cereals, other than corn, replaces a portion of the corn.

» OTHER MEMBERS OF THE B COMPLEX

Following are brief discussions of several other members of the B complex. All of them have been identified chemically and have been synthesized. At least 4 of them are nutritionally important for human beings. However, human requirements for these vitamins have not been established. Therefore it has not been feasible to propose daily dietary allowances for them. The Food and Nutrition Board has, in some cases, suggested protective amounts of the vitamins or has proposed foods in specified amounts to cover probable. needs.

Vitamin B_6 (Pyridoxine)

Vitamin B_6, proved to be essential in human nutrition, consists of 3 related chemical compounds: pyridoxine, pyridoxal, and pyridoxamine. Each compound functions in important ways to make vitamin B_6 an indispensable nutrient [12]. It is, for example, a part of an enzyme system in the body that is concerned with the utilization of proteins. Vitamin B_6 must be present for the breakdown in body tissues of amino acids from food and body proteins. It is equally important for building body proteins and also plays a role in converting tryptophan to niacin. Metabolism of the amino acid, tryptophan, is abnormal when there is a deficiency of vitamin B_6. In some manner, vitamin B_6 is also involved in the synthesis of certain highly unsaturated fatty acids in the body.

A deficiency of vitamin B_6 results in characteristic symptoms, but these are similar to those resulting from a lack of other B vitamins. A vitamin B_6 deficiency induced experimentally in adults resulted in a dermatitis commonly occurring around the eyes and at the angles of the mouth, in inflammation and soreness of the tongue and lips, in muscular weakness, nervous disorders, depression, and irritability. Infants on a proprietary milk diet, in which vitamin B_6 was lost in processing the product, developen nervous irritability and convulsive seizures. Deficiency symptoms disappeared when vitamin B_6, in any of its three forms was added to the diet.

Animal experimentation and tests on human beings indicate that an intake of 1–2 mg of vitamin B_6 daily is enough for adults [3]. This amount is readily provided by a varied diet including the foods rich in other B vitamins: liver, pork, muscle meats, whole-grain cereals (outer coats), vegetables. Few foods are poor sources. Losses of vitamin B_6 in prepared foods vary with time and temperature. Retentions in cooked meats are 50–60 percent of the amount of the vitamin present in raw cuts [18].

Pantothenic Acid

Pantothenic acid is essential in human nutrition. It is involved in certain chemical processes concerned with utilizing carbohydrates, fatty acids, and other nutrients in the body [12].

Because the vitamin is so widely distributed among foods, a deficiency has not been observed among people eating a diet of natural foods. When volunteers were fed a partially synthetic diet low in pantothenic acid, and were given a substance that inhibits the action of the vitamin, the following symptoms developed: weakness, fatigue, psychosis, unsteadiness of gait, and mental sluggishness. The subjects were quarrelsome, sullen, and petulant.

The Food and Nutrition Board reports that the average diet in the United States probably provides almost 9 mg per day, and that a 2500-calorie diet selected from both plant and animal foods will supply about 10 mg of pantothenic acid per day [3]. Many of the best food sources are those rich in the other B vitamins: liver, kidney, heart, and eggs. Lean muscle meats, legumes, and cereals are important but somewhat lesser sources than the glandular meats; milk and most vegetables and fruits are less concentrated sources than the muscle meats.

Biotin

Biotin is believed to play a role in normal human nutrition by participating in the activity of several enzyme systems [12]. Among the symptoms of biotin deficiency produced experimentally in human beings are dry scaly dermatitis, nervous symptoms, and tongue signs. The interrelationship of biotin with the functions of other B-complex vitamins is indicated by the nature of these symptoms.

Biotin is found in many foods and is synthesized by intestinal bacteria. There seems little danger of a deficiency of the vitamin unless the diet contains a large amount of raw egg white. Avidin, a protein in raw egg white, combines with biotin and prevents its absorption and use by the body. The Food and Nutrition Board suggests that human beings who consume diets containing 150–300 μg of biotin daily will undoubtedly obtain enough vitamin, and that this amount is provided by the average American diet [3]. Biotin is available in organ meats, muscle meats, milk, most vegetables, egg yolk, grains, and some fruits.

Folacin and Vitamin B_{12}

These 2 vitamins have antianemia properties in common. Both are needed in the formation of red blood cells, although their exact biochemical interrelationships are unknown. Both function as parts of enzyme systems in the body [12]. Folacin and vitamin B_{12} are essential in human nutrition and must be included in daily meals.

Folacin (Folic Acid Group) Folacin stimulates the formation of blood cells in certain anemias: the bone marrow manufactures the blood cells, but the formation process cannot be completed, and the blood cells remain immature—in the absence of folacin. There is a functional relationship between folacin and ascorbic acid. Folacin is transformed in the body into a substance related to ascorbic acid. Ascorbic acid stimulates the change. This related factor and ascorbic acid, along with folacin, are important in the prevention and arrest of certain anemias.

The human requirement for folacin has not yet been determined because a deficiency has not been induced in human beings with a diet low in folacin [3]. The intestinal synthesis of folacin, which may be important in human beings, further complicates the problem. Information on human needs is based on the response of patients with megoblastic anemia (immature red cells). Responses in varying degrees were noted with folacin doses of 125–500 μg daily. The Food and Nutrition Board has proposed that an intake of about 0.5 mg of folacin daily can be expected to cover nutritional needs of normal persons. Green leaves, liver, legumes, muscle meats, whole grains, and other vegetables are good sources of folacin.

Vitamin B_{12} This is the antipernicious-anemia vitamin, obtained originally from liver. A red crystalline substance was isolated from liver in 1948 and was named vitamin B_{12}. But as early as 1926 physicians were treating pernicious anemia successfully with liver and an extract of liver, unaware that they were dealing with a new vitamin. Vitamin B_{12} is now used routinely in the treatment of pernicious anemia. In this type of anemia the bone marrow is unable to produce red blood cells fast enough to keep ahead of their destruction. It is not because there is a lack of vitamin B_{12} in the diet, but because a person with pernicious anemia fails to absorb from the intestinal tract the vitamin that is available. Inability to absorb enough vitamin B_{12} is due, in turn, to the lack of a substance in gastric juice called the "intrinsic factor." This deficiency is overcome by the direct administration of vitamin B_{12}. The injection of about 1 μg daily controls the anemia.

The dietary requirement for vitamin B_{12} is unknown. A normal diet is believed to contain 8–15 μg daily [12]. Dietary inadequacy of B_{12} is probably rare and perhaps occurs only on strict vegetarian diets. In the limited number of cases known, the symptoms were similar in general character to those resulting from other B vitamin deficiencies. Some of the best food sources are liver, kidney, milk, muscle meats, cheese and eggs. Apparently fruits and vegetables provide none.

Choline

Choline is important in human nutrition, but because the body can make it from methionine, an amino acid, with the aid of vitamin B_{12} and folacin, it is probably not a required dietary constituent [12]. The chief function of choline in the body is related to the utilization of fat. Choline, in conjunction with methionine, vitamine B_{12}, and folacin, acts to prevent fatty livers in animals under certain conditions of diet. It is impossible to establish a dietary allowance for choline because of the body's ability to manufacture it. The amount available from this source, therefore, depends largely on the amount of methionine in the diet. Choline is widely distributed in plant and animal foods. There is no likelihood of a deficiency in average varied meals. The best food sources are liver, kidney, muscle meats, nuts, legumes, and milk.

Ascorbic Acid (Vitamin C)

Ascorbic acid is another water-soluble vitamin. It was originally known as vitamin C. Later, when it was identified chemically, it was named ascorbic acid to relate it to the dietary deficiency disease, *scurvy*. The 2 names are used interchangeably at the present time.

Functions of Ascorbic Acid Ascorbic acid has a number of important functions in the body [1,19]. Perhaps the most fundamental of them is its part in forming and maintaining a substance that binds living cells together. This substance holds the cells in proper relation to each other and to the body fluids that surround and nourish them. If this binding material is weak in the walls of small blood vessels hemorrhages may occur. This is not uncommon in the gums and in other parts of the body when there is a prolonged deficiency of ascorbic acid.

Ascorbic acid also helps build body resistance to bacterial infection when the vitamin is present in living tissue. A prolonged deficiency of ascorbic acid intake, on the other hand, lowers the ability of the body to resist infection. Persons suffering from infectious diseases such as tuberculosis have a lowered tissue concentration of ascorbic acid, suggesting increased usage or great destruction of the vitamin.

A high ascorbic acid level in the blood also hastens the process of healing wounds; this knowledge was applied extensively in

World War II. One theory holds that ascorbic acid is essential for the production of new cells and the replacement of injured tissue. Thus the high concentration of ascorbic acid in rapidly multiplying cells and tissues would explain the action of rapid healing; low concentrations would explain delayed healing.

Ascorbic Acid Deficiency Disease

Scurvy has been known since the fifteenth century. Persons afflicted were mostly men who went to sea and were deprived of fresh foods for months or even years at a time. It was not until the middle of the eighteenth century, however, that diet became the prime suspect as the cause. At that time a physician in the Royal British navy attempted to discover which, if any, foods were involved. He fed several food supplements to a group of sailors suffering from scurvy. Two of the sailors received a daily supplement of 2 oranges and 1 lemon. They were the only ones who showed improvement. Among other supplements tested were vinegar, cider, and sea water. All men had the same basic diet. As the result of this experiment, the physician recommended the regular use of citrus fruits by the British navy and merchant marine. Almost exactly 50 years later, upon the urging of another naval physician, an administrative order made it a requirement that each British seaman and marine be issued lemon or orange juice daily. As a result, scurvy disappeared from the British navy "as if by magic." Knowledge that citrus fruits would prevent and cure scurvy still did not reveal the secret of their curative property. It was not until the early part of the twentieth century that vitamin C was discovered. A few years later, the vitamin was isolated from lemons and called ascorbic acid.

People with scurvy show these symptoms: general weakness, lack of appetite, thickened and scaly skin, spongy gums, and hemorrhages in body tissues. If the condition continues, death often ensues. Outright scurvy is uncommon in this country today. Infants on sterilized formulas who do not receive a regular source of ascorbic acid sometimes develop characteristic symptoms. Soft tissues, particularly those surrounding the joints, become swollen: they are tender and painful. Elderly people on limited diets deficient in vitamin C are more apt to show characteristic symptoms: swollen, spongy, and sore gums. Hemorrhages sometimes appear in spots on the body that receive even mild pressure, indicating that the walls of blood vessels are fragile. Moderate symptoms are difficult to diagnose because most of them can be due to other causes. The best proof of scurvy lies in the cure. If intake of pure ascorbic acid removes the symptoms, lack of ascorbic acid may be assumed to be the cause. The cure is usually dramatic and complete.

Food Sources of Ascorbic Acid

Ascorbic acid is distributed unevenly in nature. It is produced by plants in the process of growth and is not present in mature seeds. The U.S. Department of Agriculture reports the percentage of ascorbic acid available from the food groups as follows: about 92 percent from all kinds of vegetables and fruits; the remaining 8 percent from meats, poultry, fish, and dairy products, excluding butter; most of the 8 percent is derived from dairy products. Dry legumes, eggs, cereals, sugars, and fats provide none, or negligible amounts. Of the 92 percent of ascorbic acid obtained from fruits and vegetables, roughly two-fifths are provided by citrus fruits and tomatoes; one-fifth each by leafy green and yellow vegetables, potatoes and sweet potatoes, and other fruits and vegetables. Considering all sources, citrus fruits and tomatoes furnish more than one-third of the amount of ascorbic acid available for diets in this country [5].

Figure 7.11, which gives specimen representative foods, bears out the importance of fruits and vegetables as sources of ascorbic acid. The foods are listed in descending order of the vitamin values per serving. It is notable that only foods in the upper half of the list (27 foods) contribute *any* ascorbic acid. In this half appear all the fruits and vegetables on the specimen representative list. Liver and milk are the only other kinds of foods that appear in this portion of the list. In the lower half of the list, composed of foods that yield no ascorbic acid, are the muscle meats, fish, poultry, eggs, cheese, cereals, fats, oils, and sugar.

It is evident from Figure 7.11 that citrus fruits are rich in ascorbic acid. They have the added advantage of being available the year around in various forms. The fresh juices of the orange and lemon are essentially equal in ascorbic acid value per serving; grapefruit and lime juices furnish about two-thirds as much; and tangerine juice yields about half as much as orange and lemon juices. One-half cantaloup yields about twice as much ascorbic acid as does a wedge of watermelon. Strawberries are more than twice as rich per serving as blackberries, blueberries, and raspberries. Orange juice furnishes four times as much ascorbic acid as the same amount of pineapple juice.

Apples, apricots, peaches, pears, and prunes offer small amounts of ascorbic acid per serving. They are important sources only when they are eaten in large amounts daily and in forms in which the vitamin has not been lost in processing. Pineapples and bananas are slightly better sources than the fruits just named but they are definitely of lesser value than citrus fruits, strawberries, and cantaloup. Strawberries and cantaloup are seasonal in many parts of the country. When they are plentiful and cheap, they provide excellent and varied sources of ascorbic acid.

Tropical fruits, not commonly available in the United States, are very concentrated sources of ascorbic acid. The ascerola cherry, which grows wild in the Caribbean area, is an example. One or two cherries provide all the ascorbic acid required by either adult or child for a day. Papayas and guavas are other excellent sources. (See Appendix G.)

The dark green and leafy kinds excel among vegetables as sources of ascorbic acid. Broccoli is an outstanding source, but the leafy "greens," especially turnip greens and collards, yield almost as much per serving. Most of the other "greens," including spinach, are about one-half as rich as broccoli in ascorbic acid. One medium-size potato, white or sweet, yields slightly less ascorbic acid than does a serving of spinach.

Tomato juice is served frequently as an alternate for orange juice. This is desirable for variety and often for economy reasons. It should be noted, however, that the two are not equal in ascorbic acid value per serving, and that more tomato juice is required to give the same amount of the vitamin as orange juice.

There is no way of knowing the precise ascorbic acid value of any individual food at the time it is eaten. Its content is affected by many factors, which include the conditions under which it was grown, the time and temperature involved in handling it, the kind and amount of processing it has undergone, and the conditions of storage before use.

Variations in Ascorbic Acid Values in Foods Varieties of fruits and vegetables also vary in ascorbic acid concentration. Strains of fruits can be bred for increased ascorbic acid content. Apples, for example,

Fig. 7.11 Servings of representative foods in order of their importance as sources of ascorbic acid. (Each bar represents an approximate ascorbic acid value for the series of foods listed below it.)

Food *	Weight or ** Approximate Measure	Ascorbic Acid Milligrams
60 mg		
Orange	1 medium	66
Cantaloup	1/2 melon	63
Broccoli	1/2 cup	56
50 mg		
Grapefruit	1/2 medium	50
Orange juice, fresh	1/2 cup (small glass)	46
Strawberries, raw	1/2 cup	44
20 mg		
Spinach	1/2 cup	27
Cabbage, shredded, raw	1/2 cup	25
Sweet potato	1 medium	24
Potato, white	1 medium	20
Tomato juice	1/2 cup (small glass)	19
Liver, beef	2 oz	18
10 mg		
Peas, green	1/2 cup	12
Pineapple juice, canned	1/2 cup (small glass)	11
Banana, raw	1 medium	10
Beans, snap, green	1/2 cup	9
Corn, canned	1/2 cup	7
Squash, winter	1/2 cup	7
3 mg		
Beans, dry, canned	3/4 cup	4
Lettuce leaves	2 large or 4 small	4
Apple, raw	1 medium	3
Apricots, dried, cooked	1/2 cup	3
Carrots, diced	1/2 cup	3
Peaches, canned	2 halves with juice	3
Milk, fluid, skim (or buttermilk)	1 cup	2
Milk, fluid, whole	1 cup	2
Prunes, dried, cooked	5 with juice	1
0 mg		
Bread, white, enriched	1 slice	trace
Cream, coffee	1 tbsp	trace
Bacon, crisp	2 slices	...
Beef, pot roast	3 oz	...
Beverage, kola type	6 oz	...
Chicken	1/4 broiler	...
Haddock	1 fillet	...
Ham, luncheon meat	2 oz	...
Pork chop	1 chop	...
Salmon, canned	1/2 cup	...
Frankfurter	1 medium	...
Butter of fortified margarine	1 tbsp	0
Cheese, cheddar	1 1/8" cube	0
Cheese, cottage, creamed	1/4 cup	0
Cornflakes, fortified	1 1/3 cup	0
Egg	1 medium	0
Macaroni, enriched, cooked	3/4 cup	0
Oatmeal, cooked	2/3 cup	0
Peanut butter	1 tbsp	0
Rice, cooked	3/4 cup	0
Oil, salad or cooking	1 tbs	0
Sausage, salami	1 slice	0
Sugar, granulated	1 tbsp	0

*Foods are in forms ready to eat. All meats and vegetables are cooked unless otherwise indicated.

**See Appendix G for further identification of these foods. On that list all foods are described more fully and both weights and measures are indicated.

ordinarily of low concentration, have been bred successfully to produce fruit of relatively high yield of the vitamin. Also, it has been shown that fruits and vegetables, such as oranges and tomatoes, ripened in direct sunlight, develop more ascorbic acid than those ripened in the shade. Such variations have entered into the average values shown in food lists and tables in this text.

Stability of Ascorbic Acid Ascorbic acid is the least stable of all nutrients. It is particularly vulnerable to oxidation, which is hastened by enzymes present in raw fruits and vegetables, and to exposure to warm temperatures, strong light, alkalies, and copper. The latter acts as a catalyst in the destruction of ascorbic acid [14]. Three general rules for handling vegetables may be evolved from these facts: move them from harvest point to the dinner table as quickly as possible; keep them cool and covered as they are moved or stored; cook them quickly without contact with alkali (such as soda in cooking water) and in a pan free from contact with copper.

In considering losses of ascorbic acid from vegetables the question is not *whether* there is loss, but *how great* is the loss. In the interim from harvest until the produce reaches the home refrigerator, a gradual loss takes place. If the vegetables are cooled immediately, are shipped in refrigerated cars or trucks, and are kept cool at the market, the loss is minimal. If, on the other hand, the produce is allowed to lie in the sun and becomes wilted and withered before it reaches the consumer, there is probably little ascorbic acid left. The same chances for preservation, and for losses, of the vitamin exist in the kitchen. Cool, crisp vegetables, used promptly and eaten raw, usually retain the most ascorbic acid. No matter how carefully they are cooked, some loss takes place. Quick cooking in a small amount of water produces the best product in terms of small losses of the vitamin. As has already been pointed out, ascorbic acid is water-soluble. Therefore, in addition to destruction of the vitamin, there can be considerable loss in the discarded cooking water. This loss is greatest when vegetables are simmered for a long time in a large amount of water.

Whole, uncut citrus fruits preserve their ascorbic acid content well even when stored at room temperature. And when cut or juiced, destruction of the vitamin is less rapid than in many other foods. The acid content of the fruit affords a measure of protection. Tomatoes have a similar advantage. Nevertheless, orange and tomato juices should be kept covered and cold and used promptly for maximum ascorbic acid content and flavor.

The public uses many frozen, canned, and dried fruits and vegetables. How do these rank with fresh forms as sources of ascorbic acid? The answer lies largely in the points already discussed—in the manner in which they have been handled before processing. The processes themselves, properly carried out to protect the vitamin, do not add greatly to the destruction. Probably as much as 90 percent of the vitamin is retained under favorable circumstances. But, once these preserved foods are reconstituted or otherwise prepared for consumption, they are subject to essentially the same additional losses in ascorbic acid as are the fresh forms of the same foods.

The ascorbic acid values in Figure 7.11 and Appendix G represent the most recent and reliable data available on the ascorbic acid content of many raw, cooked, and processed foods. It must be emphasized, however, that the values should be used with full knowledge of the multiple opportunities for ascorbic acid destruction. It would seem wise, therefore, to allow for an even greater margin of loss than is assumed in the values listed. Such a precaution is particularly desirable when meals are eaten in institutions where cooked vegetables are often held on steam tables and raw salad greens on cafeteria counters for considerable periods of time.

► *Arrange your own list of representative foods (sort cards) in order of their quantitative importance as sources of ascorbic acid.*

Enter ascorbic acid values on your meal record. Total the ascorbic acid values for the day.

The U.S. Department of Agriculture reported recently that diets in this country are not improving in ascorbic acid content as they are in certain other nutrients. The department suggests as reasons a general decline in the use of fruits and vegetables, a decline in the use of certain *kinds* of vegetables, and some shift towards *poorer sources of ascorbic acid in the choice of fruit beverages.*

► *List the various fruit and vegetable juices in Figure 7.11 with their ascorbic acid values per serving. Does this list shed any light on why ascorbic acid values of diets in this country have declined?*

Recommended Daily Allowances for Ascorbic Acid The daily dietary requirements for ascorbic acid are based on many factors. The starting point was the amount of the vitamin needed to prevent scurvy. Other considerations were subsequently added: the quantities of ascorbic acid provided for infants by human milk when mothers' intakes were adequate; ascorbic acid intakes that maintain specific functions such as wound healing; variations in blood ascorbic acid values with different ascorbic acid intakes; studies comparing the nutrition of animals that require ascorbic acid intake (man, guinea pig, monkey) with that of the many animals, such as the rat, capable of manufacturing their own [3].

On the basis of the data available, the Food and Nutrition Board has proposed allowances of 75 mg and 70 mg daily for men and women, respectively (Table 7-2). An addition of about 50 percent is made to the woman's allowance for the second half of pregnancy (100 mg) and of more than 100 percent for lactation (150 mg). The pregnancy allowance is increased in order to maintain the prepregnancy blood ascorbic acid level. The high lactation allowance is based on evidence that human milk varies in ascorbic acid content directly with the amount in the mother's diet. These allowances for adults are believed to be sufficiently liberal to cover rather wide variations in needs.

Storage of Ascorbic Acid Very little ascorbic acid is stored in the body. This fact has important bearing on daily food habits. Adequate food sources of ascorbic acid should be planned for daily consumption. Moderate excesses are believed to be beneficial; great excesses are wasteful because the body eliminates them.

How the Average Adult Can Meet His Ascorbic Acid Needs The specimen diet in Appendix B shows that it is relatively easy to obtain a diet adequate in ascorbic acid without including citrus fruits or tomatoes. Of the 78 mg of ascorbic acid provided by the diet, about two-thirds is furnished by two sources—the white potato and cole slaw—about one-fifth by the other vegetables and fruits. As previous discussion has indicated, undetermined losses of ascorbic acid from such foods, under many conditions of service, raise some question as to the dependability of the ascorbic acid values of these foods at the point of consumption. Many people who are aware of these problems prefer to be assured of an adequate intake by choosing one rich and dependable source daily.

The 4 food combinations given show ways in which a man can meet his daily ascorbic acid allowance.

MEETING DAILY ASCORBIC ACID ALLOWANCE FOR MEN: 75 mg

		Ascorbic Acid mg
	1	
Orange	1 medium	66
Beans, green	½ cup	9
Total		75
	2	
Grapefruit	½ medium	50
Sweet potato	1 medium	24
Total		74
	3	
Tomato juice	½ cup	19
Broccoli	½ cup	56
Total		75
	4	
Pineapple juice	½ cup	11
Banana	1 medium	10
Apricots, stewed	½ cup	3
Apple, raw	1 medium	3
Spinach	½ cup	27
Peas, green	½ cup	12
Corn	½ cup	7
Carrots	½ cup	3
Total		76

The first food in each combination is a popular breakfast item. The quantity of ascorbic acid each yields declines from the first through the fourth food group. With this decline, either more foods (combination 4) or more concentrated sources (combination 3) of ascorbic acid are added. Combination 4 obviously offers the most difficulty in meeting the allowance with no concentrated sources of the vitamin present.

► *What is your daily allowance for ascorbic acid? (Obtain this from Table 7-2 on the basis of your age.)*

How does your ascorbic acid intake as shown on your meal record compare with your daily allowance for ascorbic acid? In terms of food selection, explain why it falls below the allowance or exceeds the allowance. If it falls below, how could you correct it?

Ascorbic Acid Allowances for Children Ascorbic acid allowances increase throughout childhood from 30 mg daily during infancy to 100 mg daily for boys in the 16–19-year-old group (Table 7-2). Such increases are based on added needs that accompany the growth of the body and increased cellular activity. The problems of meeting the allowances for children are essentially the same as meeting those of the adult.

The 3 lists on page 160 show ways children of different ages may meet their dietary allowances for ascorbic acid. Orange juice, representing one excellent, dependable, daily source, is the sole or main item in each food group. The combinations demonstrate the increasing need for either using more than one serving of a rich source of ascorbic acid as the allowance becomes higher, or selecting one or more moderate sources to supplement the original serving.

Ascorbic Acid in Our Daily National Diet Judging by the ascorbic acid available per person per day from our total food supply, there is no doubt of the plenty of this nutrient in the United States. On this basis, 108 mg are available daily [5]. This value is higher than the daily allowance for any age or condition except lactation. It is considerably greater than for any of the ages of childhood below the teens. However, as with all other nutrients, availability and consumption are not the same thing. It is important to know how families

MEETING ASCORBIC ALLOWANCES FOR CHILDREN

Ages in Years		**4-6**		**10-12**		**16-19 (Boys)**
DAILY ASCORBIC ACID ALLOWANCES		50 mg		75 mg		100 mg
		Ascorbic Acid mg		**Ascorbic Acid mg**		**Ascorbic Acid mg**
Orange juice	½ cup	46	½ cup	46	½ cup	46
Potato	—	—	1 medium	20	1 medium	20
Banana	—	—	1 medium	10	1 medium	10
Cabbage, raw	—	—	—	—	½ cup	25
Total		46		76		101

and individuals fare with respect to ascorbic acid consumption.

Table 6-2 gives the proportion of family diets not providing recommended amounts of ascorbic acid in the United States. These data were obtained from a nation-wide dietary study made in 1955 by the U.S. Department of Agriculture in 4 geographic regions [8]. The table shows that some proportion of families in each region failed to meet the Food and Nutrition Board allowances for ascorbic acid. The deviations were 17, 19, 23, and 37 percent below the allowances in the North East, the North Central, the West and the South, respectively. Further data show that farm families in the South fared less well than the city families: only 54 percent of the former met the allowances for ascorbic acid. Income was a handicap in the total group of families. Eighty-four percent of families in the highest income group met the ascorbic acid allowances; only 70 percent of families did so in the lowest income group.

Studies of diets by age groups made by State Experiment Station investigators give additional information with respect to ascorbic acid intake [9]. Figures 7.12 and 7.13 summarize the data for persons 4–80 years of age. The diets of girls and boys up to 12 years of age more than met the dietary allowances for ascorbic acid. From 12 to 20 years, both fell below their respective allowances. After 30 years of age, the intake of men was adequate in relation to the allowances, but that of the women was marginal or low. When the individual diets of adolescents in one locality were examined (Fig. 6.5), more than one-fifth of the girls 15–18 years of age failed to attain two-thirds of their allowances for ascorbic acid. Almost the same proportion of girls in the 12–14-year-old group were similarly deficient. Ascorbic acid is the one nutrient for which the boys' records were no better than the girls'.

Assessing Ascorbic Acid Nutriture

Ascorbic acid concentration in the blood in the various age groups studied by the Experiment Stations, was generally fair to good. In many cases there was a significant correlation between blood level and the ascorbic acid intake. One interesting deviation was in the men who had higher intakes than women but lower ascorbic acid blood levels. It was suggested that men may use ascorbic acid differently than women and may have a considerably higher requirement. The mouth and gum signs associated with deficiency of ascorbic acid were found to be fairly well correlated with

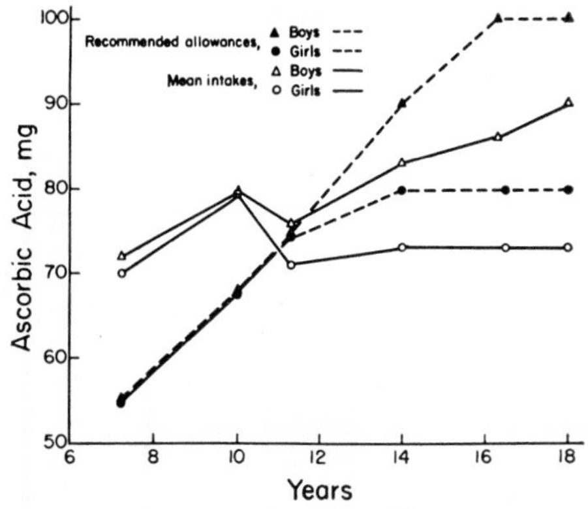

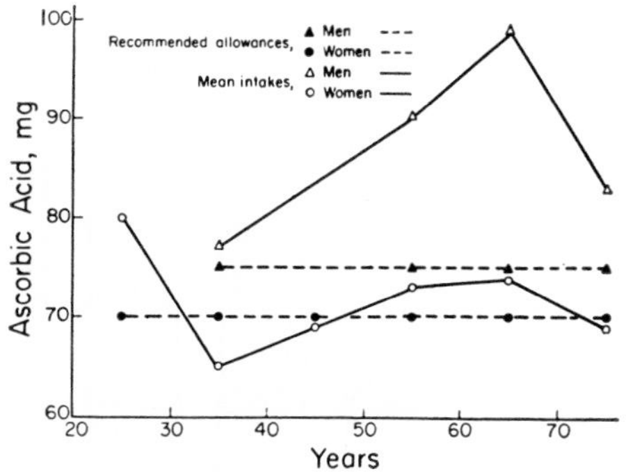

Figs. 7.12 and 7.13 Ascorbic acid intake in relation to daily dietary allowances. *(left)* Average daily ascorbic acid intake of boys and girls 4-20 years of age. *(right)* Average daily ascorbic acid intake of men and women from 20 to more than 80 years of age. (A. F. Morgan [Ed.], *Nutritional Status U.S.A.* Bull. 769. Berkeley, Calif.: University of California, Division of Agricultural Sciences, Agricultural Experiment Station, p. 37.)

the level of ascorbic acid in the blood, but they were not consistently related to the intake of the vitamin as reported on the week's diet record. Because of this observation, it has been suggested that "blood will tell" when food records will not [9]. Blood levels of ascorbic acid perhaps reflect somewhat more accurately the long-term nutritional status with respect to the vitamin; diet records reflect the current, and not always typical, vitamin intake.

» THE DIET AS A WHOLE IN RELATION TO BODY NEEDS

We have considered the nutritional needs of the body, one by one, and have found that they all can be met by proper selection of foods from the nutrient classes: proteins, fats, carbohydrates, mineral elements, and vitamins. Special attention has been given separately to certain nutritive needs in relation to the recommended daily dietary allowances proposed by the Food and Nutrition Board of the National Academy of Sciences-National Research Council.

You are now ready to coordinate these "parts" and to think of your diet as a whole in relation to your total needs. A graphic summary based on your own data is an effective device for visualizing such information, even though it involves only rough estimates of amounts of foods. You are equipped to make such a summary if you have calculated the calorie and nutrient content of one typical day's meals. If you also estimated your daily energy need and recorded your body weight at essentially the same period, the summary will have added interest.

Your own graphic summary will resemble Figure 7.14, which is based on the specimen diet in Appendix B. Its contributions are compared with accepted nutrient goals for a hypothetical young person (woman) whose daily calorie needs are estimated in Chapter 4, whose weight status is given in Appendix E, and whose dietary allowances are summarized in Appendix C.

Of the bars in Figure 7.14, some ex-

Fig. 7.14 A graphic summary of the specimen diet in Appendix B: weight status and nutrient intakes in relation to desirable goals for a young woman.

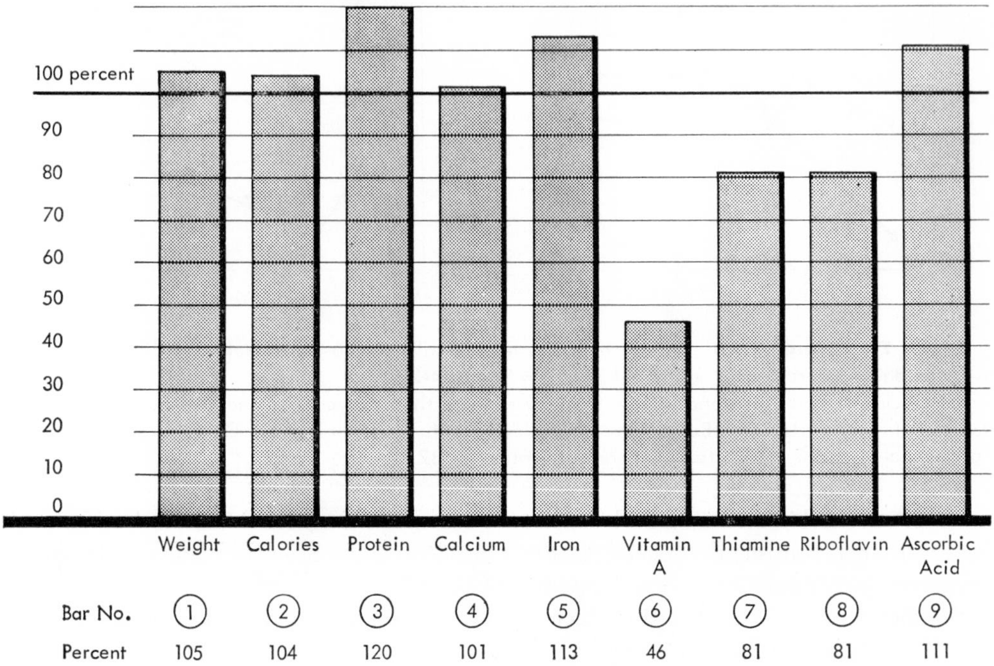

tend above the 100 percent line; some fall short of it. This may be interpreted to mean that some items are above and some below a level considered desirable. For a better understanding of Figure 7.14 it is necessary to examine the bars closely. The first 2 are concerned with body weight and calorie intake. The first shows the actual body weight of the young woman to be about 5 percent above desirable weight (medium build). The second bar shows her calorie intake from the specimen diet to be about 4 percent above estimated calorie need based on her activity record. (Her calorie *allowance* could have been used as the standard instead of the calculated value.)

The third through the ninth bars represent the intake of 7 nutrients in relation to the recommended daily dietary allowances for each. Four nutrients—protein, calcium, iron, and ascorbic acid—rise above their allowances; the remaining 3—vitamin A, thiamine, and riboflavin—fall below. Vitamin D is not represented in Figure 7.14 because no allowance has been proposed for the adult—except during pregnancy and lactation. Niacin is also omitted for reasons given in the text.

If you lack the data to prepare your own graphic summary, you may review Figure 7.14 in relation to the information on which it is based. Evaluate the Figure and characterize the diet as suggested at the end of this chapter.

How To Make Your Own Graphic Summary

Draw on cross-bar paper 9 identical bars, leaving space above to permit extensions. Each bar represents 100 percent of the following:

Bar No. 1—Your desirable weight (median) (See Appendix D.)
Bar No. 2—Estimated calorie need (See Chapter 4.)
Bar No. 3 through Bar No. 9—Recommended daily dietary allowances for protein, calcium, iron, vitamin A value, thiamine, riboflavin, and ascorbic acid

Use your own records to indicate on appropriate bars the percentages that your own data register *above* or *below* 100 percent. For example, to plot bar No. 1, divide your actual weight by your desirable weight; to plot bar No. 2, divide your total calorie intake from your personal meal record by your calculated energy need based on activity; to plot all other bars, divide the total intake of each nutrient from your personal meal record by the allowance for each corresponding nutrient.

Show on the bars which items are above and which items are below the 100-percent mark. Provide a suitable caption for the chart and a key to its contents.

Evaluation of Graphic Summary

► *Evaluate your own graphic summary (or Fig. 7.14) in terms of the subject matter covered in Section Two.*

What do your first 2 bars show with respect to your body weight and calorie intake?

If your actual weight (bar No. 1) is higher in relation to desirable weight than your calorie intake in relation to calorie need (bar No. 2) what kind of curve would you expect your weight chart to show? Is that the case? If the situation were reversed, what would be your answer?

If your calorie intake (bar No. 2) is low in relation to estimated calorie need, does it seem to prove the statement, "A low calorie diet usually means one low in dietary essentials?"

Consider each of the nutrients separately on your chart.

Which nutrients are provided adequately by your meals?

Which foods are chiefly responsible for bringing each of these bars up to 100 percent or above?

Which nutrients fall below 100 percent of the recommended dietary allowances?

Which foods are lacking and thus responsible for the deficits?

Characterize your diet as a whole.

In general, does it meet or nearly meet the recommended daily dietary allowances?

Or, is it grossly below them in several nutrients?

What major adjustments should you make in choices of foods to be assured your diet will be more nearly adequate nutritionally?

To Test Your Knowledge

In recent weeks you have undoubtedly become increasingly aware of pamphlets, advertisements, and slogans promoting food products and dietary supplements. A good test of your knowledge at this juncture is to evaluate their nutritional statements in light of current information on the topics covered.

VITAMINS—A FEW HIGHLIGHTS

	Vitamin A	Thiamine	Riboflavin	Niacin	Ascorbic Acid
WHAT VITAMINS DO FOR YOU	Helps keep outer skin and lining membranes intact and healthy to resist infection Helps to maintain normal vision; protects against night blindness Contributes to health, growth, and to good tooth formation	Helps convert sources of energy in the body into energy for work Essential to good digestion and normal appetite Necessary to a normally functioning nervous system	Helps cells use oxygen in providing body with energy Contributes to smooth skin in nose - mouth area; protects against cracking at corners of mouth Helps to keep eyes and lids healthy and vision clear	Helps translate sources of body energy into usable energy Protects body against pellagra symptoms: skin lesions, inflammation of mucous membranes (such as mouth, tongue and intestinal tract), psychic changes	Helps form a substance that binds living cells together; strengthens walls of blood vessels Helps build body resistance to bacterial infection Hastens healing of wounds
SOME OF THE BEST FOOD SOURCES	**Vitamin A Value** Liver Dark green leafy vegetables Deep yellow vegetables (most) and fruits Butter, fortified margarine, cream Egg yolk Whole milk	Lean pork Enriched and whole grain cereal products Organ meats (liver) Muscle meats Legumes Milk	Milk, cheeses Organ meats (liver) Muscle meats Whole grain, enriched cereal products Leafy green vegetables	**Niacin Equivalent** Meats, poultry, fish Peanuts, other nuts, dry beans and peas Milk eggs Enriched and whole grains (excluding corn)	Citrus fruits, juices Strawberries Cantaloup Tomatoes, juice Dark green vegetables, including "greens" Potatoes

STABILITY TO HANDLING	Stable to ordinary cooking temperatures Unstable to long exposure in air, at warm temperatures Not dissolved in cooking water	Unstable to heat, especially in alkaline solutions (soda) Dissolved in cooking water	Fairly stable to ordinary cooking temperatures, especially in acid solutions Unstable to ultra violet light (direct sunlight) Dissolved in cooking water	Stable in dry state Dissolved in cooking water	Stable in acid Unstable: destroyed by oxidation, which is hastened by warm temperature, long slow cooking, exposure to alkali and copper Dissolved in cooking water
RECOMMENDED DAILY DIETARY ALLOWANCES					
ADULTS	5000 IU 6000 IU pregnancy 8000 IU lactation	1.0–1.6 mg 1.3 mg pregnancy 1.7 mg lactation	1.5–1.8 mg 2.0 mg pregnancy 2.5 mg lactation	17–21 mg 20 mg pregnancy 19 mg lactation	75 mg—men 70 mg—women 100 mg—pregnancy 150 mg—lactation
CHILDREN (above infancy)	2000–5000 IU	0.7–1.8 mg	1.0–2.5 mg	8–25 mg	35–100 mg
STORAGE IN ANIMAL BODY	Reserves of vitamin A stored: 95 percent in liver 5 percent in muscles	Little storage except in pork tissues	Some storage in body organs such as liver, kidney, heart	Some storage, in liver and muscle	Little storage; some in liver

REFERENCES

1. Wohl, M. G., and Goodhart, R. S. (Eds.), *Modern Nutrition in Health and Disease.* 2nd ed. Philadelphia: Lea & Febiger, 1960.
2. *The Heinz Handbook of Nutrition.* New York: McGraw-Hill Book Company, Inc., 1959.
3. Food and Nutrition Board, *Recommended Dietary Allowances,* Pub. 589. Washington, D.C.: National Academy of Sciences-National Research Council, 1958.
4. McCollum, E. B., and McCollum, E. V., "Vitamins A, D, E, K," *Food—The Yearbook of Agriculture.* Washington, D.C.: U.S. Department of Agriculture, 1959. p. 130.
5. Economic Research Service, *Consumption of Food in the United States 1909–52.* Supplement for 1960 to Agricultural Handbook No. 62. Washington, D.C.: U.S. Department of Agriculture, August 1961.
6. Wilson, E. D., Fisher, K. H., and Fuqua, M. E., *Principles of Nutrition,* New York: John Wiley & Sons, Inc., 1959.
7. Council on Foods and Nutrition, "Vitamin Preparations as Dietary Supplements and as Therapeutic Agents," *J. Am. Med. Assoc.,* 169 (Jan. 3, 1959) pp. 41–45.
8. LeBovit, C., and Clark, F., "Are We Well Fed?" *Food—The Yearbook of Agriculture.* Washington, D.C.: U.S. Department of Agriculture, 1959. p. 620.
9. Morgan, A. F., *Nutritional Status, U.S.A. Bull.* 769. Berkeley: California Agricultural Experiment Station, University of California, Oct. 1959.
10. Deuel, H. J., *The Lipids—Their Chemistry and Biochemistry.* Vol. III. New York: Interscience Publishers, Inc., 1957.
11. Horwitt, M. K., "Vitamin E in Human Nutrition—An Interpretive Review," *Borden's Review of Nutrition Research,* 22 (Jan.–March 1961) pp. 1–17. New York: The Borden Company.
12. Goldsmith, G. A., "Vitamins of the B Complex," *Food—The Yearbook of Agriculture.* Washington, D.C.: U.S. Department of Agriculture, 1959. p. 139.
13. Food and Nutrition Board, *Cereal Enrichment in Perspective, 1958.* Washington, D.C.: National Academy of Sciences-National Research Council, 1958.
14. Watt, B. K., and Woot-Tsuen, W. L., "Conserving Nutritive Values," *Food—The Yearbook of Agriculture.* Washington, D.C.: U.S. Department of Agriculture, 1959. p. 483.
15. Joint FAO/WHO Expert Committee on Nutrition, *Fourth Report, 1955; Fifth Report, 1958.* Rome, Italy: Food and Agriculture Organization of the United Nations.
16. Harrell, R. F., "Mental Response to Added Thiamine," *J. Nutrition,* 31 (March 1946) pp. 283–98.
17. Phipard, E. F., "Recommended Allowances in Assessing Diets," *J. Am. Dietet. Assoc.* 36 (Jan. 1960) pp. 37–41.
18. Lushbough, C. H., "The Role of Vitamin B_6 in Human Nutrition," *Food and Nutrition News,* 29 (Jan. 1958) pp. 1; 4. Chicago: National Livestock and Meat Board.
19. Dodds, M. L., "Vitamin C," *Food—The Yearbook of Agriculture.* Washington, D.C.: U.S. Department of Agriculture, 1959, p. 150.

READINGS

Barnes, R. H., "Nutritional Contributions of the Gastrointestinal Tract," *Food and Nutrition News,* 34 (Jan. 1961) pp. 1; 4. Chicago: National Livestock and Meat Board.

Elvehjem, C. H., "Why Vitamins?" *Today's Health.* 36 (Feb. 1958) pp. 18–19; 60–61.

Flynn, H., *Venture, Voyages and Vitamins* (booklet). Chicago: National Dairy Council.

Horwitt, M. K., "Niacin-tryptophan Requirements of Man," *Nutrition News,* 22 (April 1959) p. 5. Chicago: National Dairy Council.

Krehl, W. H., "Nutrition and Health of Your Skin," *Food and Nutrition News,* 32 (Feb. 1961) pp. 1; 4. Chicago: National Livestock and Meat Board.

Lorenz, A. J., "The Conquest of Scurvy," *J. Am. Dietet. Assoc.,* 30 (July 1954) pp. 665–70.

Watt, B. K., and Stiebeling, H. K., "Keeping the Values in Foods," *Today's Health,* 36 (April 1958) pp. 48–51.

SECTION THREE

Nutrition in everyday meals

Science must be applied if it is to be useful. And the science of nutrition finds its use in providing the foundation for intelligent food selection and sound nutriture. Section Two furnishes the scientific basis for the nutrient components of an adequate diet. Section Three provides the practical interpretation. Here the emphasis shifts to foods and food groups, which are the purveyors of those nutrients. Learning to regard foods in the light of their collective contribution of nutrients is a first step in successful meal planning.

Obviously it is impractical to calculate the nutrient content of daily meals. There must be some short-cut method that serves essentially the same purpose. This has taken the form of daily food patterns. In recent years almost every country has developed a food selection guide to assist its people. Each has been influenced by the cultural background of its population and the basic food supplies available in the countries to be served. Such plans testify to the fact that there are countless ways to obtain an adequate diet and that a food pattern, applicable and useful in one country, may be entirely useless in another country.

A major purpose of Section Three is to consider a daily food pattern designed to serve the nutritional needs of people of the United States. It will be explored from the standpoints of its reliability and adaptability when applied to the needs of the individual members of the family and to the family group as a whole.

CHAPTER 8

Daily food patterns

A successful food pattern is in reality a set of "rules" for selecting nutritionally adequate, varied, and satisfying meals. It has been developed by persons with a wide knowledge of nutrient values and an acquaintance with the eating practices of the peoples who are to use the pattern. As applied to this country it promises to meet reasonably well the recommended daily dietary allowances for different ages and conditions, when it is properly interpreted and used. A reliable daily food pattern, in effect, becomes the counterpart of the allowances in terms of familiar foods that compose daily meals.

At this point in your study of nutrition you should be capable of developing your own daily food pattern. To do so you would calculate the nutrient yield of different groupings of foods until you arrived at a combination that would meet your own dietary allowances. However, in view of the fact that many such patterns have been proposed, it will be equally informative and less time-consuming to evaluate one already in use. Because such patterns are obtainable from reliable sources, one might question the need to evaluate them. Aside from the experience to be acquired from such an evaluation, this critical approach should henceforth characterize your attitude toward interpretation of all nutrition information.

Table 8-1 presents a daily food pattern of the type currently recommended for the use of individuals and families in the United States. It takes into account the meal habits of and the food supplies available to the people of this country and it is flexible enough to cover regional, seasonal, and food budget differences. The pattern is a cross-section of several such guides available at the present time [1]. It presents the foods for choice under 4 main groups: milk group, meat group, vegetable-fruit group, and bread-cereals group. A 4-group plan was presented by nutritionists of Harvard University in 1955. It was a suggested revision of the Basic 7 pattern then in common use [2]. As you discovered in Section Two, certain kinds of foods are similar in their nutrient content; it is therefore possible to select from groupings of such foods. These particular 4 food groups were chosen for the pattern because of the significant nutrient contribution each makes to the total diet (Table 8-2). They have thus earned the title *foundation* foods. It will be noted that they appear on Table 8-1 under this heading. A second heading, *additional* foods, includes the fats, sweets, unenriched cereals,

TABLE 8-1

A RECOMMENDED DAILY FOOD PATTERN

Foundation Foods

1. Milk Group:	3 to 4 glasses* milk—children 4 or more glasses milk—teenagers 2 or more glasses milk—adults 4 or more glasses milk—pregnant women 6 or more glasses milk—nursing mothers Cheese, ice cream, and other milk-made foods can supply part of the milk
2. Meat Group:	2 or more servings† Lean meats, fish, poultry, eggs, cheese with dry beans, dry peas, nuts, as alternates
3. Vegetable-Fruit Group:	4 or more servings‡ A dark green or deep yellow vegetable at least every other day Citrus fruit or other vitamin C-rich sources daily Other fruits and vegetables
4. Bread-Cereals Group:	4 or more servings§ Enriched, whole-grain, or restored

Foundation Foods form the nucleus for good daily meals. Use more than the minimum choices offered —in quantity and quality, to insure nutritional adequacy.

Additional Foods

Add fats, sweets, unenriched cereals, and flavorings within the limits of individual calorie needs to round out meals in food nutrients and in variety, flavor, and satiety value.

Provide vitamin D during the growth cycle (childhood, pregnancy, lactation) to supply 400 IU daily. This amount is furnished by one quart of vitamin D milk.

*1 glass milk: 1 cup; 8 oz (½ pt).
†meats: approximately 3 oz, cooked.
‡vegetables, cooked: ½ cup.
fruits, raw: units, as one medium-size orange.
§bread: 1 slice.
cooked cereal: ⅔ cup.
ready-to-eat cereal: 1 oz, about 1 cup.
See Appendix F for equivalent weights and measures.

and flavorings that are largely supplementary to the *foundation* foods. The relationships between all of these groups and how they, together, form a design for eating, is discussed in the pages that follow.

» TESTING THE PATTERN FOR RELIABILITY

The reliability of the daily food pattern must be judged by its performance as a planning tool in the hands of persons with little or no background in nutrition and with no particular interest in making it "work." Let us assume that a person who meets this description gives it a rigid test.

Minimum Food Choices from the Daily Food Pattern (Table 8-1)

A rigid test could consist of these measures: a) selecting the least number of servings of *foundation* foods stipulated by the pattern; b) making less than the most favorable choices allowable within these food groups; c) following directions in selecting *additional* foods. Figure 8.1 shows the results of following this procedure. It presents the selection of foods from the pattern, a calculated diet, a day's menus based on the diet, and a bar chart showing the outcome in terms of meeting or failing to meet the daily dietary allowances for a young woman. (See pp. 174, 175.)

As the test prescribes, minimum choices in amounts and kinds of *foundation* foods were made for Diet A in Figure 8.1. For example, in the milk group, 2 glasses of milk—the minimum recommended for an adult—were chosen. In the meat group, not only was the number of servings held to the minimum, but fish and 1 egg were chosen instead of lean meats. One egg is, in reality, only one-half serving in terms of protein yield. In the vegetable-fruit group, one-fourth cup of broccoli—only a moderately rich source of vitamin A value—was selected as the dark green vegetable. This amount is equivalent to one-half cup serving every other day. Canned grapefruit was chosen as the vitamin C source; applesauce and beets, both relatively poor sources of nutrients, were added as "other fruits and vegetables." Three slices of enriched white bread (4 percent milk solids) and one roll represented the bread-cereal group.

► *Suggest other ways of placing a minimum interpretation on the daily food pattern. Try to put the pattern to a more rigid test than is suggested here and yet adhere to its specifications.*

Diet A in Figure 8.1 presents the total nutrient contributions of these minimum choice *foundation* foods to a young adult's daily dietary allowances. The accompanying bar chart shows this same information graphically. The scale for Figure 8.1(c) represents 100 percent of each dietary allowance, and the solid area on each bar represents the percentage contribution from the total of minimum-choice foods to calories, protein, calcium, iron, vitamin A value, thiamine, riboflavin, and ascorbic acid. It is apparent that the nutrient allowances that are fully or almost met are those for protein, calcium, riboflavin, and ascorbic acid. Those which fall far short are iron, vitamin A, and thiamine. These nutrients were obtained in the proportions indicated by "spending" about one-half (46 percent) the calorie "budget."

What do the *additional* foods do to help meet these deficiencies? Diet A shows that they consist primarily of fat spreads and dressings, cookies, cakes, and concentrated sweets. From a look at the individual items on Diet A it is apparent that only the fats add significantly to the deficient nutrients. Vitamin A is increased by the fats to more than 80 percent of the allowance level. Iron and thiamine remain at two-thirds or less of the allowances for these 2 nutrients.

► *How could food choices have been altered to prevent the deficiencies in iron and thiamine in Diet A?*

What are the conclusions to be drawn from such a test? Is the daily food pattern unreliable because it fails to ensure that all dietary allowances will be met? The answer is "No, not necessarily." You will

Fig. 8.1 (a) Diet A: *Minimum choices* from the daily food pattern.

Nutrients Furnished in Relation to the Daily Dietary Allowances of a Young Woman

Foods	Measures	Calories	Protein (g)	Calcium (mg)	Iron (mg)	Vitamin A Value (IU)	Thiamine (mg)	Ribo-flavin (mg)	Ascorbic acid (mg)
Foundation Foods									
1. Milk Group									
Milk, whole	2 cups	330	18	570	0.2	780	0.16	0.84	4
2. Meat Group									
Haddock	3 oz	135	16	15	0.5	50	0.03	0.08	---
Egg, medium	1	80	6	27	1.1	590	0.05	0.15	0
3. Vegetable-fruit Group									
Broccoli	1/4 cup	10	2	49	0.5	1275	0.03	0.06	28
Beets	1/2 cup	35	1	18	0.6	15	0.02	0.04	6
Lettuce	2 leaves	5	1	11	0.2	270	0.02	0.04	4
Grapefruit	1/2 cup, can'd	80	1	16	0.4	10	0.04	0.02	38
Applesauce	1/2 cup	90	tr.	5	0,5	40	0.03	0.02	2
4. Bread-cereal Group									
Bread, enriched	3 slices	180	6	57	1.8	tr.	0.18	0.15	tr.
Rolls	1	115	3	28	0.7	tr.	0.11	0.07	tr.
Totals, Foundation Foods		1060	54	796	6.5	3030	0.67	1.47	82
Dietary Allowances for Young Woman		2300	58	800	12.0	5000	1.20	1.50	70
Additional Foods									
Butter*	6 tsp	210	tr.	6	tr.	920	---	---	---
Mayonnaise	2 tbsp	220	tr.	4	0.2	80	tr.	tr.	0
Tartar sauce	1 tbsp	110	tr.	2	0.1	40	tr.	tr.	0
Honey	1 tbsp	60	tr.	1	0.2	0	tr.	0.01	1
Sugar	3 tsp	51	0	---	---	0	0	0	0
Cookies	2	220	4	12	0.4	0	0.02	0.02	0
Gelatine	1/2 cup, dessert, pl.	80	2	0	0	0	0	0	0
Cupcake	1, iced	160	3	58	0.2	50	0.01	0.04	tr.
Candy	1 oz milk Choc.	145	2	61	0.3	40	0.03	0.11	0
Totals, Additional Foods		1256	11	144	1.4	1130	0.06	0.18	1
GRAND TOTALS		2316	65	940	7.9	4160	0.73	1.65	83

*or margarine fortified with vitamin A

Fig. 8.1 (b) Menus based on Diet A.

Foundation Foods (46 percent of total calories)		Calories		Additional Foods		Calories
			BREAKFAST			
Grapefruit, canned	1/2 cup	80				
Toast, enriched	1 slice	60	+	Butter*	2 tsp	70
			+	Honey	1 tbsp	60
Milk, whole	1 cup	165				
				Coffee		
				+ sugar	1 tsp	17
			LUNCH			
Egg salad sandwich						
Bread, enriched	2 slices	120	+	Mayonnaise	2 tbsp	220
Egg	1	80				
Lettuce	2 leaves	5				
Applesauce	1/2 cup	90				
Milk, whole	1 cup	165		Cookies	2	220
				Beverage		
				+ sugar	1 tsp	17
			DINNER			
Haddock	3 oz	135	+	Tartar sauce	1 tbsp	110
Broccoli	1/4 cup	10	+	Butter*	1 tsp	35
Beets	1/2 cup	35	+	Butter*	2 tsp	70
Roll	1	115	+	Butter*	1 tsp	35
				Gelatine dessert	1/2 cup	80
				Cupcake	1	160
				Beverage		
				+ sugar	1 tsp	17
			BETWEEN MEALS			
				Milk chocolate	1/4 bar	145
	Total Calories	1060			Total Calories	1256

GRAND TOTAL, CALORIES FOR THE DAY – 2316

* or margarine fortified with vitamin A

Fig. 8.1 (c) Graphic summary of Diet A: *Minimum choices* from the daily food pattern.

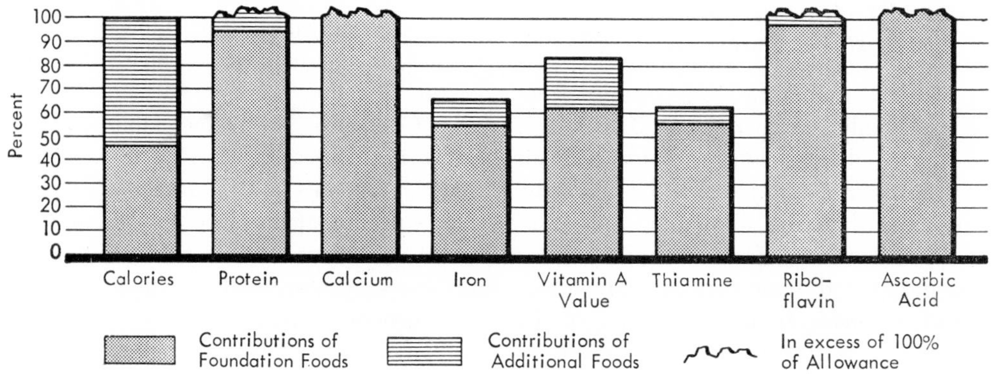

recall that the dietary allowances represent *desirable* daily intakes, not actual need. A diet that provides 80–90 percent of a nutrient would not be considered low in that nutrient. Also, in interpreting the pattern, some persons would make better choices and take larger servings of the *foundation* foods, both of which would increase the nutrient contributions. Finally, a different choice of *additional* foods could help to make a slightly better showing for the total diet.

The function of a test of this nature is not to lessen confidence in such a pattern but to show how well it performs even under minimum conditions and to demonstrate the weaknesses that may be anticipated and overcome. No daily food pattern can cover every contingency. The dietary needs of individuals differ. Also, possibilities for choice within food groups and the fact that no two foods are identical in nutrient value leave loopholes that cannot be avoided completely. Experience shows that the surest way to override them is to choose more than the minimum number of items from the *foundation* food groups and thus provide a larger proportion of the total calories from these groups than was done in Diet A. To do this constitutes a more liberal interpretation of the daily food pattern. The practical outcome of this approach is shown in Figure 8.2 (pp. 178–179).

Liberal Interpretation of Daily Food Pattern

Diet B in Figure 8.2 is planned from the same daily food pattern as Diet A, and the dietary allowances for a young woman are again used as the goals. In Diet B, however, more than the minimum number of food items is used from each *foundation* food group and somewhat more favorable choices are made from within some of the food groups. In the milk group, for example, a serving of ice cream is added to the 2 cups of milk. In the meat group, 2 servings of lean meat and 1 egg make up the choices. For the vegetable-fruit group, the total number of servings is greater than in Diet A, and carrots replace broccoli as a richer source of vitamin A value. An extra slice of bread and an extra roll are added to the bread-cereal group.

Diet B presents the total nutrient contributions of these liberal-choice *foundation* foods to a young adult's daily dietary allowances. The accompanying bar chart shows the same information graphically. The scale for Figure 8.2 (c) represents 100 percent of each dietary allowance; the solid area on each bar represents the percentage contribution from the total of liberal-choice foods to calories, protein, calcium, iron, vitamin A value, thiamine, riboflavin, and ascorbic acid. It is apparent that the nutrient allowances are fully met. Only the calorie bar is incomplete. The total day's allowances have been achieved from foundation foods alone, with 75 percent of the calorie budget "spent" in this manner.

The general character of the *additional* foods in Diet B is essentially the same as that of the additional foods in Diet A. But there is less of them in Diet B; they furnish fewer calories and they play, nutrientwise, a more minor role than those in Diet A. It will be noted from the chart in Figure 8.2 that they are needed only to complete the calorie bar. However, they furnish small amounts of some other nutrients.

Comparing the dietary tables and the charts in Figures 8.1 and 8.2 it is obvious that the amounts and kinds of foods chosen *within* the *foundation* food groups can make a vast difference in the outcome in terms of dietary adequacy. Also, it may be stated as a general principle that the larger the proportion of total calories provided by *foundation* foods the greater are the prospects for meeting the dietary allowances. And, as will be shown later, the lower the total calories in the diet the more important is it to have a high proportion of calories from *foundation* foods.

» A CLOSER LOOK AT THE FOUNDATION FOOD GROUPS

The interpretation of the daily food pattern as illustrated in Diets A and B has shown that the calories provided by the 4 *foundation* food groups carry the lion's share of nutrients. This fact is demonstrated more precisely in Table 8-2, which is a detailed analysis of Diet B. It shows that the emphasis given *foundation* foods is not arbitrary, but is fully justified by the facts.

It will be noted from Table 8-2 that each *foundation* food group furnishes one-fourth or more of the total of at least 2 nutrients provided by Diet B. The milk group, for example, contributes about one-fourth of the protein, two-thirds of the calcium, and nearly one-half of the riboflavin; the meat group supplies one-half of the protein and more than one-third of the iron and thiamine; the vegetable-fruit group provides practically all of the ascorbic acid, nearly three-fourths of the vitamin A value, and more than one-fourth of the iron; the bread-cereal group furnishes more than one-fourth of the iron and the thiamine. Each group makes important contributions of other nutrients as well. An analysis of the diets of city families in this country shows essentially the same distribution of nutrients within these food groups [3]. The nutrients supplied by the *additional* foods in Diet B provide a sharp contrast to those supplied by the *foundation* foods, as shown in Table 8-2. Despite the fact that *additional* foods

TABLE 8-2

FOOD SOURCES OF NUTRIENTS

Percentage Contributions of Food Groups to the Daily Dietary Allowances of a Young Woman*

FOODS	Percent Calories	Percent Protein	Percent Calcium	Percent Iron	Percent Vitamin A value	Percent Thiamine	Percent Riboflavin	Percent Ascorbic acid
All Foods	**100**	**100**	**100**	**100**	**100**	**100**	**100**	**100**
FOUNDATION FOODS								
1. Milk Group	20	(23)	(66)	2	13	11	(45)	5
2. Meat Group	21	(49)	4	(40)	7	(39)	22	0
3. Vegetable-fruit Group	**14**	9	14	(28)	(70)	22	16	(95)
4. Bread-cereal Group	20	16	14	(27)	0	(27)	16	0
ADDITIONAL FOODS								
All Additional Foods	25	3	2	3	10	1	1	0
Fats	18	0	1	2	10	0	0	0
Sweets	7	3	1	1	0	1	1	0

* Diet B, Fig. 8.2.

yield one-fourth of the calories, the only significant nutrient contribution is that of fats to vitamin A value—10 percent. It should be noted further that Table 8-2 bears out the fact that the daily food pattern, properly applied, is in reality a "translation" of the recommended daily dietary allowances.

► *Make a bar chart presenting the information contained in Table 8-2. Show the contributions of each of the 4 food groups and of the additional foods, as a whole, to*

Fig. 8.2(a) Diet B: *Liberal choices* from the daily food pattern.

Nutrients Furnished in Relation to the Daily Allowances of a Young Woman

Foods	Measures	Calories	Protein (g)	Calcium (mg)	Iron (mg)	Vitamin A Value (IU)	Thiamine (mg)	Riboflavin (mg)	Ascorbic acid (mg)
Foundation Foods									
1. Milk Group									
Milk, whole	2 cups	330	18	570	0.2	780	0.16	0.84	4
Ice cream	1/4 pt	130	2	76	0.1	320	0.03	0.12	1
2. Meat Group									
Pot roast	3 oz	245	23	10	2.9	30	0.04	0.18	---
Ham, sliced	2 oz	170	13	5	1.5	0	0.57	0.15	---
Egg, medium	1	80	6	27	1.1	590	0.05	0.15	0
3. Vegetable-fruit Group									
Peas	1/4 cup	28	2	9	0.8	288	0.10	0.06	6
Carrots	1/4 cup	10	tr.	10	0.3	4533	0.02	0.02	2
Lettuce	2 leaves	5	1	11	0.2	270	0.02	0.04	4
Lettuce	1/4 head	20	1	25	0.6	618	0.05	0.10	9
Celery	2 stalks	10	2	40	0.4	0	0.04	0.04	6
Grapefruit	1/2 medium	50	1	21	0.5	10	0.05	0.02	50
Baked apple	1 medium	120	tr.	8	0.4	50	0.04	0.02	3
Banana	1 medium	85	1	8	0.7	190	0.05	0.06	10
4. Bread-cereal Group									
Bread, enriched	4 slices	240	8	76	2.4	tr.	0.24	0.20	tr.
Rolls, enriched	2	230	6	56	1.4	tr.	0.22	0.14	tr.
Totals, Foundation Foods		1753	84	952	13.5	7679	1.68	2.14	95
Dietary Allowances for Young Woman		2300	58	800	12.0	5000	1.20	1.50	70
Additional Foods									
Butter*	5 tsp	175	tr.	5	tr.	767	---	---	---
French dr.	2 tbsp	120	tr.	6	0.2	0	0	0	0
Mayonnaise	1 tbsp	110	tr.	2	0.1	40	tr.	tr.	0
Sugar	3 tsp	51	0	0		0	0	0	0
Cookies	1	110	2	6	0.2	0	0.01	0.01	0
Totals, Additional Foods		566	2	19	0.5	807	0.01	0.01	0
GRAND TOTALS		2319	86	971	14.0	8486	1.69	2.15	95

* or margarine fortified with vitamin A

Fig. 8.2(b) Menus based on Diet B.

Foundation Foods (75 percent of total calories)		Calories		Additional Foods		Calories
BREAKFAST						
Grapefruit	1/2 medium	50	+	Sugar	1 tsp	17
Egg, poached	1 medium	80				
Toast, enriched	2 slices	120	+	Butter*	2 tsp	70
Milk, whole	1 glass	165		Coffee		
				+ Sugar	1 tsp	17
LUNCH						
Ham Sandwich						
Bread, enriched	2 slices	120				
Ham, luncheon	2 oz	170	+	Mayonnaise	1 tbsp	110
Lettuce	2 leaves	5				
Celery	2 stalks	10				
Milk, whole	1 glass	165				
Apple, baked	1 medium	120		Cookies	1	110
DINNER						
Pot Roast	3 oz	245				
Peas, carrots	1/2 cup	38	+	Butter*	1 tsp	35
Head lettuce salad	1/4 hd.	20	+	French dr.	2 tbsp	120
Rolls, enriched	2	230	+	Butter*	2 tsp	70
Ice cream	1/4 pt	130				
				Coffee		
				+ sugar	1 tsp	17
BETWEEN MEALS						
Banana	1 medium	85				
	Total Calories	1753			Total Calories	566

GRAND TOTAL, CALORIES FOR THE DAY – 2319

* or margarine fortified with vitamin A

Fig. 8.2(c). Graphic summary of Diet B: *Liberal choices* from the daily food pattern.

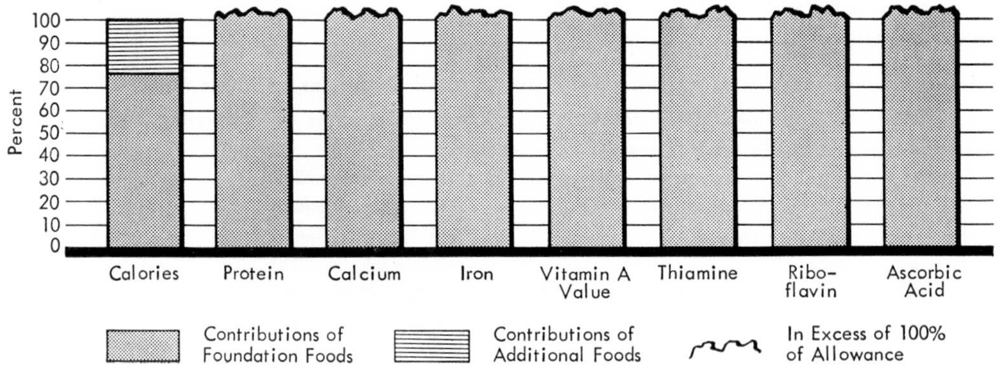

the allowances for calories and the various nutrients given on the table.

In putting the daily food pattern to use it is necessary to know more specifically the make-up of its food groups and the practical aspects of their use in meal planning [4]

Milk Group

The daily food pattern calls for specified amounts of milk to cover nutritional needs at different ages and under varying conditions. Milk "counts" when it is used as a beverage, when it is combined with other foods in prepared dishes, and when it is served over foods as cereals and desserts. To some extent milk products, such as ice cream and cheese, may be used as alternates for milk (Table 8-3). Federal and state standards have been established for the composition of milk products [5].

Milk is available in various forms: fresh fluid, evaporated, and dried. Some is whole milk, containing all of its original butterfat; some is partially or entirely skimmed. Buttermilk, for example, may be skimmed or partially skimmed milk; dry milk may be skimmed or whole milk; evaporated milk is double-strength whole milk. Any of these milks may be used as one's sole or partial milk supply, providing the total quantity is equivalent to that suggested on the food pattern. The cartons, bottle caps, cans, or packages in which these milks are sold clearly specify whether their contents are skimmed- or whole-milk products.

Labels also indicate what, if anything, has been added to the milk and state the methods of processing involved. Pasteurization, homogenization, evaporation, and drying processes are indicated, for example, and additions such as vitamin A and D concentrates and nonfat dry milk solids, are specified, with their amounts. When chocolate syrup is added to whole milk it is labelled "chocolate milk." When it is added to skim milk, it is called "chocolate drink."

TABLE 8-3

Full Equivalents of 1 Cup (8 oz) Fluid Whole Milk

½ cup undiluted evaporated milk	+	½ cup water
⅓ cup dry whole milk	+	⅔ cup water
1 cup fluid skim milk	+	¾ tbsp (1 medium pat) butter
1 cup fluid buttermilk	+	¾ tbsp (1 medium pat) butter

Full Equivalents of 1 Cup (8 oz) Fluid Skim Milk

⅓ cup dry skim milk	+	⅔ cup water
1 cup fluid buttermilk		

Calcium Equivalents of Various Dairy Foods to Specified Quantities of Whole Milk

Because the milk group makes an outstanding contribution of calcium, the various foods in the milk group are usually equated on the basis of their calcium content:

1⅓ oz (1⅓ in. cube) American or cheddar cheese	=	1 cup whole milk
¾ lb creamed cottage cheese	=	1 cup whole milk
½ cup creamed cottage cheese	=	⅓ cup whole milk
1 lb cream cheese	=	1 cup whole milk
2 tbsp cream cheese	=	1 tbsp whole milk
1 pt of ice cream	=	1 cup whole milk
½ cup of ice cream (¼ pt)	=	¼ cup whole milk

Cheeses are made from whole and from skim milk; some are hard, others are semihard or soft [6]. All are made from the curds of milk. When curds are formed in making cheese, the whey is drained off and with it part of the water-soluble vitamin content of the original milk. Thus, while cheese is a concentrated source of many of the nutrients of milk, its loss of whey prevents it from becoming a full equivalent of milk.

Ice cream is made from cream, milk and milk solids with a stabilizer, sweetening agents, flavorings, and sometimes fruits and nuts. Obviously it contains all of the nutrients of milk itself. However, the nutrients are present in different proportions in the 2 products, which prevents them from being full equivalents on a volume basis, as will be noted in Table 8-3.

One standard cup measure of milk is regarded as a serving. This represents 8 oz of fluid milk or, in liquid measure, ½ pt or ¼ qt. When the number of servings is specified in glasses as on the daily food pattern, the glasses must each be large enough to contain 1 full measuring cup of milk. About 1 oz of the hard cheeses and 2 oz of cottage cheese (¼ cup) are considered servings of these foods. For ice cream, ¼–⅓ pt is usually served the individual.

Enjoyable, safe, economical, and nutritionally adequate meals are the ultimate objective of the daily food pattern. The selection of foods within each food group should therefore be made with these points in mind. As applied to the milk group, this entails buying products of good quality and choosing forms of milk and dairy foods consistent with the limitations of the food budget, the food tastes of family members, and the nutrient values of the different products. When economy is a prime consideration, a survey of local prices of the different forms of milk will show which form, or what combination of forms, is feasible with the amount of money available.

The dairy foods purchased should be produced, handled, packaged, and sold under the jurisdiction of officially constituted agencies. State and local governments, through their Public Health Departments, largely have the legal responsibility for health protection of fluid milk supplies. Sanitary standards are recommended by the Federal Public Health Service and are used in many cases as the bases for sanitary regulations in states, counties, and municipalities. Containers and bottle caps carry a permit number issued by the local health official to each authorized dealer. Pasteurization is recognized as the only broad-scale measure that destroys all disease organisms in raw milk, if they should be present. There are small losses of water-soluble vitamins in pasteurized milk, but the public health advantage of pasteurization completely overshadows such losses.

Canned milk products are processed and handled under government supervision. The same is true of dry milks. At present, a limited amount of dry skim (nonfat dry) milk is packed under U.S. Department of Agriculture grade labels. The appearance of the official emblem on a package of such milk assures the customer of dependable quality and compliance with sanitary requirements.

Several firms are now selling cottage cheese under a U.S. inspection emblem, and certain hard cheeses bear U.S. grade designations. Grading is based on factors of flavor, body and texture, as applied to cheese [7]. Approved plants using the grading service operate under the rules for sanitation and packing specified by the U.S. Department of Agriculture.

Fresh fluid milk requires special care

in handling after it reaches the home kitchen. It should be refrigerated at once and continuously; it should be kept covered in its original container and isolated in the refrigerator from foods of strong odor; left-over milk should never be returned to the original container. These measures not only protect the milk from possible contamination but from foreign flavors that lessen the enjoyment in consumption.

Meat Group

The daily food pattern offers a double listing under the meat group: a) foods of animal origin—lean meats, fish, poultry, eggs, and cheese, and b) alternate foods of vegetable origin—dry beans, dry peas, and nuts. These general classes offer a large number of individual foods from which to choose the 2 or more daily servings indicated for this group. *Lean meat,* for example, can be selected from such available sources as beef, veal, lamb, pork—fresh or cured—and liver, heart, brains, tongue, and kidneys, called "variety meats." *Fish* choices include fish, as such, and shell fish, fresh- and salt-water varieties of fish, and fish in fresh, dried, frozen, or canned forms. *Poultry* refers to any type of fowl such as chicken, turkey, guinea hen, duck, or goose, and the livers of these birds. Meats, poultry, and fish may be prepared in many different ways: roasted, broiled, fried, or in stews, thus adding to the variety in selection. *Eggs* may be those from any kind of fowl, but data used in this text are for domestic hens' eggs. Cheese is included in the pattern because of its protein content. It therefore includes the hard cheeses and cottage cheese but not cream cheese.

The alternate sources in the meat group include all kinds of dry legumes. In this country, the common kinds, such as navy and lima beans, are usually served baked or boiled in main dishes. Also in this classification are lentils and the various kinds of split dried peas, pinto beans, chick peas, and pigeon peas so popular in Latin America. Peanuts and other kinds of nuts, as well as peanut butter, are likewise considered alternates in the meat group.

The meat group thus offers almost limitless choices from many kinds and varieties of food, prepared in many different ways. Their main common contribution is protein. From previous consideration of protein, you know that animal and vegetable sources of protein differ in quality, that it is desirable for an individual to take a portion of his daily protein from animal sources, and to include some of it in each meal (Chap. 5). This "rule," plus the importance of including the maximum in other nutrients offered by the meat group, has led to some practical pointers in applying the daily food pattern: select at least 1 serving from the lean meats daily; include 1 egg every day or at least 3–5 weekly; eat a variety meat (liver) about once a week; have 1–2 servings of lean pork weekly; and, finally, make a practice of choosing more than the minimum of 2 servings daily from the meat group as a whole.

About 3 oz of cooked fish, poultry, or lean meat (without bone) are considered 1 serving on the daily food pattern and in the tables and food lists appearing throughout the text. The same meats in the raw state weigh about 4 oz. The portions vary somewhat with the kind and cut of meat. Cooked liver, for example, is given as 2 oz; chops appear as single units and therefore usually weigh more than 3 oz.

The following quantities of other foods in the meat group are usually considered as servings: 1 egg, 1 oz of cheese, 2 oz of luncheon meat such as the bolognas, and 2 tbsps of peanut butter. It must be remembered, however, that each one provides only about one-half or less of the amount of protein in a serving of lean meat, fish, or poultry. (See Chap. 5.) Therefore, if any one of these is to be used as a full protein equivalent the amount must be doubled. The alternative is to use enough of another protein source to make up the difference. The sizes of servings are to be altered for persons whose needs differ from those of the average adult. Young children and elderly people may have smaller servings; fast-growing teen-agers may have larger ones.

Meats, as a group, are very well liked and form the basis of many meals. Therefore, if economy is a consideration it is important to know how to get the most meat for the money available. Price is not the criterion of food value, and flavor is often more a matter of how the meat is cooked than its cost per pound. One should know how to choose and cook meat to obtain the maximum food value and flavor in the particular dish to be prepared.

Considerable assistance is offered consumers in choosing meat for its safety and quality. For example, federal inspection is compulsory for all meat shipped in interstate commerce. All meat that is graded must first be inspected for wholesomeness. Meats that pass inspection carry a purple (harmless vegetable coloring) stamp, round in shape, which bears the legend "U.S. Inspected and Passed."

Beef, veal, calf, lamb, and mutton are federally graded. They bear a purple stamp in the shape of a shield with the letters U.S.D.A. and the designated grade that applies in a given case. The federal meat grader grades only whole carcasses or wholesale cuts. This is done in the interest of a fair and technically adequate appraisal of the entire animal. However, the stamping is done in such a way that the grade label appears on almost all retail cuts.

Grades have been carefully defined and they are similar for most meats. The details are beyond the scope of this text. But the U.S. Department of Agriculture, through its consumer bulletins, provides such information [7,8]. The same holds true for poultry and eggs, and to a more limited extent, for dried beans and peas, which have their own grading systems. As indicated above, all grades under the federal grading system are wholesome meats. Grades offer the customer a choice of quality. They give him an opportunity to choose a less expensive cut of meat when such a cut suits his needs. The lower grades usually have more lean, less fat (and *sometimes* less bone), and thus give more for the money than higher grades. Any good quality beef—graded or ungraded —has a red lean portion, red bones, and flaky light-colored fat.

Fresh meat, like fresh milk, needs care in the kitchen if it is to remain in top condition and of best flavor. It should be covered loosely and stored in the refrigerator. Ground fresh meats and variety meats, such as liver, keep less well than others. They should be cooked within a day or two, at the most, after purchase.

Vegetable-fruit Group

Table 8-2 shows that the vegetable-fruit group is almost the sole source of ascorbic acid in Diet B and provides more than two-thirds of the vitamin A value. But there is great variation in the yield of these vitamins from individual kinds of fruits and vegetables. It is important to know these variations and to understand the possibilities for choice within the vegetable-fruit group. This makes it possible to take advantage of the nutrient values offered and to avoid the limitations imposed by poor choices. The group as a whole is composed of a vast number of foods from which to select the 4 or more servings specified by the daily food pattern.

Dark Green, Deep Yellow Sources of vitamin A Value (Fig. 7.1).

The dark green (mainly leafy) vegetables, eaten chiefly for vitamin A value, include beet greens, broccoli, chard, collards, cress, kale, mustard greens, spinach, turnip greens, and wild greens (dandelion greens and others).

The deep yellow vegetables, also eaten for vitamin A value, include carrots, pumpkin, sweet potatoes, winter squash, and yams.

A few yellow-flesh fruits, eaten for vitamin A value, are apricots, cantaloups, mangoes and persimmons. (For a few vitamin A equivalents, see Table 8–4).

Sources of Ascorbic Acid (Fig. 7.11).

Citrus fruits, eaten chiefly for ascorbic acid, include grapefruit, grapefruit juice, oranges, orange juice.

Other good sources of ascorbic acid: cantaloups, raw strawberries, broccoli, green peppers.

Less concentrated but often significant sources of ascorbic acid in daily meals: tomatoes, tomato juice, white potatoes, dark green leafy vegetables, and other raw vegetables and fruits. (For a few ascorbic acid equivalents, see Table 8–5).

Other Fruits and Vegetables These include all of the other fruits and vegetables that are available, such as snap beans,

TABLE 8-4

EQUIVALENTS IN VITAMIN A VALUE*

Each of the following common foods in the quantity designated provides approximately the same amount of vitamin A value as does ½ cup of carrots. This amount is about twice the adult's daily dietary allowance for the vitamin.

CARROTS	**½ cup (cooked)**	**1 serving**	**Vitamin A value 9065 IU**
	Approximate quantity	Approximate servings	
Dandelion greens	⅓ cup	⅔ serving	
Spinach	½ cup (scant)	1 serving	
Sweet potato	1 medium	1 serving	
Collards	⅔ cup	1⅓ servings	
Cantaloup (orange flesh)	¾ fruit	1½ servings	
Winter squash	¾ cup	1½ servings	
Mustard greens	1 cup	2 servings	
Broccoli	2 cups	4 servings	
Apricots (dried, cooked)	2 cups	4 servings	
Tomato juice	3½ cups	7 servings	
Green peas	8 cups	16 servings	
Cabbage (shredded, raw)	113 cups	226 servings	

* Vegetables cooked unless otherwise specified

TABLE 8-5

EQUIVALENTS IN ASCORBIC ACID

Each of the following common foods in the quantity designated provides approximately the same amount of ascorbic acid as does 1 serving of fresh orange juice. This amount is about ⅔ of an adult's daily dietary allowance for this vitamin.

ORANGE JUICE	**½ cup (1 small glass)**	**1 serving**	**Ascorbic acid 46 mg**
	Approximate quantity	Approximate servings	
Cantaloup	⅓ melon	1 scant serving	
Grapefruit	½ fruit	1 serving	
Broccoli (cooked)	½ cup (scant)	1 serving	
Strawberries (raw)	½ cup	1 serving	
Cabbage (shredded, raw)	1 cup	2 servings	
Potato, white, cooked	2⅓ potatoes	2⅓ servings	
Tomato juice	1¼ cups	2½ servings	
Pineapple juice	2 cups	4 servings	
Lettuce	1¼ heads	5 servings	
Green beans (cooked)	2½ cups	5 servings	
Apple	15 apples	15 servings	
Apple juice	23 cups	46 servings	

beets, peas, summer squash, apples, bananas, cherries, pears, peaches, and plums. These fruits and vegetables furnish some vitamin A and ascorbic acid and they provide variety in color, texture, and flavor in rounding out daily meals.

Many of the fruits and vegetables mentioned above are available in the fresh, canned, dried, and frozen forms. Nutrients are well preserved in modern processing methods. Therefore, fruits and vegetables of high quality at the time of processing are good sources of the nutrients present in the foods originally.

Serving sizes of vegetables and fruits vary with the kind and form in which they are served: ½-cup servings apply to practically all cooked vegetables, cooked fruits, and fruit juices. In the case of most raw fruits, it is more practical to consider as 1 serving a single unit of the fruit, such as 1 banana or 1 potato, or some portion of a unit, such as ½ grapefruit. This plan for designating serving sizes has been used almost exclusively in Appendix G and in the lists and tables throughout the text.

It will be noted that the daily food pattern specifies a dark green or deep yellow vegetable at least every other day. This means that an individual may well eat a full serving of such a vegetable *every* day. If that is not feasible, he may choose a half serving daily or a full serving 3 to 4 times weekly. Some good sources of vitamin A value also provide significant amounts of ascorbic acid, as shown in Tables 8-4 and 8-5.

In choosing foods for ascorbic acid value it is usually safer to pick 1 excellent or 2 good sources daily rather than depend on small amounts from a number of poor sources. If lesser sources are to be used it is best that they be eaten in the raw form. Ascorbic acid is easily destroyed or lost in the handling and cooking of foods. Normal losses are presumably accounted for in Appendix G. However, there is no way of knowing the exact losses that have taken place in any given food at the time it is eaten (Chap. 7).

The condition of fresh vegetables and fruits when they reach market makes a big difference in the food value, appearance, and flavor of the foods when served. Foods that are wilted, discolored, soft, and moldy have probably lost most of their ascorbic acid. In addition, there is wastage from discards and trimming. Such foods are expensive at any price.

The federal government has determined grades and specifications for most of the fresh fruits and vegetables on the market. At present, this has been done chiefly for the wholesaler, but the consumer benefits indirectly because of the generally high quality of graded products. In addition, there are a limited number of standards developed for use at the retail level. These grades and their definitions are carefully outlined in publications of the U.S. Department of Agriculture [7]. It is important for consumers to become familiar with the characteristics that form the basis for grades. These characteristics are helpful in identifying desirable qualities in shopping for fresh fruits and vegetables which bear no grade designations [9]. Grades have also been developed for a large number of canned, dried, and frozen fruits and vegetables.

The specific suggestions made in Chapter 7 for handling and cooking vegetables and fruits in the home to preserve ascorbic acid should be reviewed at this time. The measures taken to keep foods crisp and to preserve their attractiveness and flavor are the same measures that help to retain their nutritive values [10].

► Calculate at local prices the costs of *foods in Table 8-4 that are equivalent in* vitamin A value to 1/2 cup of cooked carrots.

Do the same for foods in Table 8-5 that are equivalent in ascorbic acid yield to 1/2 cup of orange juice.

Consider the practical importance of the comparative costs of the different items. Consider also the feasibility of using the various foods in the amounts required as daily items of diet.

Bread-cereals Group

The bread-cereals group includes all of the grains that are served in *whole-grain, enriched,* or *restored* form: wheat, corn, oats, buckwheat, rice, rye. It consists of several categories of foods, as follows:

Breads: yeast breads, rolls, biscuits, buns, muffins, pancakes, waffles, crackers

Breakfast foods: ready-to-eat—flaked, rolled, puffed; to be cooked—whole, ground, rolled

Cereal foods: macaroni, spaghetti, noodles, flours, rice

The daily food pattern calls for 4 or more servings of whole-grain, enriched, or restored cereals:

Enriched flour and breads have been defined and described in earlier chapters. Essentially, enriched flour is white flour to which specified amounts of iron, thiamine, riboflavin, and niacin have been added.

Whole grains are those which retain the germ and the outer layers of the grain, and thus the nutrients contained in those parts. Whole-grain products include whole-wheat flour and the products made from it, dark rye flour, brown rice, and whole ground corn meal.

Restored grains are those to which nutrients lost in processing are restored to the approximate level contained in the original grain.

Serving sizes of grain products vary with the different forms in which they are served: in breads, for example, they are designated in small convenient units, such as 1 slice, 1 bun, or 1 pancake. In cooked cereals, the serving is about ⅔ cup; in the lighter, ready-to-eat cereals the serving is about 1 cup. Servings of cereal foods such as macaroni, spaghetti, or rice have been designated as ¾ cup when they are used as main dishes in a meal, usually combined with another food—meat, tomato, or cheese, for example. The individual variations in measures within the bread-cereal group are indicated in the separate listings in Appendix G.

In general, individual servings within the bread-cereals group can be used interchangeably in menus as long as they adhere to the whole grain, enriched, or restored categories. As shown in Table 8-2, cereals do not make a striking contribution in any 1 or 2 nutrients but a substantial contribution to several of them. Enrichment of flours and breads has done much to make cereals important sources of certain nutrients in the United States food supply. Two of these nutrients, thiamine and iron, are often difficult to obtain, as indicated in Section Two. The use of recommended amounts of enriched or whole-grain cereals in many cases may be the deciding factor in achieving adequacy in these 2 nutrients. The addition of dry skim milk in making bread also increases its nutrient contribution. In commercial bakeries it is common practice to add 3–4 percent of nonfat dry milk by weight to the flour mix. Many cereal breakfast foods are fortified with various nutrients that enhance their nutritive value.

Cereals of all kinds, including breads, are pleasantly bland foods that do not jade the appetite. They are therefore usually present in at least one form in almost every meal. Their blandness lends itself to pleasing combinations with other foods, such as fruits with breakfast foods, vegetables or cheese with macaroni, and spreads on breads. Grain products are staple articles of diet that blend with and extend the use of many other foods.

The major losses of nutrients in the processing of cereals have been taken into consideration in Appendix G. Also considered are additional losses, chiefly thiamine, which may result when cereals are cooked. Even small decreases in thiamine are taken account of in toasting bread. This amounts to a 15–20 percent loss from heat in slices of medium thickness. In thinner slices, the loss is greater.

Consumers are assisted in shopping for cereals in two chief ways: by labels on wrappings and, to a limited extent, by federal gradings of a few products. On bread wrappers, the purchaser is informed if the bread is made from enriched flour; is given the percentages of the *minimum*[1] daily requirements for thiamine, riboflavin, niacin, and iron provided by ½ lb of the bread; is told if the bread is made with milk; and is given the weight of the loaf. Containers for breakfast foods indicate which, if any, nutrients have been added to fortify or restore the cereal, how much of each nutrient is present in a specified amount of the product, and what percentage they supply of the *minimum*[1] daily requirements.

Federal grades have been established for both white and brown rice. Retail packages sometimes carry these grades. Usually 2 numerical grades are used for white rice in the retail trade; 4 for brown rice. The grades are based on such factors as the pres-

[1] Minimum standards established for industry by the Federal Food and Drug Administration. (These are lower than the Food and Nutrition Board's Recommended Daily Dietary Allowances.)

ence or absence of defective kernels and objectionable foreign material, whether or not varieties are mixed, and general appearance and color.

» ADDITIONAL FOODS

Additional foods are all those which do not fall within the *foundation* groups just described. Specifically, they include fats—table spreads, cooking fats, and oils—sugars, honey, sirups, jams, jellies, candies, soft drinks, and unenriched, refined cereals. Such foods are used alone as well as in and on foods: a) in mixtures such as baked goods, casserole dishes, "made desserts," and b) as additions to foods, such as butter to bread, sugar to fruits, dressings to salads.

When *additional* foods are combined in recipes with *foundation* foods the resulting dishes are classified in accordance with the predominating ingredients. Only if a *foundation* food is the chief ingredient, or is supplied in sufficient quantity to provide each individual with a full serving of that food, should a dish be so classed. A jello dessert, for example, with a few slices of banana, should not be considered a serving of fruit.

Additional foods are definitely a part of daily meals even though they do not merit the emphasis accorded *foundation* foods as sources of nutrients. Besides their contribution of calories and some nutrients, *additional* foods help to give meals "staying" qualities; they lend interest, and variety in flavor and texture. The use of *additional* foods need not be urged in meals because a) they are already present to some extent in *foundation* foods, such as fat in milk and meat, and natural sugars in ripened fruits; and b) calories are easy to obtain—every food provides some. The calories most needed are those which also provide nutrients in abundance.

Specific examples of *additional* foods apappear in Diets A and B of Figures 8.1 and 8.2. Their contributions, under conditions of minimum and liberal selection of *foundation* foods have been demonstrated and discussed. It is evident that the nutrient content of *additional* foods is small under all practical circumstances. It is probably rare that real nutrient deficits can be wiped out with *additional* foods. The bar chart accompanying Diet A serves as one illustration of this point: the calorie allowance was completed with *additional* foods (horizontal lines on calorie bar) and the vitamin A shortage was lessened considerably, but the more serious lacks—those in iron and thiamine—were affected very little by these additions.

» THE DAY'S MENUS

Thus far we have interpreted the daily food pattern only in terms of total amounts of foods used on a daily basis. We need now to break down these foods into meal units. The menus adjoining Diets A and B were developed from the corresponding diets. They show how the concept of *foundation* and *additional* foods carries over into meal planning. The identical foods listed on the diet forms are repeated in the menus. The *foundation* foods are listed on the left in the menus; the *additional* foods on the right. The *foundation* foods were first suitably distributed throughout the meals. The *additional* foods included are those compatible with the *foundation* foods and those needed to increase palatibility and energy value of the meals. Calories are recorded on the menus to identify the totals with the corresponding ones of the calculated diets and to emphasize the relationship between the proportion of the total calories furnished by *foundation foods* and the nutrient value of the 2 diets.

It is apparent that the daily food pattern leads directly to daily meal plans and the making of menus. Listing *foundation* foods and *additional* foods separately has 2 advantages: a) it serves as a check on the meal planner as to the number and kinds of *foundation* foods he includes, and b) it suggests the best choices of *additional* foods to supplement the former in achieving satisfactory meals (Figs. 8.1 [b] and 8. 2 [b]).

In planning meals for other persons one soon learns to know individual preferences. These should be taken into account in choosing both *foundation* and *additional* foods. The choices available are practically limitless. Variety in choice, diversity in textures in foods in a meal, interesting color contrasts in foods, may all be observed in planning nutritionally adequate meals around a daily food pattern. Never should foods be considered as isolated units in planning meals, but always in relation to other foods in the meal and in the day's meals. Foods brought together in a meal should present a composite of good flavor, texture, color contrast, and nutrition. Meal planning for individuals, to meet special situations, and for the family as a group is discussed in Chapter 9.

REFERENCES

1. Daily Food Patterns (posters), *Food for Fitness—A Daily Food Guide*. Washington, D.C.: U.S. Department of Agriculture; *A Guide to Good Eating*. Chicago: National Dairy Council; *Shield of Good Health*. Chicago: Wheat Flour Institute; *Foodway to Follow*. Chicago: American Institute of Baking.
2. Hayes, O., Trulson, M. F., and Stare, F. J., "Suggested Revisions of the Basic 7," *J. Am. Dietet. Assoc.* 31 (Nov. 1955) pp. 1103–1107.
3. Page, L., and Phipard, E. F., *Essentials of an Adequate Diet . . . Facts for Nutrition Programs*. Home Econ. Res. Rept. No. 3. Washington, D.C.: U.S. Dept. of Agriculture, 1957. (Table 5, p. 18.)
4. Phipard, E. F., and Page, L., "A Guide to Eating," *Food—The Yearbook of Agriculture*. Washington, D.C.: U.S. Department of Agriculture, 1959. p. 267.
5. *Federal and State Standards for the Composition of Milk Products*. Agricultural Handbook No. 51. Washington, D.C.: U.S. Department of Agriculture, 1959.
6. *Cheese-buying Guide for Consumers*. Marketing Bull. 17. Washington, D.C.: U.S. Department of Agriculture, 1961.
7. *Shopper's Guide to U.S. Grades for Food*. Home and Garden Bull. 58. Washington, D.C.: U.S. Department of Agriculture, 1961.
8. *U.S. Grades for Beef*. Marketing Bull. 15. Washington, D.C.: U.S. Department of Agriculture, 1960.
9. Morrison, W. W., *Tips on Selecting Fruits and Vegetables*. Marketing Bull. 13. Washington, D.C.: U.S. Department of Agriculture, 1961.
10. Watt, B. K., and Stiebeling, H. K., "Keeping the Values in Food," *Today's Health*, 36 (April 1958) pp. 48–51.

READINGS

Birdsall, J. J., Teply, L. J., and Derse, P. H., "Effects of Light on Homogenized Whole Milk and Some Fortified Milk Products," *Food Technology,* 12 (Dec. 1958) p. 670.

Cereal Glossary. Chicago: The Cereal Institute, Inc.

"Food Quality," *Food—The Yearbook of Agriculture.* Washington, D.C.: U.S. Department of Agriculture, 1959. pp. 327–457.

Institute of Home Economics, *Food for Fitness—A Daily Food Guide.* Leaflet 424. Washington, D.C.: U.S. Department of Agriculture, 1958.

Leverton, R. M., "What is Good Nutrition?" *Today's Health,* 36 (March 1958) pp. 31; 54–59.

McHenry, E. W., *Foods Without Fads: A Common-sense Guide to Nutrition.* Philadelphia: J. B. Lippincott Company, 1960.

Quality Milk—Its Importance to You and Your Community. Chicago: National Dairy Council, 1960.

Watt, B. K., and Leung, Woot-Tsuen Wu, "Conserving Nutritive Values," *Food—The Yearbook of Agriculture.* Washington, D.C.: U.S. Department of Agriculture, 1959. p. 483.

CHAPTER 9

Adapting the daily food pattern to different situations

Up to this point in Section Three we have considered a daily food pattern as a tool in planning adequate meals, with emphasis on the nutritional needs of adults. The pattern that was tested against the daily dietary allowances for a young adult (Diet B) appears to meet the needs of the "average" person in good health. However, we know that individuals differ in dietary requirements. Particularly do calorie needs vary. Some adults, for example are large, vigorous, and active; others are small, quiet, and sedentary; some are young, some are old; some are overweight and need to reduce; a few are underweight and need to build up. Many fit into still other categories. Can the daily food pattern be adapted to all of these situations? Let us first examine a few of the special problems of adult nutrition to see what adjustments are called for.

» ADAPTING THE "PATTERN" TO WEIGHT CONTROL

Many people in this country are overweight. Perhaps as much as one-fifth of the adult population is seriously so. It is said to be our most glaring nutritional fault. There are 2 chief reasons for our overweight problem: too much intake from a plentiful, "rich" food supply; too little output in terms of physical work or exercise. Even a moderate amount of our food can provide an excess of calories. The pattern of overeating often starts in childhood when parents encourage overconsumption. The expenditure of energy does not balance the intake. The fact that we are a mechanized nation has reduced the need for physical effort at all periods of life. Overweight creeps up as energy needs are lessened with age: basal metabolism gradually declines; physical activities are curtailed. The practical problem for each individual therefore becomes one of adhering to the daily food pattern to assure nutritional adequacy of his diet without exceeding his energy need.

Although the consequences of overweight have been well publicized, this information has not served to reverse the upward trend. Body bulk is increasing, especially after the early adult years. Overweight is a handicap in chronic degenerative conditions, particularly cardiovascular and renal diseases (Chap. 3). Statistics show that men who are 20 percent or more overweight, have a death rate about one-half higher than that of men with desirable weights [1]. Length of life itself is jeopardized by excess body weight. Life insurance companies regard overweight persons as greater risks than those of desirable weight and charge them higher rates accordingly. The advantages of maintaining desirable weight are a trim, compact, maneuverable body that functions in maximum health and efficiency.

In considering normal energy needs and expenditures in Chapter 4, you became acquainted with desirable weight ranges for men and women of different body builds (Appendix D) and developed your own weight chart (Appendix E). In view of the unfavorable health picture presented for the overweight person, it becomes important for any individual to stay within the weight range or zone indicated for his height and body build. In many cases it is preferable for the weight to be kept near the lower part of the range. New data show that, in terms of longevity, moderate underweight is not a health handicap, but highly to be desired [1]. For an adult to pattern his food habits and activities to maintain his body weight within the desired weight zone is the preferred type of weight control.

Prevention of Overweight

It is easier to *keep* off than to *take* off unwanted pounds. If your weight is within the range desirable for you but you are gaining steadily, you should find out the reasons for the gain.

► *Recheck your calorie intake for a representative day or two.*

Have you inadvertently added extra foods that are causing weight increase?

Are you skipping meals to cut down on total calories? Studies show that this is a futile gesture.

Do you come from a family that tends to overeat? Are your parents overweight? Do you seem to be headed for the same fate?

Recheck your activity schedule for a representative day. (See Chap. 4.)

Have you dropped an activity which has lessened your energy needs?

Are you continuing to keep a weight chart? It provides the best proof of the effectiveness of preventive measures.

Prevention is simple if you raise and answer questions such as these and then *do* something about what you learn from them. It may mean cutting out a bedtime snack, omitting dessert at lunch or dinner, or walking up a few flights of stairs daily instead of taking the elevator. Any and all of these measures are easier than trying to lose excess fat, once it has accumulated.

Weight Reduction

Unfortunately an individual often slips over into the overweight class before he realizes it. It is the purpose here to consider simple modifications of a normal diet which will help an individual return to his desirable weight range. This will be done with moderate reduction of calories and maintenance of a high nutrient level. It is assumed that the need for reducing calories is due merely to a mild maladjustment between intake of energy-yielding foods and energy expenditure by the body and that there are no deep-seated emotional problems which will serve as interfering forces. If a real overweight problem appears to exist, a physician should be consulted. He will decide if weight reduction should be attempted, how much weight should be shed, and how rapidly it should be lost.

Implementing a Reducing Diet Diet C in Figure 9.1 presents a moderately low-calorie diet with suggested menus for 1 day. The diet is based on the daily food pattern and it meets the recommended daily dietary allowances for a young woman, with the exception of the calorie allowance. One thousand calories have been cut from Diet B, which was planned for the same young woman with the same nutrient standards, but with her full calorie allowance (Fig. 8.2). It will be noted that the menus for the 2 diets are almost identical. The meat, eggs, and vegetables are the same in kind and amount. The differences are chiefly those in form and quantity of other foods.

All low-calorie diet plans designed to bring about safe and permanent weight reduction have certain characteristics in common. Let us examine Diet C in light of these generally accepted qualifications.

Characteristics of Sound Reducing Diets 1. *The diet should be built around familiar and well-liked foods.* The more nearly the meals resemble those he is accustomed to and likes, the longer will an individual be willing to continue on the diet. And unless the dieter wishes to continue, the experiment may not last long enough to measure its success in terms of weight loss. Keeping the new diet similar to the old does not mean that no changes need be made to achieve success in dieting. The degree of change depends on the quality of the food habits prior to the weight-reduction regime.

Diet C has been developed from Diet B in order to show how a person already eating a good diet can reduce his calorie intake and yet continue to eat his customary foods. This can be done either at home or in a restaurant. Actually, the changes are almost imperceptible to the casual observer.

For the person who starts a reducing diet with poor food habits, there may be many changes. If, for example, he is accustomed to meals low in *foundation* foods, overbalanced in sweetened beverages and high calorie desserts, his appetite must be retrained. Even in such a situation care must be exercised to retain the best features of the original diet and to preserve a nucleus of favorite dishes. Food is comforting; familiar foods are like old friends. Eating a reducing diet should be a pleasure, not a chore. Even more than usual care should be taken to make the food attractive and tasty. Meals eaten at the family table or elsewhere in a pleasant atmosphere are usually the ones that contribute most to permanent weight loss.

The numberless crash reducing diets that consist entirely of 2 or 3 foods are not recommended. Unpalatable, limited combinations of foods, such as tangerines and clams or lamb chops and grapefruit, soon pall and the reducing regime quickly ends. The individual foods in combinations of this character are usually appetizing in themselves and contribute their nutrient share to a varied diet. But neither used alone nor with 1 or 2 other foods are they nutritionally adequate or satisfying to the dieter. Variety, rather than sameness, is desirable in low calorie diets. The very monotony of such extreme, unnatural diets is responsible in part for their short lives. When they have ended, the inclination is to return to former food patterns and to habits of overindulgence. The only really successful reducing diet is one on which a person can live happily until the desired weight loss has been realized. (See Chap. 10 for a discussion of diet theories as promoted by food faddists and quacks. Many of their publications and nostrums apply to weight reduction.)

► *Each member of the class calculate one of the well-known fad reducing diets composed of 2 or 3 foods.*

Allow for enough of the total food combination to provide 1000 calories. Indi-

Fig. 9.1 (a) Diet C: A low-calorie diet based on Diet B.

Nutrients Furnished in Relation to the Daily Dietary Allowances of a Young Woman

Foods	Measures	Calories	Fat (g)	Protein (g)	Calcium (mg)	Iron (mg)	Vitamin A Value (IU)	Thiamine (mg)	Ribo-flavin (mg)	Ascorbic acid (mg)
Foundation Foods										
1. Milk Group										
Milk, skim	2 cups	180	tr.	18	596	0.2	20	0.20	0.88	4
2. Meat Group										
Pot Roast	3 oz	245	16	23	10	2.9	30	0.04	0.18	---
Ham, sliced	2 oz	170	13	13	5	1.5	0	0.57	0.15	---
Egg, medium	1	80	6	6	27	1.1	590	0.05	0.15	0
3. Vegetable-fruit Group										
Peas	1/4 cup	28	tr.	2	9	0.8	288	0.10	0.06	6
Carrots	1/4 cup	10	tr.	tr.	10	0.3	4533	0.02	0.02	2
Lettuce	2 leaves	5	tr.	1	11	0.2	270	0.02	0.04	4
Lettuce	1/4 head	20	tr.	1	25	0.6	618	0.05	0.10	9
Celery	3 stalks	15	tr.	3	60	0.6	0	0.06	0.06	9
Grapefruit	1/2 medium	50	tr.	1	21	0.5	10	0.05	0.02	50
Apple, raw	1 medium	70	tr.	tr.	8	0.4	50	0.04	0.02	3
4. Bread-cereal Group										
Bread, enriched	2 slices	120	2	4	38	1.2	tr.	0.12	0.10	tr.
Roll, enriched	1 yeast	115	2	3	28	0.7	tr.	0.11	0.07	tr.
Totals, Foundation Foods		1108	39	75	848	11.0	6409	1.43	1.85	87
Dietary Allowances for Young Woman		2300			800	12.0	5000	1.20	1.50	70
Additional Foods										
Butter*	3 tsp	105	11	tr.	3	tr.	460	---	---	---
Mayonnaise	1/2 tbsp	55	6	tr.	1	0.1	20	tr.	tr.	0
French Dr.	1 tbsp	60	6	tr.	3	0.1	0	0	0	0
Totals, Additional Foods		220	23	tr.	7	0.2	480	tr.	tr.	0
GRAND TOTALS		1328	62	75	855	11.2	6889	1.43	1.85	87

*or margarine fortified with vitamin A

cate the amount of each food represented.

Calculate the nutrient content of this 1000-calorie diet.

Evaluate each diet from the standpoint of: nutrient adequacy, palatability, probable length of time the individual would remain on the diet.

2. *Meals should be satisfying.* Successful reducing diets must be satisfying—they must allay hunger. Otherwise the dieter is constantly unhappy and periodically "breaks over." Diet "breaks" may be so costly in terms of added calories that the effects of the diet itself are nullified.

Testing reducing diets on adult subjects has revealed some of the ways of making low calorie diets satisfying. One way is to divide the food fairly evenly among the meals of the day. This means a substantial breakfast, which is something chronic dieters seldom enjoy. Many omit breakfast entirely. Protein foods at break-

Fig. 9.1 (b) Menus based on Diet C.

Foundation Foods (83 percent of total calories)		Calories		Additional Foods		Calories
			BREAKFAST			
Grapefruit	1/2 medium	50	+	Sugar substitute, if desired		0
Egg, poached	1 medium	80				
Toast, enriched	1 slice	60		Butter‡	1 tsp	35
*Milk, skim	1 cup	90				
				Coffee or tea with sugar substitute, if desired		0
			LUNCH			
Ham Sandwich (open face)						
Bread, enriched	1 slice	60				
Ham, luncheon	2 oz	170	+	Mayonnaise	1/2 tbsp	55
Lettuce	2 leaves	5				
*Celery	3 stalks	15				
*Apple, raw	1 medium	70		Coffee or tea with sugar substitute, if desired		0
			DINNER			
Pot Roast	3 oz	245				
Peas and carrots	1/2 cup	38	+	Butter‡	1 tsp	35
Head lettuce salad	1/4 head	20	+	French Dr.	1 tbsp	60
Roll, yeast	1 roll	115	+	Butter	1 tsp	35
				Coffee or tea with sugar substitute, if desired		0
			BETWEEN MEALS			
Milk, skim	1 cup	90				
	Total Calories	1108			Total Calories	220

GRAND TOTAL, CALORIES FOR THE DAY - 1328

*Some or all of the foods with an asterisk may be taken between meals if the person dieting is better satisfied when he eats more often.

‡or margarine fortified with vitamin A.

fast help to sustain a satisfactory level of blood sugar for several hours following the morning meal [2].

Proteins, with their relatively slow digestion, absorption, and metabolism, may contribute to a steadier supply of glucose in the blood than do carbohydrates. Low blood sugar is associated with hunger, fatigue, weakness, and inability to concentrate. A good breakfast is important irrespective of the total calorie level of meals for the day. But it has special importance for sustaining vigor and efficiency during a reducing regime when total daily calorie intake is below energy expenditure. A comparison of the breakfasts in Diets B and C show that they follow the same menu pattern. Both provide a liberal amount of animal protein in the form of milk and egg. Each would be considered a substantial meal.

Diets moderately high in fat and high

in protein have also been found to be more satisfying to reducers than conventional low calorie diets. When diets of 1000–1400 calories contain upwards of 80 g of fat and 80–90 g of protein, dieters are, for the most part, contented with their meals and remain on their diets consistently [3].

It will be noted that Diet C provides 62 g of fat and 75 g of protein. Although these amounts do not meet the suggested levels, they are probably higher in fat and protein than traditional reducing diets. Changing the pint of skim milk in Diet C to whole milk would add 20 g of fat, thus raising the fat content of the diet to the desired level. A second egg would raise the protein above 80 g and further increase the fat. Either or both changes would, of course, call for other adjustments if the original calorie level of Diet C were to be maintained.

Some dieters are better satisfied with their reducing regime if a portion of their food is reserved for eating at times of the day when they crave to eat, notably at bedtime. This arrangement has been suggested for Diet C. Such snacks may be substantial foods, such as a portion of the day's milk or fruit. Or, if the dieter is satisfied with going through the motions of eating, the snacks may be foods, such as celery, which furnish almost no calories but which give pleasure in chewing and swallowing and a temporary relief from hunger.

► *Suggest ways of increasing the fat level of Diet C to about 80 g without altering the total calories or lessening the nutrient value of the diet.*

Suggest ways of increasing the protein level of Diet C to about 90 g without altering the total calories or lessening the nutrient value of the diet.

3. *The diet should be adequate nutritionally.* A nutritionally adequate diet with lowered calorie yield can mean improved health and a greater sense of well-being for the overweight person. On the other hand, reducing diets that are too low in calories and are inadequate in nutrient content are a hazard to health. Individuals who remain on them for prolonged periods of time lose strength and vitality and some become actually ill. As stated earlier, Diet C meets the recommended daily dietary allowances in all respects except in calories. The specifications for the daily food pattern are met, with the exception of 1 serving from the bread-cereal food group.

The majority of the calories (83 percent) in Diet C are provided by the *foundation* foods. In Diet B, which yields about 1000 more total calories, 75 percent of the calories come from foundation foods. This difference demonstrates the point made in Chapter 8 that the lower the total calorie level of the diet, the larger the proportion of calories that must be provided by foundation foods if the diet is to be nutritionally adequate.

Empty calories must be kept to a minimum in a reducing diet. Figure 9.2 shows how 2 foods may furnish a similar number of calories, but in one food they are provided by pure carbohydrate in the form of sugar.

The 6-oz. serving of soft drink yields only calories; the same amount of skim milk furnishes significant amounts of protein, calcium, riboflavin, and other nutrients, and somewhat fewer calories. It is apparent that in choosing foods for a reducing diet one must know not only calorie values of foods but also what such foods contribute to the nutritional adequacy of the diet.

The *additional* foods in Diet C are confined to those which enhance the palatability of the *foundation* foods, largely fats. Concentrated sweets such as jellies, jams, candies, rich desserts, and sweet sauces are omitted. When the desired weight loss is accomplished, such items can be added experimentally in small amounts to determine what quantities, if any, can be added without gain in weight.

A high protein diet, useful in the ways already mentioned, is also needed to prevent losses of nitrogen from the body. When total energy intake is low and proteins must be burned for fuel, nitrogen is sacrificed in the process and the usual result is a negative nitrogen balance (Chap. 5). Amounts of protein usually considered sufficient in a normal diet should therefore be raised when total calories are reduced if nitrogen requirements are to be met. An increase from 1 g of protein per kg (2.2 lbs) of body weight to 1½ g is suggested as desirable for the daily intake on a reducing diet—a basis comparable to the 90 g suggested earlier. Controlled studies with subjects on moderately low calorie diets of supposed adequate nutrient content have shown not only losses of body nitrogen, but negative balances in calcium and phosphorus as well.

Special liquid-formula diets which claim to be fully adequate nutritionally may be superior to the inadequate fad diets referred to previously. However, when judged on the basis of the long-term objectives of a successful reducing program, they are equally vulnerable [4]. Neither type is designed to develop and maintain good eating habits that assure stable body weight and fit into a normal living program. Many of the liquid-formula diets provide too few calories for any reasonably active adult. A sudden drop from the calories provided in a varied and liberal diet to the low calorie level of a formula diet may be dangerous to health, despite the adequate nutrient content of the formula. This is true especially if the formula is continued to the point of causing a precipitous drop in body weight.

► *Draw up several basic diet "rules" for reducing body weight safely which you think would work for you.*

How would you change Diet C to more nearly meet your own food preferences without lessening its nutritive value or changing radically the proportion of calories provided by foundation foods.

Develop a series of suggestions for re-

Fig. 9.2 More than calories are needed. A comparison of the nutrients and calories supplied by the same amounts of soft drink and skim milk.

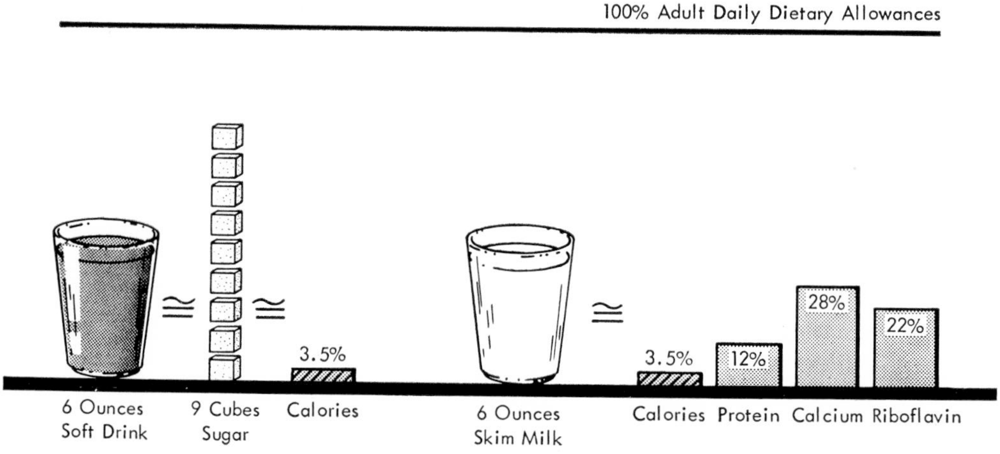

ducing weight for the person who eats his meals away from home: a) when he lives in a dormitory or other institution where there are planned meals; b) when he has free choice of foods, as in a restaurant.

4. *Calorie yield must be low enough to cause weight loss.* When foods supply less energy than the body needs, it uses its own stored fats as fuel. This is the principle upon which reducing diets are based. It is only by holding to a diet with a calorie deficit until excess fat is used up that a reducing regime can be considered successful. Of all the characteristics of a reducing diet discussed here, the low calorie feature is the most difficult to put into practice and the one most exacting in terms of successful weight loss.

The total weight loss to be sought depends on how much one varies from desirable weight. Let us assume that, originally, your weight was within the normal range for your height and body build (Appendix D) on about 2300 calories (Diet B). Later you began to gain weight, and now you are 10 lbs above the upper limit of your desirable range. This may not represent a serious excess at present, but if the upward trend continues it can lead to an amount that will be difficult to lose.

A modest goal for weight reduction is advised. Two pounds a week, or less, is a reasonable objective. One pound of body fat has the value of 3500 calories. Therefore, a daily deficit of 500 calories would result in a 3500-calorie loss in 1 week, ($500 \times 7 = 3500$). If a 2-lb weekly loss is the goal, the current daily diet should be curtailed by 7000 calories a week or 1000 calories daily. That would mean cutting the 2300-calorie diet to about 1300 calories. How one may eliminate 1000 calories from the day's food intake and yet continue to eat from the same menu is shown in the specimen diets B and. C. Table 9-1 lists the changes made in Diet B to reduce its calorie yield to that of Diet C.

If adhered to faithfully, Diet C should result in a loss of 1½–2 lbs in body weight per week. The amount will vary from week to week and may tend to lessen as the desired weight level is approached. Variation in water retention is often a factor in irregular weekly weight loss, even on a consistently low calorie intake. The 1000-calorie deficit plan can be applied to the regular

TABLE 9-1

CALORIE REDUCTIONS IN DIET B TO EQUAL CALORIES OF DIET C

Changes Made	Calories "Saved"
Skim milk was substituted for whole milk (1 pt)	150
Bread and rolls were cut from 6 to 3 servings	235
Butter was cut from 5 to 3 tsp	70
Mayonnaise was cut from 1 tbsp to ½ tbsp	55
French dressing was cut from 2 tbsp to 1 tbsp	60
Artificial sweetener was substituted for sugar (3 tsp) [5]	51
Banana was omitted	85
Raw apple was substituted for sweetened baked apple	50
Dessert omitted from lunch and dinner	240
Total calories "saved"	996

diet at any calorie level. However, this should be done judiciously, for there is a calorie limit below which it is impossible to maintain dietary adequacy. Only with nuitritional knowledge, skillfully applied, can an adult meet his dietary allowances on a diet of less than about 1000 calories daily.

Weight loss may be aided by moderate exercise such as walking or housework. Strenuous exercise, which creates a greater appetite, may defeat its own purpose. This gradual method of weight reduction is not spectacular. It employs no extreme measures, it offers no short cuts. It doesn't claim to be effective without effort. Beware of the schemes that promise you can "eat all you want" [6]. Don't be taken in by the quick, painless processes advocated by those selling "reducing salts" for the bath or special devices for rolling off fat. Take appetite depressants only under a physician's order and supervision.

The result of overeating—the pounds of excess body fat—should serve as its own best motivating force for weight reduction. This may take the form of concern for health, "the doctor's orders," which often is the most effective one. Another major motive is personal appearance, the unsightliness of accumulated fat. Underlying concerns have to do with the fit of clothes, social acceptance, and qualifications for jobs. Whatever the motive, it must be sufficiently strong to carry a person through a period of adjustment to a calorie level that will insure the desired weight loss. One is more apt to be successful if he quietly makes up his mind to lose weight and goes about it without fanfare. Success in weight reduction is itself a powerful motivator. The reward of conscientious dieting is tangible evidence of weight decline. And one way to sustain interest in hewing to the diet line is by weighing regularly and keeping a weight chart. Weekly weighings are sufficient. (See Chap. 4 for the correct method of taking height and weight, and for directions for starting a weight chart.)

► *Make a list of foods from Appendix G that would qualify as low-calorie desserts. Group them by approximate calorie values to suggest the types most suitable for reducing diets.*

Select from Appendix G the apple desserts and arrange them in order of their calorie value per serving, from fresh raw apple to apple pie. Indicate in each case how the calorie value of each has been increased above that of the fresh apple. How could the calorie value of each be increased still more? Consider the relative usefulness of these apple dishes in reducing diets.

Maintenance Diets

If weight reduction proceeds according to plan, desirable weight is reached eventually. It is then that a maintenance diet should be planned to yield just the amount of energy needed by the body. This usually means a somewhat more liberal supply of calories than the reducing diet afforded, but fewer calories than yielded by the original diet that permitted the weight gain. Expansion of the diet should be on an experimental basis until a level is found that provides a balance of energy, and thus a constant weight level. The calorie intake level might be raised 100 calories at a time; one continues experimenting with intake levels until the zero point is reached, beyond which weight gains again take place. Each increase in calories will have to be tried at least a week before the result is known. Foods added should still be in the moderate calorie range and give the dieter maximum satisfaction if the appetite training just experienced is to bear fruit in terms of permanent food habits.

Building-up Diets

The foregoing discussion of weight control has been devoted largely to dietary treatment of overweight. This is because overweight, not underweight, is a health problem in this country. Yet there are many underweight people. They need to know how to plan a diet in which energy intake *exceeds* energy output. It is only by living on such a diet, at least temporarily, that an underweight person can store enough body fat to put him in the desirable weight range. Obviously, nutrient intakes should remain high—high enough to meet the dietary allowances. Calories must be increased. If a person wishes to gain about 2 lbs per week he should add approximately 1000 calories daily until he has achieved his weight goal. Thus we have the reverse of the reducing diet. More *additional* foods can be eaten but this should not be overdone. An adequate diet and good food habits are still the long-term objectives.

Modifying a 2300-calorie diet *upward* instead of *downward* means adding rather than subtracting sources of food energy. How can this be done without throwing the diet out of balance? Again moderation is urged. Eating larger servings of foundation foods, using whole milk instead of skim milk, more spreads, sauces and dressings, real sugar instead of a substitute, adding simple desserts—these are good ways to start. If one has difficulty gaining weight he often has appetite and capacity problems as well. In that case, small and frequent meals may help to accomplish the purpose of the build-up diet.

► *How would you add 1000 calories to Diet B to achieve a total of 3300 calories? Re-plan the day's meals and snacks to make them into a practical plan for gaining weight.*

What proportion of the calories in your build-up diet are provided by foundation foods?

Overweight in Children

The subject of overweight children and dietary treatment thereof will be touched upon only briefly. Children who are inclined to overeat and who tend to be overweight can be helped by some of the simple expedients described for adults, with emphasis on normal physical activity. When obesity exists or simple measures fail, a physician's advice should be sought. Overweight in childhood is often the forerunner of obesity in later life. And experience has shown that long-standing obesity has the least chance of being treated effectively.

There is some evidence to indicate that body weight is more easily controlled in children when the diet is liberally supplied with nutrients, even if calories are fairly high. Iowa children of normal weight, for example, who were eating a nutritious diet, had a slightly higher calorie intake than did overweight children in the study. The latter, on diets inferior in nutritive value, maintained their overweight status despite the lower energy value of their diets.

» ADAPTING THE "PATTERN" TO DIETS OF OLDER PERSONS

Basal energy metabolism decreases slightly but steadily throughout adult life. Also, activities tend to be less strenuous with advancing years. Both are factors in lowering the recommended daily calorie allowances for men from 3200 calories per day at 25 years of age to 2550 calories at 65 years of age, and in lowering those for women from 2300 at 25 years of age to 1800 calories at 65 years of age. The problem of meal planning for good nutrition of older persons, therefore, is largely one of keeping nutrients *up* and calories adjusted in line with desirable body weight. Dietary studies made in this country on thousands of mature men and women show that in general, this adjustment is not being made satisfactorily. There is much overweight in the aging population, showing calorie intakes in excess of needs, and many clear-cut nutrient shortages indicating poor food choices [7, 8].

Kinds of Food Needed

There is general agreement that, if the diet in early adult life is nutritionally adequate, its general character need not be altered in later years. Protein, mineral and vitamin allowances remain high (Appendix C). If body weight is within the desired range, Diet B may well serve as a guide to general content and menu plan. If the individual is overweight and calories must be reduced, Diet C offers a guide to meals high in *foundation* foods and low in *additional* foods. If the individual is underweight, Diet B may serve as the nucleus for a diet more ample, particularly in *foundation* foods.

Dietary studies show that older people, particularly women, use less than recommended amounts of milk, which accounts for their notably low calcium intake (Chap. 6). They sometimes object to drinking milk because of the bulkiness of the fluid. In that case milk may be used in the preparation of foods. Milk, in dry or liquid form, can be added to casserole dishes, soups, and desserts. Diets low in vitamin A and ascorbic acid, which are common among older people, indicate failure to use adequate amounts of fruits and vegetables. If this is due to poor teeth or ill-fitting dentures, these foods may be served cooked, or even pureed, and combined with other foods. Difficulty in chewing may also serve to curtail the use of meat. Ground or chopped meats circumvent this problem, and eggs, cheese, and cottage cheese provide protein alternates that are easy to eat.

Strengthening the diets of older people can best be achieved by increasing consumption of *foundation* foods. Increasing the intake of *foundation* foods means decreasing the intake of *additional* foods if calorie levels are to be maintained or lowered. Consumption of fats and high fat mixtures can well be curtailed in the later years. Processes of digestion slow down and fat digestion enzymes can handle fat less well than formerly. It is advisable not to tax the mechanism unduly. Sweets also may well be taken in small amounts. They satisfy the appetite easily and fail to yield the nutrients the body needs. Menus for aging individuals are planned in the same way as those for younger adults: to provide the maximum number of *foundation* foods compatible with attractive, edible meals.

Food vs. Pills

Older people should be encouraged to enjoy the ordinary foods of the garden and market instead of "health" foods, special dietary supplements and nutrient concentrates in "pills," which are often advocated. Common foods are cheaper and provide all the nutrients needed under ordinary circumstances. In one study aging people were reported to be taking a variety of "pills" to supplement their diets. However, investigation of the diets proved that the nutrients supplied by the pills were not the ones lacking in their diets [9]. In the main they were the ones already provided amply by the meals; the lacking nutrients could easily have been furnished with a slight adjustment in food choices.

Food Habits

The present state of nutrition of older people depends on their food habits of a lifetime. Poor food habits sometimes leave scars that cannot be erased. Moreover, if people have eaten poorly since childhood the inclination to continue doing so is strong, even though there is great need for change. Often the changes indicated are not drastic: perhaps a regular food source of ascorbic acid or adding milk to the diet is all that is needed. Appetite is often a stumbling block to the eating of adequate meals. Poor appetite may be influenced by many things: living and eating alone, which can lead to introspection and a negative outlook; shopping for one person and cooking in small quantities under unfavorable conditions; limited funds to buy attractive foods and those requiring a minimum of preparation.

In general it may be said that the chief nutrition problem of aging persons lies not in the changing physiological needs of such persons but in devising practical ways of providing them with appetizing, nutritious meals. Many older persons need dietetic and social consultation and aid [10]. They require meals hearty enough to keep up their health and vigor. And, so far as possible, the meals should be eaten in company, which helps them enjoy the food and diverts their attention from real or imaginary ills.

» ADAPTING THE "PATTERN" TO THE GROWTH CYCLE

The daily food pattern given in Chapter 8 takes account of the special needs for growth in 3 ways: a) by specifying varying quantities of milk for different ages and conditions; b) by signifying a regular source of vitamin D; c) by leaving flexible such matters as serving sizes of *foundation* foods and the kinds and amounts of *additional* foods. Let us see how the pattern may be applied in meeting the daily dietary allowances in different segments of the growth cycle [11].

Pregnancy and Lactation

The growth cycle begins long before a child is born. During the prenatal period the baby is nourished solely from his mother's blood. All elements for building and nourishing the baby must come from the mother's food or from her body. The fetus takes priority over the mother with respect to certain nutrients but is spared from harmful excesses by maternal protective mechanisms [12].

Meeting Dietary Allowances The recommended daily dietary allowances and their significance for pregnancy and lactation have been considered for each of the nutrients at appropriate points in Section Two. For convenience, these allowances are summarized in Table 9-2 in comparison with those for the nonpregnant woman of child-bearing age. The increased dietary needs of pregnancy and lactation are indeed striking.

Pregnancy All dietary allowances in pregnancy are increased above the prepregnancy level. Protein, iron, riboflavin, and ascorbic acid are raised by one-fourth to one-half; the calcium allowance is practically doubled; and an allowance is established for vitamin D. The critical need for increasing these nutrients arises during the second half of pregnancy. But, unless the diet has been excellent before pregnancy, the change should be made as soon as pregnancy is

TABLE 9-2

PREGNANCY AND LACTATION: PROGRESSIVE INCREASES IN DAILY DIETARY ALLOWANCES

	Age in years	Calories	Protein g	Calcium mg	Iron mg	Vitamin A IU	Thiamin mg	Riboflavin mg	Ascorbic acid mg	Vitamin D IU
Nonpregnant woman	25	2300	58	800	12	5000	1.2	1.5	70	
Pregnancy, second half		2600	78	1500	15	6000	1.3	2.0	100	400
Lactation		3300	98	2000	15	8000	1.7	2.5	150	400

recognized. If the mother's diet has been fully adequate before pregnancy, the food changes required to meet her new allowances are relatively minor, as will be shown.

The daily food pattern calls for an *addition* of 2 glasses (1 pt) or more of milk daily to the prepregnancy diet and specifies a source of vitamin D that will provide 400 IU. If the prepregnancy diet represents liberal choices from the food pattern and its pint of milk is fortified with vitamin D, the shift to an adequate pregnancy diet may be made merely by adding the additional pint of vitamin D milk. But, even within the framework of the food pattern, the selection of foods may vary widely and the results may be quite different, as demonstrated in Diets A and B. Therefore, the exact additions to be made in building up to a pregnancy diet depend on the content of the original diet before pregnancy.

Using Diet B as the base for a pregnancy diet, Table 9-3 shows what is needed to convert it into a satisfactory pregnancy diet. The total calories and nutrients from Diet B have been transferred to line 1 of Table 9-3. On line 4 are the recommended dietary allowances for the latter half of pregnancy—our objective in this case. By adding values for 2 cups of vitamin D skim milk (line 2) to Diet B values, the dietary allowances for pregnancy are fully or nearly met, with the exception of calories (lines 3 and 4). The shortage in calories is desirable. Undue weight gain in pregnancy is discouraged by physicians. If there is need to keep calories still lower, the 2 cups of vitamin D skim milk may be added to the low-calorie Diet C instead of to Diet B.

But nutritional adequacy is not enough. The total selection of foods must fit into carefully planned meals if they are to be enjoyable and satisfying. As an example, the extra 2 glasses of milk may easily be integrated into the menus suggested for Diet B or C. Meals for the pregnant woman should not be noticeably different from those for other members of the household, and should be enjoyed at the family table.

The daily food pattern offers considerable leeway in the choice and preparation of foods. The meals need not be monotonous. The extra milk, for example, may be taken as a beverage or in cooked foods. Cheese and ice cream may be used in part as alternates for milk (Chap. 8). Practical suggestions for wide choices from the meat, vegetable-fruit, and bread-cereals groups are given in Chapter 8. It is particularly important that a high proportion of the calories be supplied by *foundation* foods.

Despite the ease with which a pregnant woman may obtain an adequate diet from wholesome, familiar foods, the latter are often supplanted in part with multiple

TABLE 9-3

MEETING THE DIETARY ALLOWANCES FOR PREGNANCY

	Calories	Protein g	Calcium mg	Iron mg	Vitamin A IU	Thiamin mg	Riboflavin mg	Ascorbic acid mg	Vitamin D IU
1. Diet B, nutrient contributions	2319	86	971	14.0	8486	1.69	2.14	95	200
+									
2. Vitamin D skim milk, 2 cups	180	18	596	0.2	20	0.20	0.88	4	200
3. Totals	2499	104	1567	14.2	8506	1.89	3.02	99	400
4. *Allowances Latter Half of Pregnancy*	2600	78	1500	15.0	6000	1.30	2.00	100	400

mineral and vitamin preparations. The use of calcium pills (usually in capsule form with phosphorus and vitamin D) in place of milk is a common substitution. The chief problems involved in this practice are: a) the likelihood that the amount of calcium supplied by the pills fails to meet the calcium allowance; b) failure to obtain from the pills the important other nutrients supplied by the milk; c) the cost of the pills vs. the cost of the milk; and d) the difficulty of preparing tasty and satisfying meals with milk excluded or present in very small amounts.

Figure 9.3 demonstrates the first and second of these problems in substituting calcium pills for milk. It shows the calcium, phosphorus, and vitamin D yields of 6 calcium capsules and of 1 qt of whole milk in relation to the dietary allowances for a pregnant woman for these 3 nutrients. It shows, in addition, the "bonus" in other nutrients from the milk not supplied by the pills.

The results are arresting: a commonly used brand of calcium capsules taken in maximum dosage supplies only one-third of the daily calcium allowance of the pregnant woman. From your knowledge of calcium distribution in foods, you realize the virtual impossibility of obtaining the additional two-thirds (1000 mg of calcium) needed daily to meet the calcium allowance for pregnancy if milk is eliminated from the diet. A similar comparison on the basis of phosphorus and vitamin D yields shows that the capsules provide about 25 percent of the estimated need for phosphorus, but 500 percent of the vitamin D allowance—an excess that may be a liability, as has been pointed out in Chapter 7.

A quart of milk, on the other hand, supplies about three-fourths of the calcium and phosphorus allowances, and 100 percent of the vitamin D allowance. The bonus is 24, 26, 46, and 84 percent of the recommended allowances for thiamine, vitamin A, protein, and riboflavin, respectively. Milk is often limited in pregnancy diets because it is thought to be fattening. If gaining weight is a problem, skim milk, which yields only one-half the calories of whole milk, may be used in place of whole milk. If skim milk is used, vegetables and fruits must be chosen with special care for their vitamin A value.

In the considered opinion of many physicians who are doing research on the nutrient needs of pregnancy, supplementation of the pregnancy diet with pills and special concentrates is ill advised [13,14]. They point out that excessive intakes above the recommended dietary allowances do not bestow protective benefits. One research group has said, on the basis of studies at Vanderbilt University, that "the common obstetric routine of broad-spectrum nutritional supplementation is questioned both as to need and as to dosage level. It is felt that the essential nutrients can be readily obtained from food sources" [15].

A new awareness of dietary interrelationships, a benefit to be derived from foods, as such, and not from isolated nutrients, may well serve as an added deterrent. One physician investigator says: "The principal lessons to be learned by surveying the mass of new information on interrelationships of nutritive factors are a humble respect for nutritive balance in foods and a healthy skepticism of indiscriminate administration of single supplements" [16].

On the basis of the information presented here, any price paid for calcium pills is high providing the mother can take and enjoy milk and other common foods. Excessive nutrients of any kind are financially extravagant, wasteful of nutrients, and in the case of certain vitamins, may actually be harmful to health.

In spite of the ease with which the dietary allowances for pregnancy can be met by eating everyday foods, many women fail to attain them. Considerable effort has been made to determine what, if any, relationship exists between the diet of the mother, the course of her pregnancy, and the nutrition and health of the baby. A study at Harvard University showed that in a group of pregnant women, 94 percent of those whose diets were rated "excellent" or "good," in that they met or practically met the dietary

Fig. 9.3 Calcium pills and milk: A comparison of their nutrient contributions.

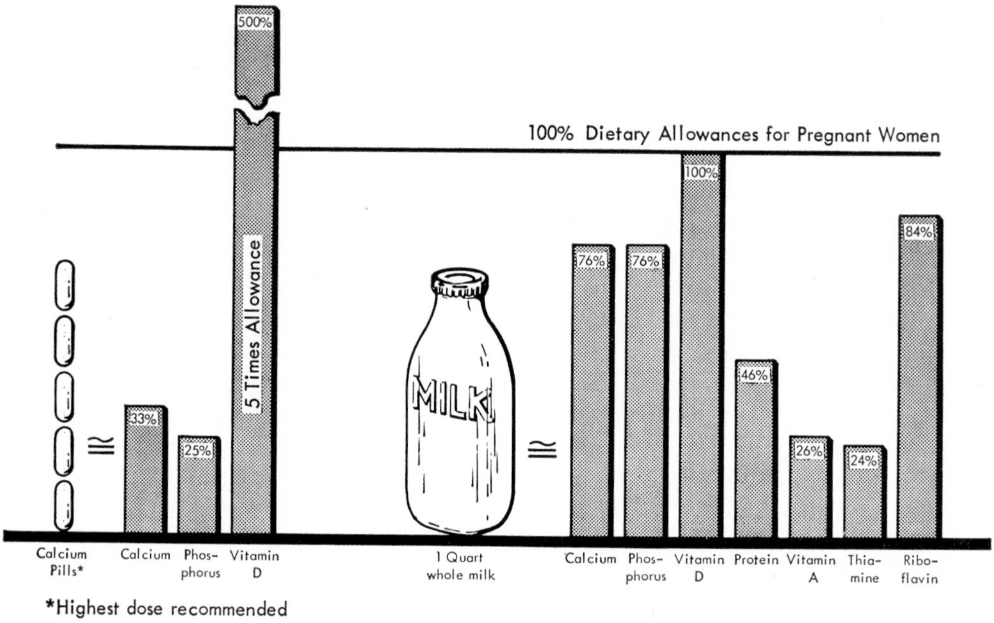

allowances, gave birth to babies who were classed as "excellent" or "good." In contrast, 67 percent of the infants born to women whose diets during pregnancy were "very poor" were in the least favorable physical condition at birth. The investigators point out that the poor diets in their series of 216 women were faulty not only during pregnancy, but were chronically poor prior to conception. They comment: "It seems very probable that the mother's nutritional state at the time she enters pregnancy, as well as the quality and quantity of her diet during pregnancy, may be an important factor in determining the condition of the infant at birth" [17].

Lactation The adequacy of the pregnancy diet not only determines the mother's ability to supply nutrients to the fetus but also determines her ability to produce breast milk of adequate quantity and concentration to meet the needs of the infant later. The adequacy of the lactation diet of the mother determines whether there will be a continuing supply of high quality milk. And good nutrition of a breast-fed baby is most readily attained when the baby receives an ample amount of mother's milk of high nutrient content.

The most obvious difference between the daily food patterns for pregnancy and for lactation lies in the 6 or more glasses of milk recommended for nursing mothers (Table 8-1). Other differences are obscured by the "or more" phrase in the recommendations for *foundation* foods. The need for the added foods is borne out by the high dietary allowances for lactation in comparison with those for the pregnant and nonpregnant adult, as shown on Table 9-2. Using the totals for a pregnancy diet (Table 9-3, line 3) as the base, let us see what is needed to convert an adequate pregnancy diet into a satisfactory lactation diet. All dietary allowances except iron and vitamin D are increased 25 percent or more. Calcium and vitamin A are raised by one-third and ascorbic acid by one-half above the pregnancy level.

Two ways are shown in Table 9-4 of increasing the nutrient level from a pregnancy to a lactation diet. In method 1, 2 cups of *whole* milk and ½ cup of orange juice are added to the pregnancy diet. All nutrient allowances for the lactation diet are thus met. In method 2, 2 cups of *skim* milk and ½ cup of broccoli are added to the pregnancy diet. The skim milk supplies the extra calcium needed and the broccoli provides the vitamin A and ascorbic acid. (Any one of the "greens" might have been used in place of the broccoli for vitamin A value but not for ascorbic acid.) The second method offers a generally more liberal nutrient supply in relation to lactation allowances, with a saving of nearly 200 calories. As in pregnancy, it is desirable to keep calories low enough to prevent undue weight gain. The extra 2 cups of milk proposed for methods 1 and 2 need not carry 200 units of vitamin D. However, this modest surplus is not considered an excess. Had the pregnancy diet been inadequate in one or more nutrients, the problem would have been much more difficult. It would undoubtedly have been necessary to add several foods to meet the dietary allowances for lactation.

Meals during lactation should continue to be inviting and enjoyable, with wide choices made from the various categories in the daily food pattern. The discrepancy in calories between calculated totals and recommended allowances as shown on Table 9-4 may easily be bridged by larger servings, if desired. If the larger servings are from the *foundation* food groups, they will provide a comfortable surplus of nutrients to take care of varying individual needs. Die-

TABLE 9-4

TWO WAYS OF MEETING DIETARY ALLOWANCES FOR LACTATION

	Calories	Protein g	Calcium mg	Iron mg	Vitamin A IU	Thiamin mg	Riboflavin mg	Ascorbic acid mg	Vitamin D IU
1									
1. Pregnancy Diet Table 9-3, line 3	2499	104	1567	14.2	8506	1.89	3.02	99	400
+									
2. Vitamin D whole milk, 2 cups	330	18	570	0.2	780	0.16	0.84	4	200
+									
3. Orange Juice, ½ cup	60	1	13	0.3	250	0.11	0.03	46	—
4. Totals	2889	123	2150	14.7	9536	2.16	3.89	149	600
5. *Lactation Allowances*	3300	98	2000	15.0	8000	1.7	2.5	150	400
2									
1. Pregnancy Diet Table 9-3, line 3	2499	104	1567	14.2	8506	1.89	3.02	99	400
+									
2. Vitamin D skim milk, 2 cups	180	18	596	0.2	20	0.20	0.88	4	200
+									
3. Broccoli, cooked, ½ cup	20	3	98	1.0	2550	0.05	0.11	56	—
4. Totals	2699	125	2261	15.4	11,076	2.14	4.01	159	600
5. *Lactation Allowances* (Table 9-2)	3300	98	2000	15.0	8000	1.7	2.5	150	400

tary supplements are to be avoided here, as in pregnancy, unless there is reason, determined by a physician, for eliminating certain foods from the diet. In that case, supplements should be prescribed that supply the specific nutrients that are missing.

► *Show various ways in which Diet A in Figure 8.1 for an adult (inadequate in iron and thiamine) may be made into one which meets the daily dietary allowances for pregnancy.*

Building on this pregnancy diet, show ways to meet the daily dietary allowances for lactation, other than those used in Table 9-4.

Childhood

Here we are largely concerned with applying the daily food pattern to the diets of children who are old enough to eat regularly at the family table. Planning the diets of infants is the province of the physician. Whether a baby is fed from the breast or bottle, other foods are added daily to his diet of milk. Such additions serve 2 purposes: they assure the nutritional adequacy of his diet, and they accustom him, gradually, to the common foods he will eat throughout his life. The physician in charge indicates the foods to add, when they are to be added, and the forms in which they are to be fed. By the end of the first year, the baby is usually on a daily 3–5-meal schedule and he is eating a variety of foods covered by the daily food pattern. By the time he is 2 years old, he is routinely eating his meals with the family, and few adjustments need be made in family menus to suit his needs.

Adapting the daily food pattern (Table 8-1) to the requirements of children of different ages is largely a matter of adjusting a) the number of servings of milk; b) the sizes of servings of other *foundation* foods; and c) the quantities and kinds of *additional* foods commensurate with total energy requirements. Table 9-5 shows one example of the way a family's menus may be adapted to the needs of 3 age groups—

TABLE 9-5

SAMPLE MEALS, FROM THE SAME MENUS, FOR THREE AGES OF CHILDHOOD MEALS BASED ON THE DAILY FOOD PATTERN

5 Years Old*	10 Years Old*	15 Years Old* (Boy)
Breakfast	**Breakfast**	**Breakfast**
Orange	Orange	Orange
Whole-grain cereal: ½ cup	Whole-grain cereal: ⅔ cup	Whole-grain cereal: 1 cup
Milk: ⅓ cup	Milk: ½ cup	Milk: ¾ cup
Toast: 1 slice	Toast: 2 slices	Toast: 3 slices
Butter:† 1 tsp	Butter:† 2 tsp	Butter:† 3 tsp
Milk: 1 glass	Milk: 1 glass	Jam: 2 tbsp
		Ham: 1 slice
		Cocoa: 2 cups
Dinner	**Lunch**	**Lunch**
Creamed eggs: ½ cup	Creamed eggs: ½ cup	Creamed eggs: 1 cup on toast
Green cabbage: ¼ cup	Cole slaw: ¾ cup	Cole slaw: 1 cup
Roll: 1	Roll: 1	Rolls: 2
Butter:† 1 tsp	Butter:† 1 tsp	Butter:† 2 tsp
Stewed fruit: ⅓ cup	Stewed fruit: ½ cup	Stewed fruit: 1 cup
Cookie: 1	Cookie: 1	Cookies: 2
Milk: 1 glass	Milk: 1 glass	Milk: 2 glasses
Supper	**Dinner**	**Dinner**
Meat patty: 1 (small)	Meat patty: 1 (large)	Meat patty: 2 (large)
Baked potato: 1 (small)	Baked potato: 1 (medium)	Baked potato: 1 (large)
Butter:† 1 tsp	Butter:† 1 tsp	Butter:† 1 tbsp
Carrots: ¼ cup	Carrots: ½ cup	Carrots: ¾ cup
Bread: 1 slice	Bread: 2 slices	Bread: 3 slices
Butter:† 1 tsp	Butter:† 2 tsp	Butter:† 3 tsp
Tomato: 2 slices	Tomato: 2 slices	Tomato: 3 slices
Applesauce: ½ cup	Apple pie: 1 slice	Apple pie: 1 large slice
Milk: 1 glass	Milk: 1 glass	Milk: 1 glass

* Approximate ages.

† Or margarine fortified with vitamin A.

5-, 10-, and 15-year-old children, all eating from the same table and enjoying almost identical foods.

Let us test the meals of the 10-year-old child to see a) how closely they adhere to the daily food pattern, and b) whether they meet the recommended daily dietary allowances for 10–12-year-old children (see Diet D, Fig. 9.4).

Daily Food Pattern The list of foods on the extreme left in Diet D, in the quantities used, meets the amounts and kinds specified for children by the daily food pattern: *Milk group*—the 3½ glasses (cups) of vitamin D milk used for drinking, with some additional milk in the creamed eggs, meets the specification of "3 to 4 glasses of milk for children." *Meat group*—the meat patty and creamed egg satisfy the minimum of "2 or more servings" in this group. Both are liberal servings, however, and both provide animal proteins. *Vegetable-fruit group*—the "4 or more servings" required for this group are liberally met with 4 servings of vegetables and 2 servings of fruit. Equally important, a deep-yellow vegetable, carrots, and a rich source of ascorbic acid (orange) are included. *Bread-cereal group*—the 4 slices of enriched bread, 1 enriched roll, and 1 serving of oatmeal fully satisfy the recommendation for "4 or more servings" in this group. These foods, together with suitable *additional* foods, are combined in the menus that accompany Diet D.

Daily Dietary Allowances The calculations for Diet D show that the *foundation* foods alone, in the kinds and amounts suggested for the 10-year-old, meet the daily dietary allowances proposed for children in this age bracket, except for calories. Because of growth requirements, the nutrient needs of children are proportionately higher in terms of body size than those for adults. Comparing the allowances for the 10–12-year-old group with those for adults (Appendix C), the former are as high or higher in nearly every nutrient than those at the various levels of adulthood, except pregnancy and lactation. They are strikingly similar to those of the 25-year-old woman, except for calcium, which is one-third higher for the child; calories, protein, thiamine, riboflavin, and ascorbic acid are also slightly higher for childhood.

The allowances for children are high, but they are met with relative ease, as shown in Diet D. The higher calorie allowance for the child is a favorable factor. It gives the meal planner a liberal calorie "budget" within which to allocate his "expenditures" for the nutrients. In addition, the higher milk quota for children called for by the daily food pattern makes it possible to attain the greater daily allowance for calcium needed for growth, and results in a desirably high proportion (75 percent) of calories "spent" for *foundation* foods.

It is safe to assume that by adjusting quantities of foods in line with total energy needs, the nutrient allowances of the 5-year-old and the 15-year-old are similarly met by the meals suggested (Table 9-5). Characteristics of meals at the different age levels represented will be discussed briefly. In Section Two, the significance of the recommended daily dietary allowances for the different nutrients in childhood is analyzed and ways to attain them are demonstrated with small groupings of foods. In addition, data are reported on the adequacy of diets in childhood with respect to these same nutrients. It is pertinent for students to review this information in connection with the present problem of applying the daily food pattern to planning meals for children. Figures 9.5 and 9.6 in particular should be considered in relation to Figures 3.4 and 3.5. The former are reminders of the growth

Fig. 9.4 (a) Diet D: A child's diet, based on the daily food pattern.

To Meet the Daily Dietary Allowances of Children 10-12 Years of Age

Foods	Measures	Calories	Protein (g)	Calcium (mg)	Iron (mg)	Vitamin A Value (IU)	Thiamine (mg)	Riboflavin (mg)	Ascorbic acid (mg)	Vitamin D (IU)
Foundation Foods										
1. Milk Group										
Milk, whole vitamin D	3 1/2 cups	578	32	998	0.4	1365	0.28	1.47	7	350
2. Meat Group										
Meat Patty	1 large	245	21	9	2.7	30	0.07	0.02	---	---
Egg, creamed	1/2 cup	190	9	103	1.2	928	0.07	0.25	tr.	50
3. Vegetable-fruit Group										
Coleslaw	3/4 cup	75	2	36	0.5	60	0.05	0.05	38	
Carrots	1/2 cup	20	1	19	0.5	9065	0.04	0.04	3	
Tomato	2 slices	15	1	8	0.5	820	0.04	0.03	18	
Potato, baked	1 medium	90	3	9	0.7	tr.	0.10	0.04	20	
Orange	1 medium	70	1	63	0.3	290	0.12	0.03	66	
Prunes, stewed	1/2 cup	160	1	21	1.5	733	0.03	0.06	1	
4. Bread-cereal Group										
Oatmeal	2/3 cup	100	3	14	1.1	0	0.15	0.03	0	
Bread, enriched	4 slices	240	8	76	2.4	tr.	0.24	0.20	tr.	
Roll, enriched	1, yeast	115	3	28	0.7	tr.	0.11	0.07	tr.	
Totals, Foundation Foods		1898	85	1384	12.5	13,291	1.30	2.29	153	400
Dietary Allowances for Children 10-12 Years of Age		2500	70	1200	12.0	4500	1.30	1.80	75	400
Additional Foods										
Sugar	1 tsp	17	0	0	0	0	0	0	0	
Butter**	2 tbsp	210	0	0	0	920	0	0	0	
Cookies*	1, assorted	110	2	6	0.2	0	0.01	0.01	0	
Apple pie*	1/8 of 9" pie	290	3	8	0.4	193	0.04	0.02	1	
Totals, Additional Foods		627	5	14	0.6	1113	0.5	0.03	1	
GRAND TOTALS		2525	90	1398	13.1	14,404	1.35	2.32	154	400

*Pie and cookies are borderline foods with respect to classification as foundation foods. Each food of this type should be judged on an individual basis, depending on the kind and quantity of ingredients. They are classed here as additional foods. This is sound procedure, particularly in children's diets, because such foods, high in fat and sugar, usually have a disproportionately low yield of nutrients to calories.

**or margarine fortified with vitamin A

and development that take place in a well-nourished boy between the ages of 2 and 17 years. The latter provide the evidence that nutrients in common foods supply the building material to support this growth.

Preschool Age By the time a child is 2 years old he will, ideally, have learned to know and like most of the common foods that will be available to him throughout life. He may be less interested in food than formerly due to the slower growth rate and the many distractions at this age. A *smaller* appetite, however, should not necessarily be interpreted as a *poor* appetite, and a less eager eater should not be allowed to develop

Fig. 9.4 (b) Menus based on Diet D.

Foundation Foods (75 percent of total calories)		Calories		Additional Foods		Calories
			BREAKFAST			
Orange	1 medium	70				
Oatmeal	2/3 cup	100	+	Sugar	1 tsp	17
+ milk, whole	1/2 cup	83				
Toast, enriched	2 slices	120		Butter*	2 tsp	70
Milk, whole	1 glass	165				
			LUNCH			
Creamed eggs	1/2 cup	190				
Coleslaw	3/4 cup	75				
Roll, enriched	1, yeast	115	+	Butter*	1 tsp	35
Prunes, stewed	1/2 cup	160				
Milk, whole	1 glass	165				
				Cookie	1	110
			DINNER			
Meat Patty	3 ounces	245				
Potato, baked	1 medium	90	+	Butter*	1 tsp	35
Carrots, cooked	1/2 cup	20				
Tomato, raw	2 slices	15				
Bread, enriched	2 slices	120	+	Butter*	2 tsp	70
Milk, whole	1 glass	165				
				Apple pie	1/8	290
			BETWEEN MEALS			
		Food for snacks may be taken from the regular meals, as bread, butter, fruit.				
	Total Calories	1898			Total Calories	627

GRAND TOTAL, CALORIES for the DAY — 2525

*or margarine fortified with vitamin A

into a problem eater because of over-anxious adults.

The preschool child's meals will be chosen from the daily food pattern. Ordinarily, he will have about 3 cups of milk daily. The variety of meats, vegetables, fruits, and cereals recommended is practically unlimited. Only the amounts and sometimes the forms of the foods are adjusted to meet his needs. On Table 9-5, for example, only minor changes in the menus of the 10- and 15-year-olds are made for the 5-year-old. Other than smaller servings, the chief adjustments involve these substitutions: cooked cabbage instead of raw; applesauce instead of apple pie; and plain milk instead of cocoa. These changes would not necessarily be made in all cases. Foods should be prepared simply for preschool-age children. They prefer them that way and they learn to enjoy individual foods for their own distinct flavors.

School Age The meals of the school-age child are merely an extension of the preschool diet. On entering school, he has many new interests, the regular companionship of other children, and usually more

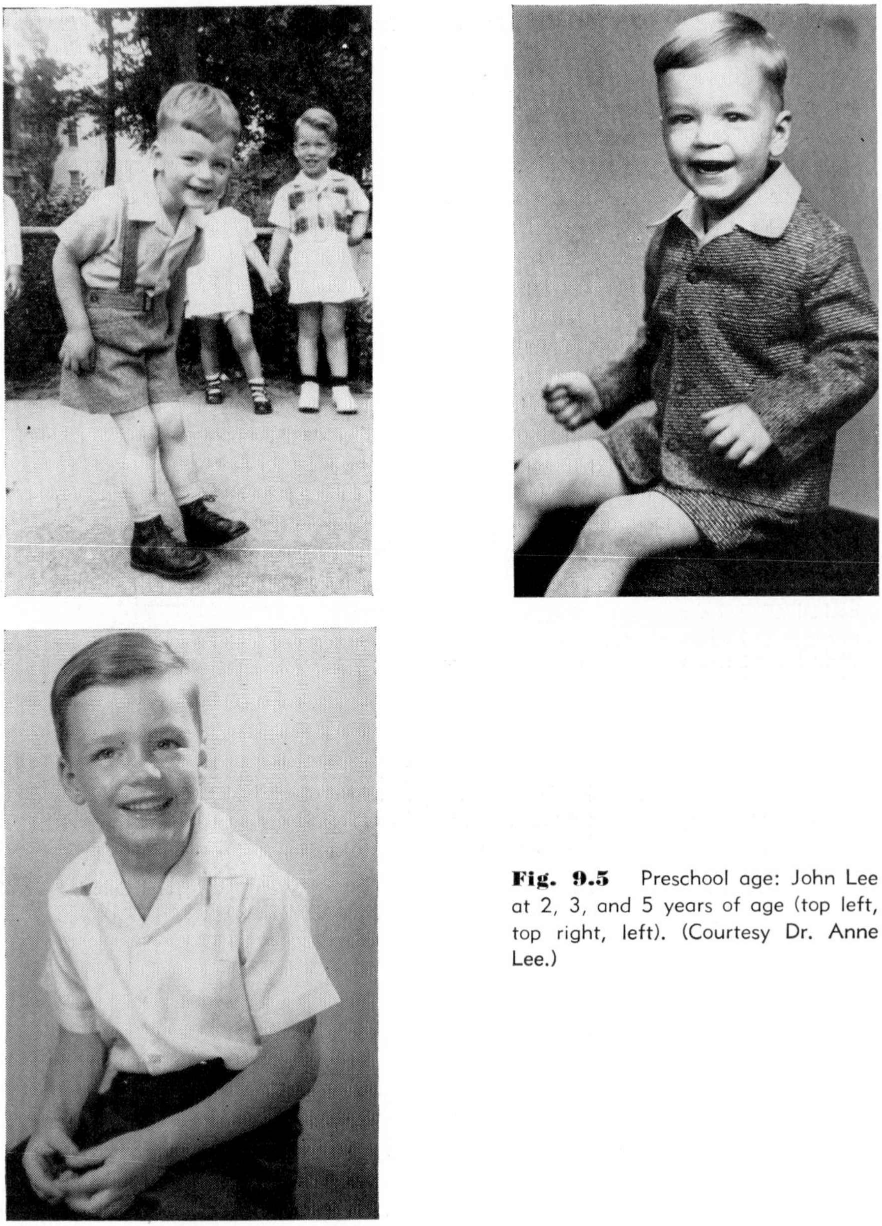

Fig. 9.5 Preschool age: John Lee at 2, 3, and 5 years of age (top left, top right, left). (Courtesy Dr. Anne Lee.)

outdoor activities—all of which help to create a new outlook on food. If a child eats lunch at school, this is a new development in the day's meal schedule. The lunch should continue to be the same ample, well-balanced meal to which he is accustomed, whether he eats it at home, carries it from home, or buys it at school. Often the school nutrition program and/or the school lunch will acquaint him with new foods and stimulate an interest in foods, their preparation, and their association in meals.

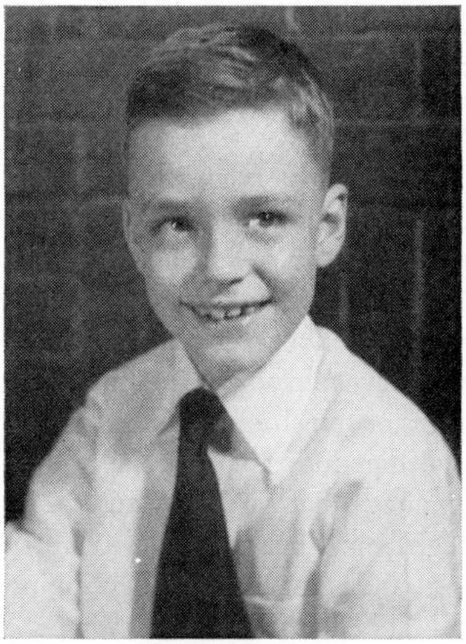

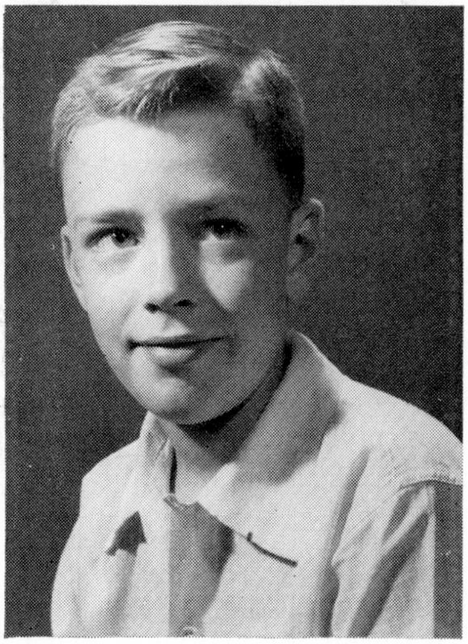

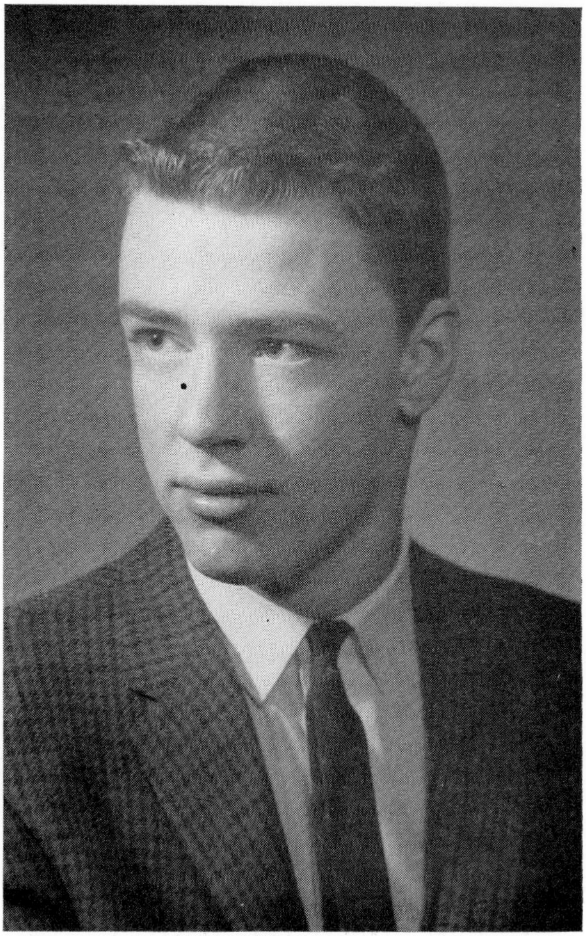

Fig. 9.6 School age: John Lee at 8½, 12, and 17 years of age (top left, left, above). (Courtesy Dr. Anne Lee.)

Good food habits at this period are sometimes maintained with difficulty [18]. A child's early and hurried breakfast, lunch away from home, the pressure of outside activities, and the consequent encroachment on sleep, may lead to appetite problems—either over- or undereating. Cooperation of the home and school in maintaining a moderate, well-planned schedule goes far in keeping him well nourished at this period.

Adolescence and the Teens

A comparison of the meals for the 3 age levels of childhood in Table 9-5 shows that those for the 15-year-old boy differ from the others chiefly in the following: more milk and milk-made dishes; larger servings of most foods—meat, eggs, vegetables, fruits, and cereals; and foods added, such as a breakfast meat and jam. The additional milk is called for specifically on the daily food pattern under "4 or more glasses" for teenagers. The larger servings of the other foods are required to meet the much higher calories and nutrient allowances at this period.

A study of the recommended dietary allowances from the 4–6-year-old age level to the late teens shows that the calorie allowance more than doubles in the case of boys (Appendix C). The same is essentially true for protein, vitamin A, thiamine, riboflavin, and ascorbic acid. The rise is only slightly less for calcium and iron. For boys in their teens, the allowances are higher than for adult men; for girls at this age, the allowances are higher than for any other period except pregnancy and lactation [19]. Thus a child about 5 years of age has a diet that yields approximately 1700 calories; by the time he is 10–12 years of age, it has risen to 2500 calories; and, in the case of a boy in his midteens it has increased to about 3500 calories. If the diet is to be nutritionally adequate, the foods must be carefully selected to assure that a corresponding increase in nutrients accompanies the rise in calories. This means strong emphasis on *foundation* foods.

In the face of these high calorie and nutrient needs, surveys of teen-agers' diets show that they are less adequate than those of any other age group. Specific nutrient inadequacies have been discussed in Section Two. In general, it may be said that boys' diets in this age group are more nearly adequate than are the girls', but their intakes are, on the average, below allowance levels in thiamine and ascorbic acid. Girls' diets are grossly deficient in calcium and iron, are lacking in thiamine, riboflavin, and ascorbic acid, and are borderline in calories and protein.

Adolescent boys and girls are growing physically at a rapid rate and developing emotionally as well. It is a period of transition to adult life. For many, it is a time of stress. These changes call for vigor, stamina, and a wholesome outlook on life that come only with good health. For girls, it is significant as a preliminary step to motherhood. One-third or more of all first-born children today are born to mothers in their teens. The greatly increased nutrient needs of pregnancy have already been discussed. The difficulties of transforming an extremely poor teen-age diet into a nutritionally adequate pregnancy diet are obvious. The course of a girl's pregnancy, her own nutritional status, and that of her developing baby are all at stake. The importance of good food habits throughout childhood and adolescence, carried on into adulthood, is apparent.

Teen-age boys usually eat better than do girls of the same age, chiefly because they have better appetites and therefore consume more food. Boys' diets are low in ascorbic acid largely because they tend to shun the vegetable-fruit group in favor of more substantial fare. Girls, on the other hand, consume small total quantities of food and take less milk, meat, and enriched cereals than specified by the daily food pattern.

Breakfast The poor food habits of teen-agers take many forms. One is that of slighting or skipping breakfast. This is particularly true of girls, and they give various reasons for it: they are not hungry in the morning; there isn't time to eat; they don't like the foods for breakfast; and they don't like to cook their own meal and eat it alone when mother doesn't get up or has already gone to work.

Another reason they give for skipping a meal is to cut down on calories and thus try to control weight. The likelihood of accomplishing just the opposite has been suggested earlier in this chapter. Figure 9.7 is a graphic representation of how the "no-breakfast" habit can work to increase rather than decrease total calories for the day. The most serious outcome of the slighted breakfast is its adverse effect on the vitality and performance of the persons who skip the meals (Chap. 2). A well-balanced breakfast that supplies about one-fourth of the daily calorie allowance and includes a serving of animal protein will usually provide its share of the needed nutrients and will help start the day with vigor. Overweight among teen-age girls is not uncommon, despite their efforts to combat it. Their greatest hope for doing so successfully lies in eating a relatively low-calorie, high-nutrient diet based on the same principles as outlined for weight control in adults.

Fad Diets Teen-agers are addicts of fad diets. Again, girls are the worse offenders, particularly in their use of fad reducing diets. They often try to live for considerable periods of time on diets drastically low in calories and nutrients. Sometimes they succeed in keeping themselves extremely thin, as they wish to be, and as a result they are under par physically. In other cases they fail to stay long on the low-calorie diet and soon gain back the weight they may have lost. The dangers of fad diets to health and

Fig. 9.7 Eat Breakfast—Lose Weight! (Courtesy Quaker Oats Company.)

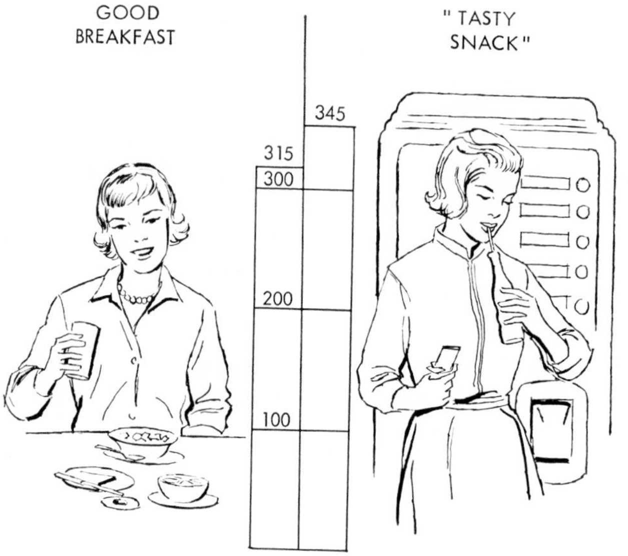

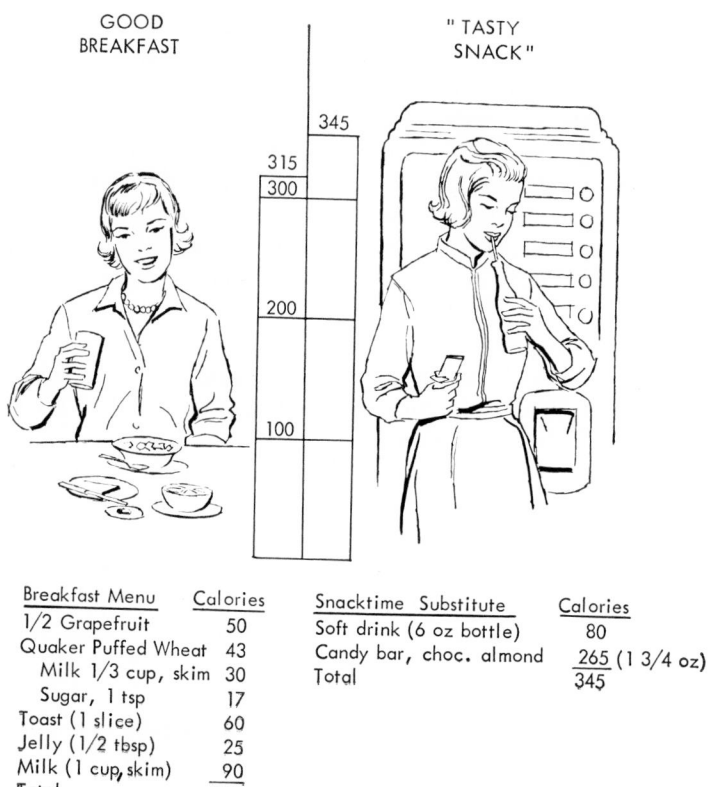

Breakfast Menu	Calories
1/2 Grapefruit	50
Quaker Puffed Wheat	43
Milk 1/3 cup, skim	30
Sugar, 1 tsp	17
Toast (1 slice)	60
Jelly (1/2 tbsp)	25
Milk (1 cup, skim)	90
Total	315

Snacktime Substitute	Calories
Soft drink (6 oz bottle)	80
Candy bar, choc. almond	265 (1 3/4 oz)
Total	345

stamina have been dealt with earlier. Such diets are particularly hazardous for young women who are still growing and who must look ahead to greater physical stresses during the reproductive period.

Diets of Athletes For the most part, a teen-ager engaged in sports improves his diet under the motivation of increasing his skill in athletic performance. This is the case when he is encouraged to follow a scientifically acceptable eating pattern, to eat regular meals, and to gain in weight and strength as a phase of his normal growth and development. In such circumstances it is to be regretted that only the relatively few who participate in athletics receive this type of motivation and guidance.

Unfortunately, in some schools, students' ideas of sound nutrition and their food habits are distorted when coaches advocate obsolete ideas with respect to special dietary needs of athletes. This practice persists, even though such theories have been shown to be without foundation in the light of modern medical and nutrition knowledge. A scientist writing recently in a professional journal explains that "The nutritional needs for athletes are really no different from non-athletes; the appetite will take care of any extra calorie need. Training tables for convenience may well be desirable, but the foods served may be the same as for the others—a well-balanced varied diet" [20].

The scientist just quoted—a physician—points out, for example, the fallacy of feeding extremely high protein diets to athletes to replace "muscular substance" supposedly "lost" in heavy muscular exercise. Energy, not protein, needs are increased with exercise. A boy's muscles are growing, but a diet that meets his daily allowance for protein supplies all that he requires. This physician also explodes the theory that the size and composition of the meal eaten immediately before the usual athletic contest of short intense duration, is of paramount importance to the performance of the athlete. He questions vitamin supplementation of diets already adequate, and the use of various proposed "energy aids." He suggests that for the usual regime 3 ample meals daily are desirable for the athlete; for a sports program that is long and exhausting, 5 smaller meals may be more satisfactory.

Coaches sometimes expose athletic teen-agers to negative diet theories that amount to taboos of wholesome foods. One such theory alleges that milk "cuts the wind" and therefore interferes with athletic performance. Despite lack of evidence to substantiate this theory, the practice continues in some quarters. Teen-agers are placed on diets devoid of milk throughout the athletic season, with tea as its usual replacement. The effect of this substitution on the nutritional value of the diet is obvious, particularly if its becomes a habit.

Encouraging boys to adopt drastic reducing diets in order to qualify for lower weight classifications in boxing or wrestling is another practice that has negative implications for nutrition. Boys who must lose 5–25 lbs in a few weeks when they would normally be gaining weight steadily, dehydrate their bodies on low fluid intake and live on diets of 400–500 calories daily. Furthermore, they must maintain this reduced weight status throughout the wrestling or boxing season. Boys consciously starve themselves to achieve these subnormal standards. Thus we have the compelling motivation of athletics acting in reverse. Medical authorities condemn this practice [21].

A well-known veteran coach collaborating with scientific authorities has this to say: "In order to obtain the energy and dexterity necessary for a winning team, week after week, an adequate diet is essential not only on days of a game, but every day. Long-term conditioning is important. In brief periods of very strenuous physical exercise, muscular efficiency depends on energy reserve and training, not on composition or size of the pre-exercise meal . . . there are no magic foods which produce super power or agility. The same meat, milk, eggs, vegetables, fruits, enriched and whole-grain breads and cereals that are fundamental to the health of every person are needed by the athlete" [22].

Snacks Snacks are a part of the food pattern of practically every teen-ager. And the character of snacks can determine whether the total day's diet is nutritionally adequate. If snacks are planned as part of the day's food and in reality represent small extra meals, they can be an asset. If, on the other hand, they consist of a succession of tidbits, they usually contribute little except calories. Studies made on the diets of adolescents in different localities show that snacks vary greatly in kind and amount but, in general, contribute more to the calorie allowance than to the nutrient allowances.

An important nutritional problem of the teens is to obtain enough to eat to satisfy appetite and to support normal growth and activity. The teen-ager whose meals are not satisfying often forms the habit of consuming enormous quantities of food between meals. The first remedial step is to try shifting the emphasis to well-balanced, ample, and satisfying meals. Snacks will then merely supplement and augment the regular meals.

Recognizing the tremendous physiological requirement for food at this age, the home and the school, through the school lunch, should do their utmost to see that regular meals meet the day's dietary allowances. If this is accomplished, the adequacy of the total diet need not hinge on the quality of snacks. Adolescents like to eat snack foods that are popular with their friends. Often these foods contribute little to body needs. When their regular meals are, in themselves, adequate, adolescents have more leeway to follow the mode in choosing snacks. As part of his nutrition education, however, an adolescent should learn to think of his total daily food intake as a unit in relation to dietary allowances, and to evaluate each addition in terms of its nutrient contribution, whether taken at mealtime or between meals.

Snacks for All

The snack habit is not confined to youth. People of all ages enjoy eating more than the traditional 3 times daily. Some do it from habit; others to gain weight; and still others to lose weight. Apparently some individuals can feel satisfied with less food, and thus lose weight, if they eat 5 or 6 times daily instead of 3 times; others merely eat more food by eating frequently, and thus gain weight. The important consideration is the total food consumed in 24 hours in relation to energy need.

In planning menus that involve snacks, 2 rules should apply: a) plan snacks as carefully as you plan regular meals, and within the framework of the daily food pattern; and b) confine selection of snacks to *foundation* foods if the total calorie allowance is low.

Figure 9.8 shows 3 groupings of food that can be used for snacks. Some or all in each group qualify as *foundation* foods. They represent low and moderately high calorie content and they show that foods and drinks, often regarded as interchangeable, vary greatly in nutrient contributions. The first grouping (A), consisting of an equal amount (¾ cup) of a kola-type bev-

Fig. 9.8 Snacks vary in calorie and nutritive content: Percentage contributions of various snacks to the total daily dietary allowances of a young woman. (Only 50 percent of 100 percent scale shown.)

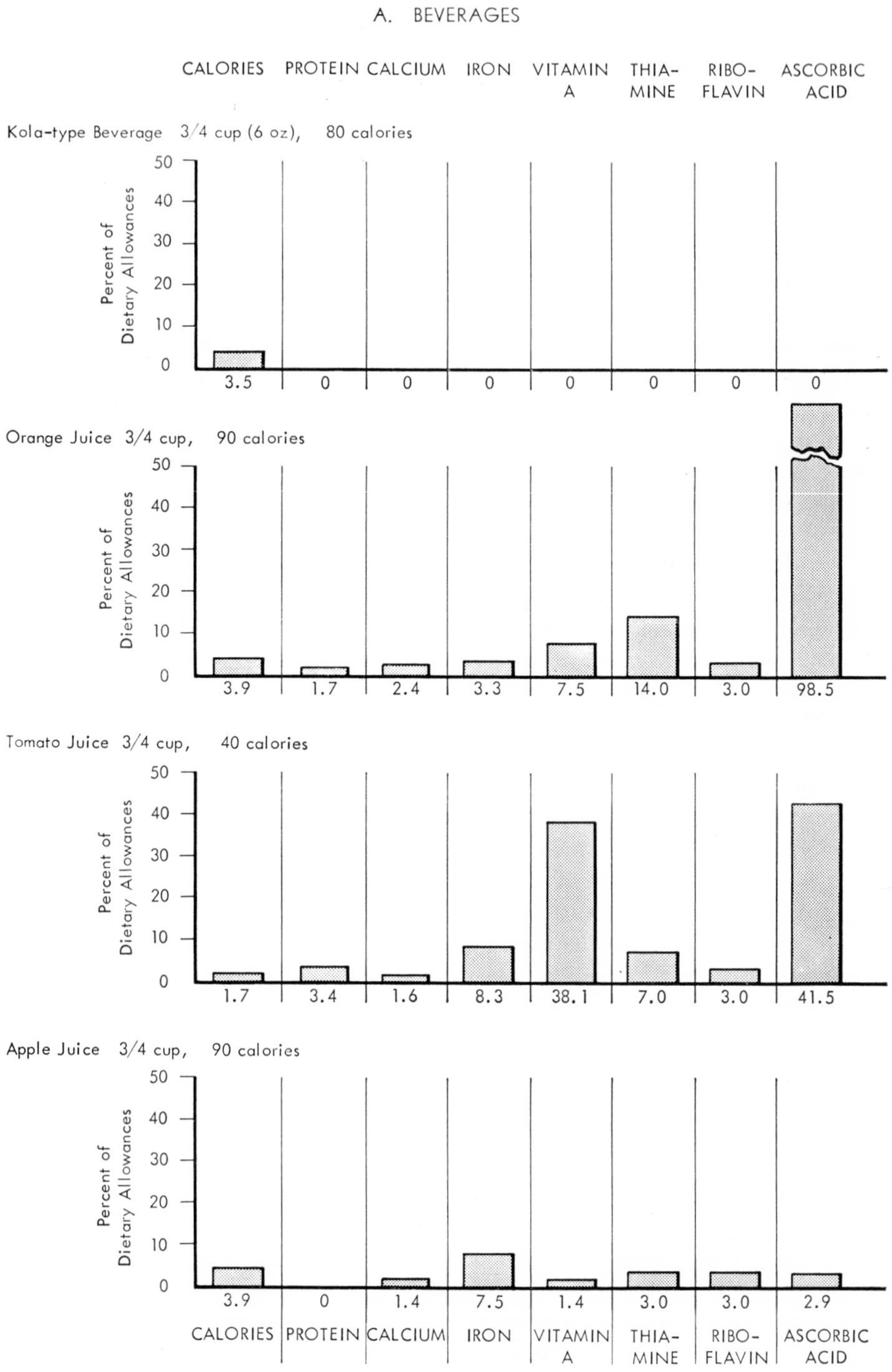

Fig. 9.8 (Continued)

B. FRUITS AND VEGETABLES

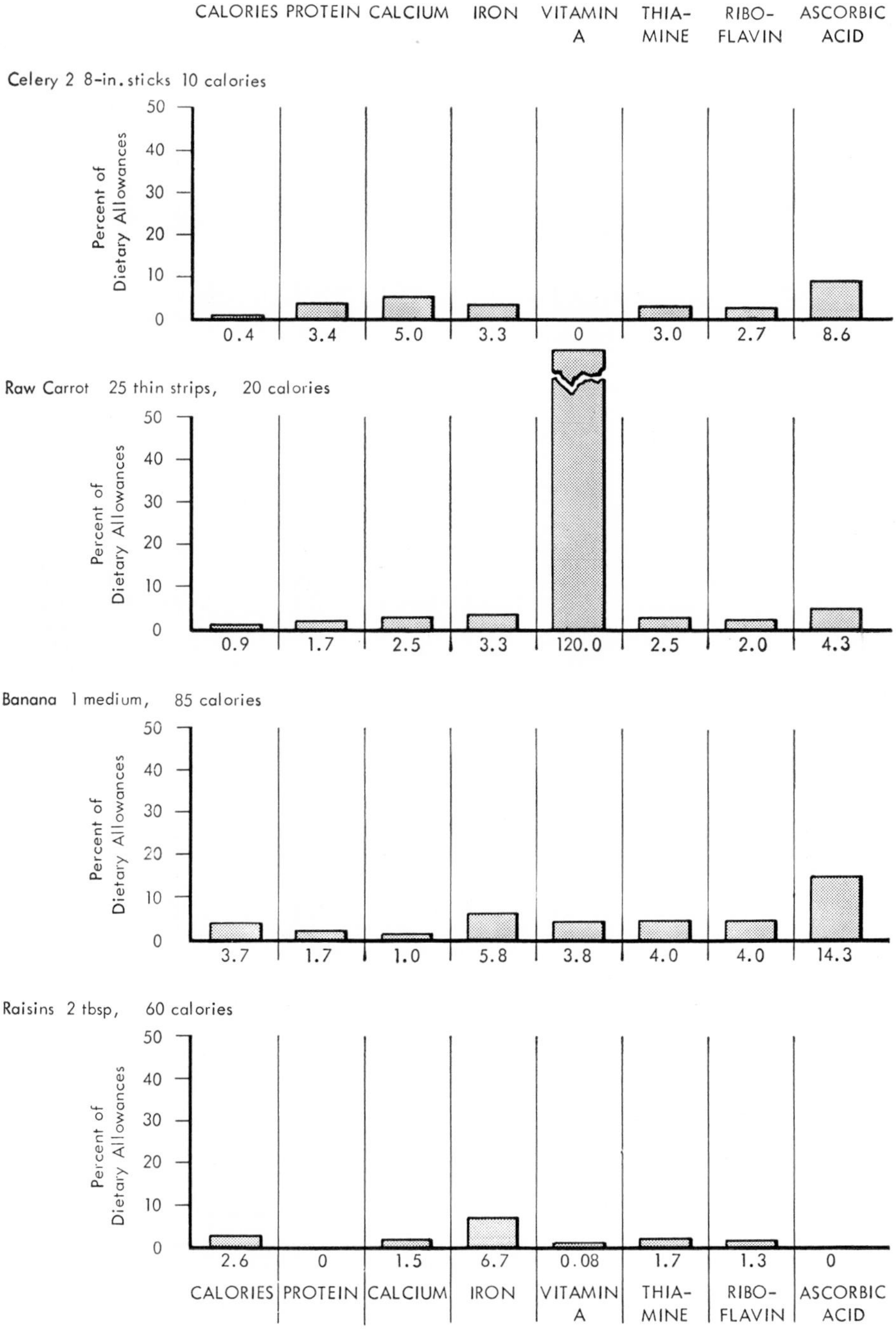

Fig. 9.8 (Conclusion)

C. SUBSTANTIAL SNACKS

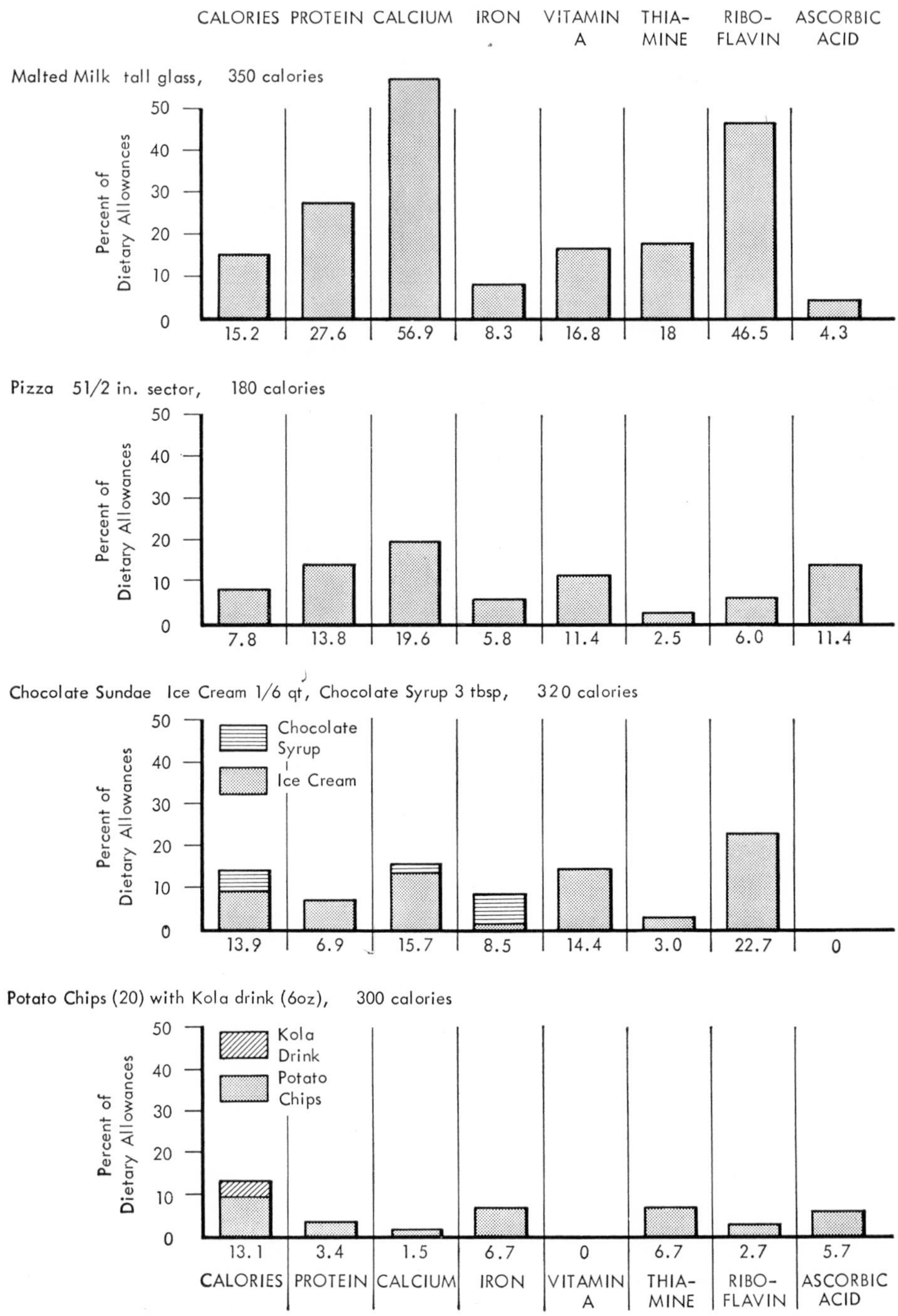
CALORIES PROTEIN CALCIUM IRON VITAMIN A THIAMINE RIBOFLAVIN ASCORBIC ACID
Malted Milk tall glass, 350 calories
Percent of Dietary Allowances
0 10 20 30 40 50
15.2 27.6 56.9 8.3 16.8 18 46.5 4.3
Pizza 51/2 in. sector, 180 calories
7.8 13.8 19.6 5.8 11.4 2.5 6.0 11.4
Chocolate Sundae Ice Cream 1/6 qt, Chocolate Syrup 3 tbsp, 320 calories
Chocolate Syrup
Ice Cream
13.9 6.9 15.7 8.5 14.4 3.0 22.7 0
Potato Chips (20) with Kola drink (6oz), 300 calories
Kola Drink
Potato Chips
13.1 3.4 1.5 6.7 0 6.7 2.7 5.7

erage and 3 fruit and vegetable juices, presents interesting contrasts. Orange and apple juices and the kola drink yield essentially the same food energy—80–90 calories. But the general picture of their nutrient contribution as shown by the height of the bars, is quite different. Orange juice provides a significant amount of several nutrients, particularly ascorbic acid; apple juice is a relatively poor source of practically all of the nutrients; the kola drink furnishes none. Tomato juice, which yields about one-half as many calories as the other 3, makes an excellent showing and is strikingly higher in vitamin A than are the other 2 juices.

The second grouping (B), consists of raw fruits and vegetables that also suggest low-calorie snacks. The range in energy yield is from 10 calories for the celery to 85 calories for the banana. If the purpose is to keep the calories to a minimum, the celery has the advantage because of its contributions, though small, of all nutrients except vitamin A value (bleached celery). Carrots, on the other hand, with only a few more calories, supply more than the total daily allowance for vitamin A value as well as some of the other nutrients. The banana makes the best contribution of ascorbic acid; raisins provide slightly more iron than any other food in this group. Thus, low-calorie snack foods may be evaluated in terms of the dietary needs and preferences of the individual.

In the third grouping (C) are popular snack foods in the higher calorie range: malted milk, chocolate sundae, potato chips with a kola drink and pizza. The first 3 furnish 300–350 calories each; the pizza about one-half that amount. If the calories from such snacks represent a substantial proportion of the total calories for the day, it is particularly important to consider their nutrient yield. The malted milk obviously yields the highest nutritive values, but the pizza (cheese type) also makes important contributions. If the quantity of pizza were doubled to equal the calorie value of malted milk, it would present an impressive picture on the chart. In the chocolate sundae, the ice cream contributes well to nutrient allowances except those for iron and ascorbic acid; the chocolate syrup supplements chiefly the iron. Potato chips make a fair showing of nutrients except in vitamin A. Its beverage accompaniment, a kola drink, provides only calories. This combination, which has essentially the same energy value (or more) as the other 3 snacks, compares unfavorably with them in practically every nutrient.

It should be pointed out that all sections of the chart are developed on the same scale and are therefore comparable. Bases for calculation are the total daily dietary allowances for a young woman. Only the lower half of the 100-percent scale is used because values fall largely in that area. The main purpose here is not to relate nutrients to the allowances but to compare the nutrient contributions of one food with another.

The Coffee Break A more formal aspect of the daily food snack, which has penetrated the business world particularly, is the "coffee break." The refreshment usually consists of coffee, with or without cream and sugar, taken alone or with a sweet breadstuff of some kind. The calorie yield may be rather high if a frosted sweet roll with butter is eaten, or it may be nil if the "break" consists only of black coffee. Whatever may be the accompaniment, the nutrient yield is usually low. This fact has two disturbing aspects: a) the finding that among young office workers the coffee break has been substituted to a large extent for breakfast, and b) the fact reported earlier

(Chap. 2) that the coffee break does not replace a good breakfast in terms of body performance during the morning work hours.

► *Compare some of your own favorite snack foods on the basis used in Figure 9.8.*

What proportion of your total daily calories is taken as snacks? Do your snacks do "their share" in furnishing nutrients?

» ADAPTING THE "PATTERN" TO FAMILY MEALS

Up to this point nutrient needs have been considered for the young adult, the aging person, the individual trying to control his weight, and those who are in the growth cycle of pregnancy, lactation, and childhood. We have seen that the daily food pattern, properly applied in each situation, results in meals that meet the daily dietary allowances for each. But these individuals do not ordinarily eat alone. They are, in varying combinations, the components of families who eat at the same table and partake of the same menu. Family meals, therefore, are in effect the summation of the meals of several individuals, all with different needs and tastes. Providing such meals successfully takes time and effort on the part of the homemaker and requires either a knowledge of nutrition or some reliable practical plan, such as the daily food pattern, for use as a guide.

Planning Family Menus

The characteristics and content of a nutritionally adequate day's food supply have been explored. Particular emphasis has been placed on planning the day's menus as a unit and on making *foundation* foods their basis. The meal planner may pinpoint the adaptation of the daily food pattern further by setting up skeleton menus for breakfast, lunch, dinner, and between-meal foods. She will develop her own skeleton menu plans based on the particular habits of her family. They will take into account such individual meal needs as packed lunches and regular bedtime snacks. Skeleton meal plans are merely a "crutch" for the planner in interpreting the daily food pattern from day to day. They serve as reminders to make meals varied and nutritious. They are flexible in that for the most part, they suggest the general content of meals, not specific foods.

Table 9-6 illustrates the adaptation of skeleton menu plans to actual menus for breakfast, lunch, dinner, and snacks. The skeleton plan is shown on the left in each column under the headings of the 3 meals and snacks. The menus on the right are those from Diet B, Chapter 8.

The selection of foods, within the framework of the daily food pattern, depends on such factors as the food preferences of the family, the ages and occupations of its members, work schedules, meal habits, and the family budget. The majority of households adhere more or less closely to the 3-meal-a-day plan. To serve meals at regular hours, fairly evenly spaced throughout the day, and similar in energy yield, are good rules to follow. Such a plan provides greater comfort and satisfaction for family members than does haphazard eating and meals that are alternately heavy and light. Meals for a mixed family of children and adults may well be planned with the children chiefly in mind. By the time children reach preschool age, they are usually eating a full variety of foods. Most simple methods of preparation, preferable for children, may be equally acceptable for

TABLE 9-6

SKELETON MENU PLANS

Applied to One Day's Menus

BREAKFAST		LUNCH		DINNER		BETWEEN-MEAL SNACKS	
Skeleton Plan	Menu*	Skeleton Plan	Menu*	Skeleton Plan	Menu*	Skeleton Plan	Menu*
Fruit	Grapefruit	Main dish such as: Sandwich Substantial soup Casserole	Ham sandwich	Main dish such as: Lean meat Fish, fowl Casserole	Pot roast	Fruits Juices Milk drinks Other	Banana
Main dish such as: Cereal Egg Meat	Poached egg	Vegetable	Lettuce Celery	Vegetable	Carrots and peas		
Milk	Milk, whole	Milk	Milk, whole	Salad or relishes	Lettuce salad Fr. dressing		
Breadstuff (enriched)	Toast	Breadstuff (enriched)	Bread in sandwich	Breadstuff (enriched)	Rolls		
Beverage	Coffee			Beverage	Coffee		
		Dessert such as Fruit Cookies Puddings	Baked apple Cookies	Dessert such as: Fruit Cake Pie Frozen desserts	Ice cream		

* Menu from Diet B for young adults.

adults. Quantities of food are, of course, adjusted to suit energy and nutrient needs.

Meals planned on a daily unit basis should be projected in advance and the period planned for may well be synchronized with the shopping schedule. Preplanning for several days or a week saves time, effort, and sometimes money. It gives opportunity to anticipate the foods that can be the basis for more than one meal. It still permits substituting one comparable food for another at the market to take advantage of good "buys." Long-range planning pre-supposes a carefully developed market list using the skeleton menu plans as a guide.

Planning to meet the specifications of the daily food pattern for each member of the family is the most challenging aspect of the job. Specifically, it involves estimating the number of servings of each food needed by each individual in the family group for a specified period and transferring the total to the market list in units to be purchased. One simple example: if 4 full-size (¼ lb raw) hamburgers and 2 half-size (⅛ lb) hamburgers are needed for a meal, the total amount of meat to be purchased is 1¼ lbs. Milk offers little or no problem in estimating purchases because of the specificity of the daily food pattern and the easy identification of serving units. Fresh vegetables probably present the greatest difficulty because of the variation in size of units (heads of broccoli, cabbage, etc.), the difference in the amount of trimming needed before use, and the shrinkage in cooking. Facility in buying just enough of the foods needed, but not too much, can best be acquired through experience. Some homemakers use a chart on which they record the numbers of servings they find can be obtained from average market units of foods, as purchased. They gradually build up a body of information that serves as a convenient reference in shopping. Such a chart can be extended to include frozen and canned foods and, if desired, cost per serving as well. The U.S. Department of Agriculture publishes useful information on the amounts to buy per serving of many foods.

Table 9-7 was developed to assure that enough foods from each food group are provided for every member of the family. The plan, worked out for a 1-week period, is based on the daily food pattern; properly followed, it provides the nutrients to meet the daily dietary allowances for all members of the family. Quantities of foods are specified for each age level for both sexes and for pregnancy and lactation. These quantities of foods, expressed in market units of pounds and quarts, are merely translations, on a weekly basis, of the daily servings indicated on the food pattern. Quantities are adapted to age, size, activity needs, and to special conditions. With this type of breakdown, a weekly shopping guide may be tailored to fit a family of any size or composition, merely by adding up the amounts in each food group that will fit the family to be served.

These amounts are only approximations, of course. Needs within age levels vary greatly. Ranges in amounts of foods take care of certain differences in needs (explained in the footnotes to Table 9-7), but individual variations in growth rate and activity must still be allowed for in each family group. Despite slight shifting to fit specific situations, the totals in any given case will provide helpful and important guide lines in furnishing the raw materials for adequate family meals.

► *Make up a weekly shopping list for a hypothetical family of specified size and composition from Table 9-7.*

Price the list on 2 levels: one in which the most economical kinds and forms of

TABLE 9-7
A WEEKLY SHOPPING GUIDE**
Based on the Daily Food Pattern
(Quantities* for one week)

Kinds of food	For children 1–6 years	For children 7–17 years	For girls 13–19 years	For boys 13–19 years	For women		For men, all ages	Totals for week for hypothetical family
					All ages	Pregnant and nursing		
Milk, cheese, ice cream (milk equivalent)†	6 qts	6–6½ qts	7 qts	7 qts	3½ qts	7–10 qts	3½ qts	
Meat, poultry, fish‡	1½–2 lbs	3–4 lbs	4½ lbs	5–5½ lbs	4–4½ lbs	4–5 lbs	5–5½ lbs	
Eggs	6 eggs	7 eggs	7 eggs	7 eggs	6 eggs	7 eggs	7 eggs	
Dry beans and peas, nuts	1 oz	2–4 oz	2 oz	4–6 oz	2 oz	2 oz	2–4 oz	
Grain products (flour equivalent)† Whole-grain, enriched, or restored	1–1½ lbs	2–3 lbs	2½–3 lbs§	4–5 lbs	2–2½ lbs	2–3 lbs	3–4 lbs	
Citrus fruits, tomatoes	1½–2 lbs	2½ lbs	2½ lbs	3 lbs	2½ lbs	3½–5 lbs	2½–3 lbs	
Dark-green and deep-yellow vegetables‖	¼ lb	½–¾ lb	¾ lb	¾ lb	¾ lb	1½ lbs	¾ lb	
Potatoes	½–1 lb	1½–2½ lbs	2 lbs	3–4 lbs	1–1½ lbs	1½–3 lbs	2–3 lbs	
Other vegetables and fruits	3½ lbs	5½ lbs	6 lbs	7 lbs	4–6 lbs	6–6½ lbs	5–7 lbs	
Fats, oils	¼–⅓ lb	½–¾ lb	¾ lb	1–1¼ lbs	½ lb	½–¾ lb	¾–1 lb	
Sugars, sweets	¼–⅔ lb	¾ lb	¾ lb	1–1¼ lbs	½–1 lb	¾ lb	1–1½ lbs	

* When a range is given, unless otherwise noted, the smaller quantity is for younger children, for adults over 55, or for pregnant women.

† For flour equivalent, count 1½ lbs of breads as 1 lb flour. See milk equivalents, Table 8-3.

‡ To meet iron allowance needed by children 1–6-years-old, girls 13–19, and pregnant and nursing women, include weekly 1 large or 2 small servings of liver or other organ meats.

§ The larger quantity is for the younger girls.

‖ If choices within the group are such that the amounts specified are not sufficient for the number of servings suggested on the daily food pattern, Table 8-1 increase the amounts and use less from the "other vegetables and fruits" group.

** *Nutrition up to Date up to You.* (Bulletin) Washington, D.C.: U.S. Department of Agriculture.

foods are purchased within the framework of the plan; one in which no effort is made to economize.[1]

Over and above the mechanics of meal planning is the consideration of the enjoyment factor in eating: the two are entirely compatible. Too often nutritious meals are associated with what one "ought" to eat, not with the foods one most enjoys. The meal planner has the task of reconciling individual preferences in foods as to flavor, texture, aroma, appearance, and even temperature, but experience in feeding a family group soon helps her to assemble in meals those foods which give maximum pleasure and satisfaction. This is achieved most successfully when the children have learned to taste all foods served, to like most of them, and to leave without comment the ones they dislike, and when adults in the household obviously enjoy the foods that make up wholesome meals. A friendly, relaxed atmosphere at mealtime creates the ideal setting for practicing good food habits.

The Food Budget [23]

Fortunately, the cost of a food does not reflect its nutritive value. Some foods are *cheap* at almost any price because of their high yield of nutrients. Others are *expensive* at any price because of their low nutrient yield. Such contrasts in food values have been pointed out repeatedly in the foregoing pages. On a low food budget it is obviously not economical, nutritionally speaking, to skimp on *foundation* foods and to overemphasize high-calorie, low-nutrient *additional* foods, even though the latter may cost less. Because the *foundation* foods carry more than their share of nutrients per calorie, they are regarded as economical. In general, however, these are also the foods in the higher price range. How can we reconcile these apparently contradictory facts and arrive at practical procedures for obtaining a diet that meets the daily dietary allowances at low cost? A few guide lines are here suggested.

The lower the food budget, the more important it is to plan meals carefully and shop for foods prudently. In interpreting the daily food pattern, economies can be effected in several ways, including the following:

1. Wise selection within the food groups: choosing less-expensive but equally nourishing sources of food such as certain cuts of meat, forms of milk, kinds and forms of vegetables and fruits; avoiding specially cooked and prepared foods and those out of season
2. Buying adequate amounts of *foundation* foods within the specifications of the daily food pattern—but not to excess when money is scarce
3. Including somewhat more than the pattern designates, but not excessive amounts, of breads and cereals in their most economical forms. Home-baked products and breakfast foods to be cooked are usually economical
4. Marketing carefully: buying in quantities that permit savings on purchases but in amounts compatible with storage space and ability to use economically
5. Controlling waste: storing shelf foods and leftovers carefully to

---

[1] The U.S. Department of Agriculture issues regularly estimates of average weekly food costs in the United States for individuals of different ages. These estimates represent current costs of providing a nutritious diet on a low, moderate, or liberal food budget. Write the Office of Information, U.S. Department of Agriculture, Washington 25, D.C.

make maximum use of the foods and to preserve the nutrients

6. Taking advantage of special sales on foods *if* they can be used to advantage and if they are really bargains

Food takes almost 20 percent of the total consumer income in the United States. This includes money spent for meals away from home as well as for food purchased for home meals. The percentage of individual family incomes spent for food of course varies greatly. In general, the percentage is much higher among low income groups than among high income groups. In other words, the poorer the family, the larger the proportion of the income that goes for food. In 1950, for example, high income families spent, on the average, only 15 percent of their income for food, but low income families spent about 45 percent. Despite this difference, in most cases the actual outlay for food was much less in low income families.

Families in the United States typically spend their food money in approximately this manner:

more than	50	percent for milk, meat, eggs
about	20	percent for vegetables and fruit
about	10	percent for grain products
about	10	percent for fats, oils, sugars, sweets
about	10	percent for spices, vinegar, leavening agents, coffee, tea, other beverages
	100	percent

Certain broad boundaries for food expenditures are automatically established in applying the daily food pattern to family meal planning. But it is the person who plans, buys, and prepares the family's food who exercises the greatest control. True, there is a low cost limit below which an adequate diet cannot be purchased. However, above this limit but still well within the low-cost zone, one can purchase a diet that is nutritionally adequate and as satisfying and enjoyable as one that costs far more. This may be done if knowledge and ingenuity are applied in practicing the types of economies outlined above.

» GENERAL APPLICATION OF THE DAILY FOOD PATTERN—A SUMMARY

Having tested the daily food pattern under various conditions, what may we conclude about its usefulness to the meal planner? Can it be turned over to a layman without advice or warnings? How can the user be safeguarded?

As stated at the outset, no daily food pattern is applicable to all situations. Many different food combinations can achieve an adequate diet; there are considerable differences in the nutrient needs of individuals and great variations in the nutrient values of foods within the food groups. The fact remains that the use of a carefully developed pattern, designed with available food supplies and prevailing dietary customs in mind, is far better than hit-and-miss planning, or no planning at all. Properly interpreted and applied, a food pattern encourages good food habits. It is important, therefore, to recognize the inherent weak points in any pattern and to take steps to strengthen them so far as possible.

In passing the daily food pattern (Table 8-1) on to a person who has had no experience in applying such a "formula" and has no basis for making decisions with respect to nutritional values, the following points may serve as a nucleus for helpful suggestions you can make.

1. *Choose more than the minimum number of servings of foundation foods.*
   The "or more" phrase on the pattern indicates that more than the minimum number of servings is nutritionally desirable, with the possible exception of the bread-cereal group when calorie intake is restricted. The larger the proportion of calories supplied from *foundation* foods, the greater the prospects for obtaining an adequate diet.
2. *Select foundation foods carefully.*
   Some nutrients are more difficult to obtain from the diet than others, chiefly because they occur in small amounts in most foods. Here are a few good rules to observe in obtaining them: Use organ meats frequently—at least once a week; choose the major representatives of the meat group more regularly than the alternates; make lean pork a weekly or semiweekly item; in choosing a dark green vegetable as a source of vitamin A, be sure it qualifies as such; use citrus fruits and tomatoes often as sources of ascorbic acid.
3. *Count only full servings.*
   In following the food pattern, estimate the number of servings correctly. Do not count as servings trivial amounts such as a leaf of lettuce, a radish, or a slice of apple. Note serving sizes indicated on the food pattern and in Chapter 8. Large servings may count for 2 if the amount warrants it. In other words, 2 servings of 1 vegetable can count the same as 1 serving each of 2 different vegetables. Or, 2 servings of meat may take the place of 1 serving of meat and 1 of a meat alternate.
4. *Use foundation foods as the framework for daily meals.*
   Use the day as a unit in planning meals. Build meals around the *foundation* foods. Enter them first in developing menus. Complete the menus for each day with *additional* foods within the limits of the calorie allowance.
5. *Use additional foods to supplement meals.*
   Include *additional* foods to round out meals, to lend variety in flavor and interest, and to increase satisfaction. Additional foods are insignificant sources of nutrients in relation to their high yield of calories and should therefore not be allowed to dominate the diet. They must be kept in line with the body's energy needs for activity and growth.
6. *Plan on variety in meals for food value and enjoyment.*
   Variety in itself does not assure nutritional adequacy. But with variety, the likelihood of including some of the hard-to-get nutrients is greater than if the choice is confined to a random few foods. Variety in foods and food combinations adds interest and pleasure to meals.

► *Analyze the 6 summary statements regarding the application of the daily food pattern. Criticize the suggestions. What would you delete? How would you alter them?*

What suggestions would you add to protect the user of the daily food pattern?

REFERENCES

1. Lew, E. A., "New Data on Underweight and Overweight Persons," *J. Am. Dietet. Assoc.*, 38 (April 1961) pp. 323–27.
2. Orent-Keiles, E., and Hallman, L. F., *The Breakfast Meal in Relation to Blood Sugar Values.* Circular 827. Washington, D.C.: U.S. Department of Agriculture, 1949.
3. Young, C., "Planning the Low Calorie Diet," *Am. J. Clinical Nutrition,* 8 (Nov., Dec. 1960) pp. 896–900.
4. Council on Foods and Nutrition, "Formula Diets and Weight Control," *J. Am. Med. Assoc.* 176 (May 6, 1961) p. 439. (Editorial, p. 442.)
5. Food and Nutrition Board, Food Protection Committee, *The Safety of Artificial Sweeteners.* Pub. 386. Washington, D.C.: National Academy of Sciences-National Research Council, 1957.
6. Fisher, K. H., and Swift, R. W., "Calories and Body Weight," *Food—The Yearbook of Agriculture.* Washington, D.C.: U.S. Department of Agriculture, 1959. p. 101.
7. Swanson, P., "Nutritional Needs after 25," *Food–The Yearbook of Agriculture.* Washington, D.C.: U.S. Department of Agriculture, 1959. p. 311.
8. Beeuwkes, A. M., "Studying the Food Habits of the Elderly," *J. Am. Dietet. Assoc.*, 37 (Sept. 1960) pp. 215–18.
9. Gillum, H. L., "What Should Oldsters Eat?" *Today's Health,* 36 (July 1958) pp. 53–55.
10. Whitehouse Conference on Aging, *The Nation and Its Older People.* Washington, D.C.: U.S. Department of Health, Education and Welfare, April 1961.
11. Hunscher, H. A., Leverton, R. M., and Cederquist, D., "The Life Cycle and its Diet—a symposium on recent findings in human nutrition," *J. Home Econ. Assoc.*, 49 (Feb. 1957) pp. 101–115.
12. Macy, I. G., and Kelly, H. J., "Food for Expectant and Nursing Mothers," *Food —The Yearbook of Agriculture.* Washington, D.C.: U.S. Department of Agriculture, 1959. p. 273.
13. May, C. D., "Vitamin Supplements," *Pediatrics.* 23 (May 1959) p. 833.
14. McCollum, E. B., "Symposium on Prenatal Nutrition," *J. Am. Dietet. Assoc.*, 36 (March 1960) p. 236–41.
15. McGanity, W. J., Bridgforth, E. B., and Darby, W. J., "Effect of Reproductive Cycle on Nutritional Status and Requirements," *J. Am. Med. Assoc.*, 168 (Dec. 20, 1958) pp. 2138–45.
16. Hepner, R., *Maternal Nutrition and the Fetus, J. Am. Med. Assoc.*, 168 (Nov. 29, 1958) pp. 1774–78.
17. Burke, B. S., Stevenson, S. S., Worcester, J., and Stuart, H. C., "Nutrition Studies during Pregnancy; V. Relation of Maternal Nutrition to Condition of Infant at Birth: Study of Siblings," *J. Nutrition,* 38 (Aug. 1949) pp. 453–67.
18. Lowenberg, M. E., "Between Infancy and Adolescence," *Food—The Yearbook of Agriculture.* Washington, D.C.: U.S. Department of Agriculture, 1959. p. 296.
19. Storvick, C. A., and Fincke, M. L., "Adolescents and Young Adults," *Food—The Yearbook of Agriculture.* Washington, D.C.: U.S. Department of Agriculture, 1959. p. 303.

20. Stare, F. J., "Diets For Athletes," *J. Am. Dietet. Assoc.*, 37 (Oct. 1960) p. 371.
21. Mayer, J., and Bullen, B., "Nutrition and Athletic Performance," *Postgraduate Medicine*, 26 (Dec. 1959) pp. 848–56.
22. Upjohn, B. S., Shea, J., Stare, F. J., and Little, L., "Nutrition of Athletes," *J. Am. Med. Assoc.*, 151 (March 7, 1953) 818–19.
23. *Food—The Yearbook of Agriculture*. Washington, D.C.: U.S. Department of Agriculture, 1959: Waugh, F. V., "What Your Money Buys," p. 557; Page, L., and Cofer, E., "Your Money's Worth," p. 567; Cofer, E., and Clark, F., "Food Plans at Different Costs," p. 576.

READINGS

Cohn, C., "Meal-eating, Nibbling and Body Metabolism," *J. Am. Dietet. Assoc.*, 38 (May 1961) pp. 433–36.

Eppright, M., "Adolescent Nutrition," *Today's Health*, 36 (May 1958) pp. 42–44.

Family Fare—Food Management and Recipes. Home and Garden Bull. 1. Washington, D.C.: U.S. Department of Agriculture, 1960.

Food for Families with School Children. Home and Garden Bull. 13. Washington, D.C.: U.S. Department of Agriculture, 1962.

Food for the Family. New York: Metropolitan Life Insurance Company, 1957.

Food for the Family with Young Children. Home and Garden Bull. 5. Washington, D.C.: U.S. Department of Agriculture, 1961.

Food Guide for Older Folks. Home and Garden Bull. 17. Washington, D.C.: U.S. Department of Agriculture, 1961. (Rev. 1962.)

The Food Way to Weight Reduction. Chicago: National Dairy Council, 1961.

Leverton, R. M., *Food Becomes You*. 2nd ed. Ames: Iowa State University Press, 1960.

———, *A Girl and Her Figure*. Chicago: National Dairy Council, 1959.

Macy, I. G., "Diet for Mothers-to-be," *Today's Health*, 36 (Aug. 1958) pp. 37; 45–48.

Maddox, G., *The Safe and Sure Way to Reduce*. New York: Random House, Inc., 1960.

Metheny, N. Y., Hunt, F. E., Patton, M. B., and Heye, H., "The Diets of Preschool Children," I. Nutritional Findings and Family Marketing Practices; II. Factors in Food Acceptance. *J. Home Economics*, 54 (April 1962) pp. 297–308.

Mitchell, H. S., "How to Eat Well and Reduce Sensibly," *Today's Health*, 36 (Sept. 1958) pp. 56–61.

Myers, M. L., and Stare, F. J., "Formulae, Fads, and Fatness," *Food and Nutrition News*, 33 (Nov. 1961) pp. 1, 4. Chicago: National Livestock and Meat Board.

Page, L., and Fincher, L. J., *Food and Your Weight*. Bull. 74. Washington, D.C.: U.S. Department of Agriculture, 1960.

Spurling, D., Krause, M., Callaghan, M., and Huenemann, R., "Poor Food Habits are Everybody's Concern" (Survey of 10,000 high-school student diets), *J. Home Econ.*, 46 (Dec. 1954) pp. 713–15.

Steele, B. F., Clayton, M. M., and Tucker, R. E., "Role of Breakfast and of Between-meal Foods in Adolescents' Nutrient Intake," *J. Am. Dietet. Assoc.* 28 (Nov. 1952) pp. 1054–57.

You Can Reduce. Chicago: National Livestock and Meat Board.

CHAPTER 10

Food fads and quackery

A chapter on food fads and quackery at this stage in a nutrition text *should* be superfluous. Your own knowledge of nutrition should be your protection against them. However, because the food faddists and quacks are so clever and convincing in their approach, you need to know how they operate and what help you can expect from public and private agencies in counteracting their false teachings. A warning of the problem and ways to meet it have thus become a necessary phase of nutrition education.

Superstitions and old sayings about foods have been with us always. *Fish and milk should not be eaten in the same meal; feed a cold and starve a fever; tomatoes clear the brain,* are familiar samples. All have been passed along from one generation to another, all have been proved false in light of the newer knowledge of nutrition. Gradually they have lost momentum and are dying out. This is true chiefly because no one has had a personal stake in perpetuating them. The same cannot be said of the selfishly motivated food fads and quackery of today.

The success of the food-faddist movement is due largely to the receptiveness of the public—a receptiveness born of a new awareness of food as a factor in health. Findings of research in nutrition and medicine, reported in the public press, stimulate this interest and curiosity. The public clamors for more. Food faddists and quacks seize upon and distort isolated aspects of the findings and move in to satisfy the demand. Unfortunately, their glamorous, irresponsible approach is more appealing to many people than the factual advice available from authentic sources [1].

The activities of faddists and quacks cover a wide range. Some specialize in the lecture-consultation-publication field, with emphasis chiefly on "health" foods and nutrient concentrates. These are the promoters of food fads—the professional food faddists. Others add to their activities the manufacture and sale of special brews and concoctions purported to prevent such conditions as cataracts, arthritis, and cancer. For convenience in discussion, this latter group will be referred to as food *quacks.* If there is any real difference between the faddists and the quacks, it is largely one of degree.

» FOOD FADS

Professional food faddists are not always easily identifiable. They often advocate what sounds like a good normal diet.

The practiced ear, however, will detect the symbols of food faddism that are invariably present, such as yoghurt, black strap molasses, brewer's yeast, and "liquid vegetables." These are usually harmless additions to any diet. It is when they are promoted in place of everyday familiar foods and out of all proportion to their nutritive values that they become fads.

Yoghurt, a fermented milk, is urged upon the public as a miracle food. Actually it has the same food value as any other sour milk of the same butterfat content. Unfortunately, the public buys it as a miracle food and pays four times as much for it as for the same amount of buttermilk. Table 10-1 shows the comparison in nutrient yield of 1 cup of yoghurt and 1 cup of buttermilk. It is apparent that they are practically identical in food value when made from milk of the same butterfat content. (The buttermilk shown on Table 10-1 has a higher butterfat content than the buttermilk in Appendix G.)

Blackstrap molasses is another product promoted as a miracle food by faddists. It is obvious from Table 10-2 that it does not qualify as such. It has no protein, fat, vitamin A or ascorbic acid. Its calcium content is of little importance if milk is taken in recommended amounts. It would require nearly ½ cup of blackstrap molasses daily to provide an adult with enough calcium to meet his dietary allowance for that mineral element. Blackstrap molasses is the residue from a third extraction in sugar making. As shown on Table 10-2, average servings of several foods commonly included in well-selected diets provide as much or more iron than molasses. Almost all the foods supply much more of the B vitamins, and some of them significant amounts of protein, vitamin A, and ascorbic acid entirely lacking in molasses. As demonstrated earlier in the text, *all dietary allowances of the average person can be met with suitable amounts of a variety of palatable foods.*

"Liquid vegetables" are the juices of raw vegetables put through a special juicer. There is no justification for most people to take their vegetables in this form. Chewing is good for the teeth and gums, and residue is needed as a digestion aid. Consuming vegetable juices in the large quantities recommended by health faddists is expensive because of the enormous quantities of the original vegetables required and the cost of the juicer. It is also time-consuming to prepare the vegetables and extract the juices. And, in certain disease conditions, the liquid intake may be excessive and the sodium content of the vegetable juice may be harmful in the quantity taken.

The practice of grinding grains at home, advocated by some faddists, can be examined in the same way and similar con-

TABLE 10-1

YOGHURT NOT A MIRACLE FOOD

Buttermilk and Yoghurt Have the Same Food Value*

Food	Measure	Calories	Protein g	Calcium mg	Iron mg	Vitamin A IU	Thiamin mg	Riboflavin mg	Ascorbic acid mg
Yoghurt	1 cup	120	8	295	0.1	170	0.09	0.43	2
Buttermilk	1 cup	110	9	285	0.1	172	0.10	0.44	2

* Both milks of about 2 percent butterfat content.

TABLE 10-2

BLACKSTRAP MOLASSES NOT A MIRACLE FOOD
Common Foods That Equal or Excel Blackstrap Molasses in Food Nutrients

Food	Measure	Calories	Protein g	Calcium mg	Iron mg	Vitamin A IU	Thiamin mg	Riboflavin mg	Ascorbic acid mg
Blackstrap molasses	1 tbsp	45	...	116	2.3	...	0.02	0.04	...
Hamburger	3 oz	245	21	9	2.7	30	0.07	0.02	...
Liver, beef	2 oz	120	13	5	4.4	30,330	0.15	2.25	18
Pot roast	3 oz	245	23	10	2.9	30	0.04	0.18	...
Baked beans	¾ cup	250	12	129	3.3	105	0.10	0.08	4
Broccoli	½ cup	20	3	98	1.0	2550	0.05	0.11	56
Mustard greens	½ cup	15	2	154	2.1	5025	0.04	0.13	32
Peas, green	½ cup	55	4	18	1.5	575	0.20	0.11	12
Bread, white, enriched	4 slices	240	8	76	2.4	trace	0.24	0.20	trace
Prunes, stewed	5 medium, juice	160	1	21	1.5	733	0.03	0.06	1

clusions reached. Grains need not be ground fresh daily to preserve their nutrients, as the faddists advocate; the mills for home-grinding are expensive and the job laborious. Satisfactory whole-grain products are available on the market at a reasonable price. And finally, enriched breads and cereals are an excellent substitute.

Other typical food fads can be disposed of similarly. Brewer's yeast, for example, is a good source of iron and B vitamins. It may be useful when a physician recommends it as a dietary supplement. It is *not* needed in the diet of a normal individual eating an adequate diet. Thus "miracle" foods, seen through the eyes of a nutritionist, lose their glamor, and their magic disappears in the light of scientific fact.

» FOOD QUACKERY

Usually the food quack has a product to sell. Such products are offered as important dietary supplements, based on "secret formulas." They are sold at high prices and are urged upon the public with half-truths and outright misinformation. The quack uses many methods to make sales. A common one is the personal approach through door-to-door selling or the lecture platform. High pressure sales tactics are used and extravagant promises are made that the products offered prevent and cure disease.

The Quack Salesman's Story

The salesman's appeals to customers fall into a recognizable pattern. Following are typical fallacies that salesmen use to create a market for their products:

Fallacy 1: worn-out soils cause deficient diets. According to the quacks, soils in this country are depleted of nutrients, and the foods grown on such soils are "devitalized." People living on "devitalized" foods become malnourished. The quacks maintain, further, that only organic fertilizers can correct the deficiencies of such soils; that inorganic fertilizers will "poison" them. Some quacks sell food supplements alleged to make good the so-called deficiencies of the foods grown on the poor soils. Others sell foods that they claim have been grown on soils enriched with organic fertilizers. Still others sell organic fertilizers and equipment, which the customer can use to grow his own foods.

The truth of the matter is that the composition of the soil has little effect on the composition of the plants grown on it. Hereditary factors control the composition of foods as they do the size and shape of plants. Poor soils produce poor crops—a low yield—but their nutritive value is not diminished (except in iodine, and possibly fluorine). Thus the quack's approach to sales through the soil depletion fallacy represents a tremendous hoax. (See Chap. 6.)

Fallacy 2: modern foods are overprocessed and require the consumer to use nutrient supplements [2]. Food quacks also base the sales promotion of their dietary supplements on the myth that foods today are ruined by overprocessing. They refer to the milling of grains, the canning and freezing of foods, and the pasteurization of milk. They refuse to recognize the fact that the enrichment of flour and fortification of breakfast foods restore much of the nutriment lost by milling, and that milling removes the outer husks of grain which many people cannot tolerate. Modern methods of canning and freezing foods preserve nutrients. Pasteurization of milk renders it safe from pathogenic bacteria, and nutrient losses are negligible. Again the public is exploited by the use of misleading facts.

Fallacy 3: all disease is traceable to inadequate diet. The sales arguments that probably have the gravest implications are these: that almost everyone suffers from dietary deficiencies; that it is practically impossible to prevent deficiencies with a diet of common foods; and that such deficiencies are the cause, not only of minor physical ills, but of serious organic diseases. The fact is that foods wisely chosen from the ample and varied supply available here, can provide all of the nutrients needed for optimum nutrition, and that highly advertised and heavily sold vitamin and mineral supplements are superfluous under all normal conditions. The special dietary supplements offered for sale are reputed to provide every known nutrient required to correct the assumed deficiency conditions and, in addition, to yield "secret benefits" not yet recognized by the medical profession. Such "off the cuff" diagnoses by unqualified persons, the promotion of erroneous concepts of food-health relationships, and promises of prevention and cure of major disease conditions, constitute a cruel deception of the public that has deplorable consequences.

» DANGERS OF FOOD FADDISM AND QUACKERY

The dangers of food faddism and quackery may be summed up as follows:

1. They undermine public confidence in the nutrient value of staple foods and in the science of nutrition.
2. They promote self-diagnosis and self-medication by selling "cures" direct to the consumer.
3. They make "do-it-yourself medicine men" of the consuming public. Time-consuming and unnecessary chores are advocated, as in the making of yoghurt, grinding grains, growing vegetables in "organic gardening" projects.
4. They cheat the public by selling people things they do not need at inflated prices. Often the people who buy, under high-pressure salesmanship, are those who can least

afford to do so. It is estimated that the American public spends at least one-half billion dollars annually on "nutrition nonsense": unneeded nutrient compounds, mixtures, "health" foods, equipment, and utensils.

5. They encourage postponement of medical diagnosis. Food supplements are offered as "cure-alls" for serious disease. This practice creates in the purchaser a false sense of security in his new-found "remedy." Competent medical attention may be sought too late.

» YOUR OWN APPROACH TO FADDISM AND QUACKERY

How can you, a person with an introductory knowledge of nutrition, identify false diet theories? First, exercise intelligent skepticism. Look for the signs of food faddism and quackery. Ask yourself these questions: Are extravagant promises made for quick "cures" of diseases that "baffle" the medical profession? Are the "cures" unorthodox, "secret formulas," and miracle concoctions? Are they sold direct to the public, by-passing the medical profession? Do the promoters claim to be "persecuted" by the medical profession, who, they claim, is afraid of competition, and do they urge "medical investigation"? Do they claim to have many professional degrees, often from unknown universities? Do they advertise widely, particularly with testimonials from people in remote places? Do they try to discredit orthodox medical treatment such as X-ray and surgery? Do they state or imply that it is impossible to choose an adequate diet from the American food supply; that meals must be reinforced with a variety of food supplements or with those favorities of the faddists such as yoghurt, brewer's yeast, and blackstrap molasses? If the answer is "yes" to some or all of these questions, the chances are great that the theories are unsound.

How can you help to counteract the influence of faddists and quacks? One way is to steer clear of fad diets yourself. Show by example that your study of nutrition has convinced you that dietary needs can usually be met with a nutritionally adequate diet and that special foods and supplements are unnecessary and wasteful. In contacts with other adults, encourage the same type of skepticism you yourself practice. Help them to know reliable sources, not only for authentic information on nutrition, but also for advice in identifying misinformation and its perpetrators. The greatest hope for eventually ridding the public of food fads lies in an informed next generation. Children at every age need to learn to like wholesome foods and to know how to choose them in quantities and combinations to make satisfying, appetizing meals. Good, well-established food habits are the best defense against faddism.

It should be recognized that there are legitimate cases of food allergy that may require the elimination of specified foods from the diet for a time, and which, in certain instances, may suggest the substitution of carefully selected dietary supplements during an observation period. But this procedure should be undertaken only under the guidance of a highly trained physician, especially equipped to diagnose and treat allergies. It is not the province of the quack who makes it his business to promote the erroneous impression that practically everyone suffers from multiple allergies that may be quickly and completely eliminated by the nostrums he sells.

» RELIABLE NUTRITION INFORMATION

Nutrition information changes with new research findings. It is therefore important to know professional organizations and agencies that keep abreast of nutrition research and can be called upon for their most recent bulletins on pertinent subjects or for answers to specific nutrition questions. Publications and/or nutrition information are available from the following sources:

The nutritionist with your state health department, located at the state capital, or with your county or city health department

The nutrition specialist, extension service, located at your state agricultural college

The food and nutrition departments of colleges and universities in your locality

Nutrition and Consumer-Use Research Service, U.S. Department of Agriculture (for publications)

You will note that public libraries are not listed here. Unfortunately, such libraries must stock books that the public requests. The result is often a mixture of the sound and unsound in nutrition reading matter on their shelves with little or no way for the uninformed person to tell the difference between them. The public is not protected legally against misleading and incorrect information appearing in journals and books. The fact that a book is popular and becomes a best seller bears no relationship to its authenticity as a source of nutrition information. Actually its very daring in promoting an unfounded or unorthodox concept may alone be responsible for phenominal sales. Before obtaining nutrition materials from public libraries it is well to ask for recommended titles from one of the individuals or agencies listed above.

» PROTECTION OF THE PUBLIC

Several public and private agencies serve as guardians against food quacks and their fraudulent and misleading claims [3]. You, as an individual, can promote their effectiveness by reporting suspected violations. Each of the organizations listed here renders a distinctive type of service. This service is described briefly.

Food and Drug Administration, U.S. Department of Health, Education and Welfare, Washington, D.C. This public agency operates under the Food, Drug and Cosmetic Act [4]. It is concerned with violations of federal labelling laws when the products are involved in interstate commerce. False or misleading statements that appear on containers or accompany them are construed as misbranding. Excluded are statements in pamphlets, magazines, and books and those made on radio, television, or the lecture platform which are not associated directly with the sale of the product.

Federal Trade Commission, Washington, D.C. As related to food quacks, this public agency has authority over false and misleading matter that falls into the category of commodity advertising if it uses the U.S. mails or crosses state lines. The privileges of free speech and press provide immunity for the offender who manages to circumvent the law by using other methods to reach the public with the same information.

The U.S. Post Office, Washington 25, D.C. The Post Office Department has the responsibility to prevent fraudulent or false advertising that solicits money by mail for products marketed by mail order. This department can take legal action against offenders, but it must prove *intent* to defraud.

Federal Communications Commission, Washington 25, D.C. This public agency has the responsibility of reviewing radio and television broadcasts at 3-year intervals as part of its function in granting licenses to operate. Both programs and advertising material can be considered in this review, as they may promote, or fail to promote the public interest. Its potential power lies in its ability to withhold licenses on the basis of findings.

Better Business Bureau: a national organization with offices in most cities. This organization, sponsored by responsible businessmen in a community, is on the alert for unorthodox or illegal trade practices [5]. It cooperates with local, state, and national law-enforcement bodies to suppress improper business methods. This includes the many such methods employed by the food quacks. The public may obtain information about questionable companies or practices and may report irregularities to their local bureaus.

American Medical Association, 535 North Dearborn Street, Chicago, Illinois. The Association's *Bureau of Investigation* exposes many quacks—their programs, publications, and the products they sell. It serves the medical profession by publishing such information in the Journal of the American Medical Association. It serves the public by answering special inquiries, directed to the bureau, concerning these pseudoscientists.

The association's *Council on Foods and Nutrition* helps advertisers to state their claims for the foods they sell, suitably and correctly, by issuing printed suggestions that serve as guide lines in preparing advertising copy, and by counselling with advertisers in preparing their material.

References appended to this chapter elaborate the work of the agencies named here and point out problems that confront those agencies which have law enforcement powers.

Other Efforts to Control Food Faddism and Quackery

In addition to the formal methods taken to control food faddists and quacks, many other efforts are being made. Professional societies in nutrition, dietetics, public health, and medicine are carrying on campaigns through their official journals and other printed materials. Some are extending their influence through lectures, discussion groups, and workshops.

As a result of all types of activity, food faddism has been discredited to some extent; a number of the food quacks have been apprehended and have served prison terms, or paid fines—or both. But many have escaped the law. They know the loopholes; they are crafty and hard to catch. In some cases their faithful followers have paid the fines imposed and thus helped them back into their profitable businesses.

It is obvious that the general public is unaware of the dangers of food faddism and quackery. They can be made aware only if they understand:

1. The serious dangers to health and life of placing confidence in the promises of untrained and irresponsible "medicine men."
2. That we have in this country the safest, most abundant and varied food supply in the world [6]; and that vitamin and mineral supplements are not only unnecessary but wasteful, in most cases, if meals are well chosen from that vast supply.

REFERENCES

1. Mitchell, H. S., "Don't Be Fooled By Fads," *Food—The Yearbook of Agriculture.* Washington, D.C.: U.S. Department of Agriculture, 1959. p. 660.
2. Council on Foods and Nutrition, "Vitamin Preparations as Dietary Supplements and as Therapeutic Agents," *J. Am. Med. Assoc.,* 169 (Jan. 3, 1959) pp. 41–45.
3. Mitchell, H. S., "Food Fads—What Protection Have We?" *J. Home Econ.,* 53 (Feb. 1961) pp. 100–103.
4. Janssen, W. F., "Food Quackery—A Law Enforcement Problem," *J. Am. Dietet. Assoc.,* 36 (Feb. 1960) pp. 110–13.
5. Mott, M. H., "Better Business Bureaus Fight Food Faddism," *J. Am. Dietet. Assoc.,* 39 (Aug. 1961) pp. 122–23.
6. Larrick, G. P., "The Nutritive Adequacy of Our Food Supply," *J. Am. Dietet. Assoc.,* 39 (Aug. 1961) pp. 117–21.

READINGS

Bell, J. N., "Let 'em Eat Hay," *Today's Health,* 36 (Sept. 1958) pp. 22–25; 66–68.

Food Facts Talk Back: food information, fallacies and facts (booklet). Chicago: The American Dietetic Association, 1957.

The Medicine Man (16 mm film; black and white; 27 min., exposé of quacks). Chicago: American Medical Association. (On free loan.)

Olson, R. E., "Food Faddism—Why?" *Nutrition Reviews,* 16 (April 1958) pp. 97–99.

CHAPTER 11

Nutrition in action around the world

A gigantic nutrition experiment has been going on in the world for centuries. Human beings around the globe, including ourselves and our ancestors, are the subjects. The test materials are the typical diets of the different countries; the standard of measurement is the nutritional well-being of the peoples. The findings of this vast experiment are relatively clear cut and unvarying from generation to generation. They show a distinct relationship between the amounts and kinds of food supplies and the energy and stamina of the populations that live on them [1]. Plentiful and nutritionally adequate diets produce peoples who are well developed, vigorous, and long lived. Scanty and poorly balanced diets produce undersized races whose peoples are short lived and below par physically. History has observed these effects and modern nutrition research has confirmed them (Chap. 2).

The broader implications of nutritional status are also apparent. It has been said that good nutrition is the best guarantee of an able, energetic population [2]. Hungry peoples are apt to be unsatisfied and restless; they often lack initiative and sustained purpose. Well-fed peoples, with vigor and stability, tend to channel their energies into constructive endeavor. The President of the United States epitomized this concept when he said recently that "intelligence and skill can only function at the peak of their capacity when the body is healthy and strong; that hardy spirits and tough minds usually inhabit sound bodies." Thus the goal of better nutrition around the world envisages not only improved physical health but also a more productive and satisfying existence for all.

At the present time, no country, including our own, has reason to be complacent with respect to its national diet. No individuals, including ourselves, can afford to be content with our nutritional status. Just as many peoples of the world are underfed, a few are overfed. Some diets lack certain nutrients; others are deficient in different respects. There is hope for improvement if each nation sees its own nutritional strengths and weaknesses in relation to accepted standards of adequacy and joins with other nations in a world-wide effort to raise the level of nutrition for all peoples.

» WORLD NUTRITION PROBLEMS TODAY

A major nutrition problem of two-thirds of the inhabitants of the world is that of obtaining enough food to sustain life and for normal activity and health. Some of these peoples constantly fend off actual starvation; others suffer from less acute, chronic undernutrition. The problem is most critical in countries where food production is far below need, where the poor economy of the country permits little importation of food, and where the typical diet is limited to a few basic items. Clear-cut evidence of the malnutrition that inevitably results from such conditions is the presence of recognizable symptoms of dietary deficiency disease in the people. Such evidence is presented in Figure 11.1. The shaded portions on the world map represent the sections where children suffer from *kwashiorkor,* an unmistakable indication of an unsatisfactory food supply.

As pointed out in Chapter 5, the onset of kwashiorkor is associated particularly with a protein intake that is low in quantity and quality. But the diet is often inadequate in total amount of food as well, and may be deficient or unbalanced with respect to several nutrients. Table 5-2 gives the calorie and protein yields of food supplies of a number of countries. It will be noted that the countries on the list that obtain the fewest calories from their diets also obtain the smallest amounts of total protein and the smallest quantities of animal protein. It is significant that these same countries fall within the shaded areas of the map in Figure 11.1, which represent the geographical distribution of kwashiorkor throughout the world.

Inadequate Food Supplies

In these vast areas the average calorie value of the diet is only two-thirds to three-fourths of that of the diet in better-fed regions. Calorie-deficient food supplies are also lacking in various nutrients. Many people living on such diets do not develop outright deficiency diseases, but they are plagued with low vigor and inefficiency, with short life spans and with high death rates. There is little hope for improving the situation materially until there is a sufficient, well-balanced food supply for all [3].

The most serious complicating factor in the nutritional outlook for these countries is their soaring populations, brought about largely by the control of infectious disease. It is ironical that as the population of a country mounts and its total needs thus increase, land that is used for growing food must be taken out of production to provide additional living space. Unless steps are taken to meet this problem, the outcome will be *less* food to feed *more* people.

The Need for Increased Local Food Production

Increased local production of essential foods and expanded facilities for developing and using all such food supplies appear to offer the major sources of relief from hunger. This calls for the application of modern methods of agriculture to make possible greater yields from an ever-shrinking acreage. It also requires such measures as raising animals for meat and milk and poultry for meat and eggs, developing ponds and streams for domestic fish, and cultivating gardens for native vegetables and fruits.

Countries in need of help are being aided in the application of such methods. In many cases this means revamping farming methods that have been in practice for centuries and launching new endeavors. Some countries have already made encouraging progress. Eventual success in terms of improved nutrition will depend on whether rate of production of food is sufficiently accelerated to catch up with rate of population increase.

In some countries, even where food is

abundant, certain existing national habits are a barrier to good nutrition for the population as a whole [4]. For example, peoples may use domestic animals as pets rather than for food—while they are starving for protein. They may reject fish from local streams or refuse milk because of hidebound eating habits, often based on ancient taboos. Analysis of the forces that give promise of effecting change in such situations and of ways to apply them thus becomes part of the process of solving world nutrition problems (Chap. 1).

Where Food Supplies Are More Plentiful

The unshaded areas of the map (Fig. 11.1) show the parts of the world where the food situation is less grim. The diets of many of the populations that live in these sections are relatively varied in character and yield the needed calories. Gross forms of dietary deficiency diseases have largely disappeared here. The peoples in some of the countries have increased in body size from generation to generation, and their life spans have been lengthened. The plentifulness of food supplies has undoubtedly been a major factor in such changes.

In the United States, which lies in this favored region, there is unprecedented variety and abundance of food, and the supply has increased in nutrient content over the years. But availability of food is not an automatic guarantee of dietary adequacy [5]. Even where there are food surpluses, some people do not get enough to eat, or fail to eat the right kinds of food. And even the many people who habitually overeat often have unbalanced diets because of inadequate amounts of certain nutrients and more than they need of others.

Overeating, coupled with reduced energy need due to mechanized living, has resulted in excess body fat in a considerable

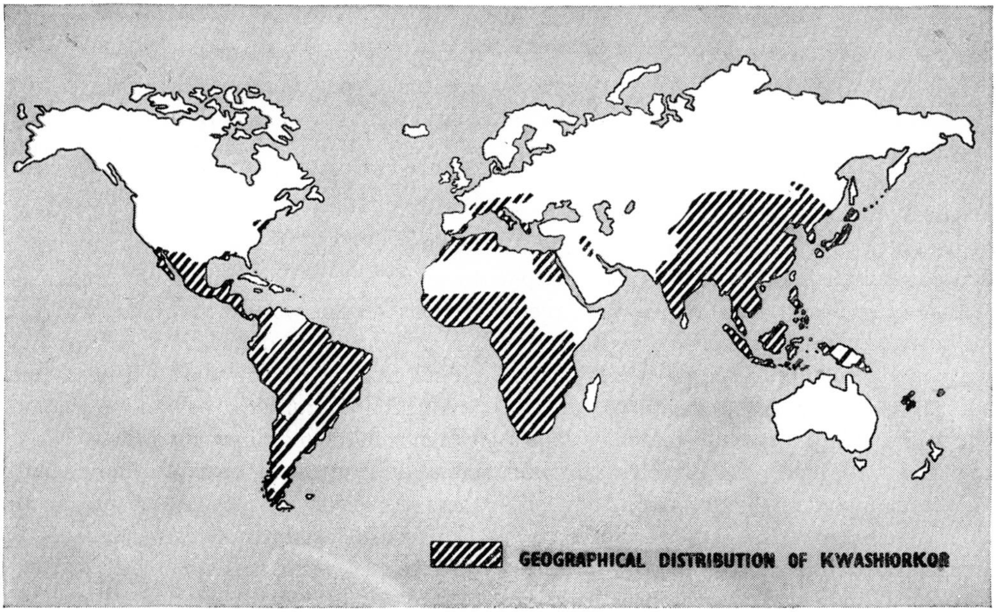

Fig. 11.1 The distribution of kwashiorkor throughout the world. (Courtesy Food and Agriculture Organization.)

segment of the population in this country. Overweight is a form of malnutrition associated with the onset of degenerative diseases such as those of the blood vessels. Nutrition problems can exist in the midst of affluence. Survival, and even evidences of nutritional progress, do not necessarily indicate the achievement of optimal health, nor do they suggest a relaxation of vigilance in working toward that goal.

The ample food supply of the United States is due largely to the efficiency of its agricultural operations. And increased production of food is due more to improved yields than to the use of more land for farming. In the 20 years prior to 1957, average per acre yields and production of milk per cow, eggs per hen, and meat per unit of feed increased by one-third. During the same period, the output per man-hour of farm labor was doubled. There seems reason to believe that such progress has not reached its limit [6].

Steps to Abundance

The working bases for continued production increases lie in research that makes possible new technologies, in conservation practices that preserve natural resources such as soils and water, and in the application of research findings to the practical operation of growing, handling, and marketing foods. These steps, which pave the way for abundance, apply to all foods: meat, milk, fish, poultry, eggs, cereals, vegetables, and fruits. The technically underdeveloped countries will increase their own supplies of these important foods when they are able to adopt modern methods. The mechanization of farms and the use of fertilizers, pesticides, improved harvesting methods, rapid transportation of products to market, and safe, efficient ways of preserving, packaging, distributing, and merchandising foods, are important elements in providing a plentiful food supply [2].

» WORLD NUTRITION PROBLEMS OF THE FUTURE

The number one nutrition problem of the future will continue to be that of providing nutritionally adequate diets for the peoples of the world. Research in food production will proceed, and new ways of applying the findings will be sought constantly. In the developing countries, emphasis will still be placed on increasing the quantities of food produced to keep pace with population growth. In the countries with more abundant food supplies, continued attention will be given to the prudent use of abundant food supplies and to ways of keeping total intake in line with energy needs. Even these latter countries, however, cannot ignore the possibilities of eventual food shortages. They must give consideration to the fact that ultimately food production limits may be reached while the population trend continues upward.

Figure 11.2 shows the race between food production increases and population increases from 1952 to the present in 7 sections of the world and in the world at large. Where the dotted lines on the individual charts lie below the solid lines, food production is running behind population. When the dotted lines dip still lower or cross downward through the solid lines, these are signs of losing the race. Figure 11.2, considered in its entirety, presents an unfavorable prospect, with a half or more of the world regions giving, rather than gaining, ground. It also proves that average data on the food-population situation for

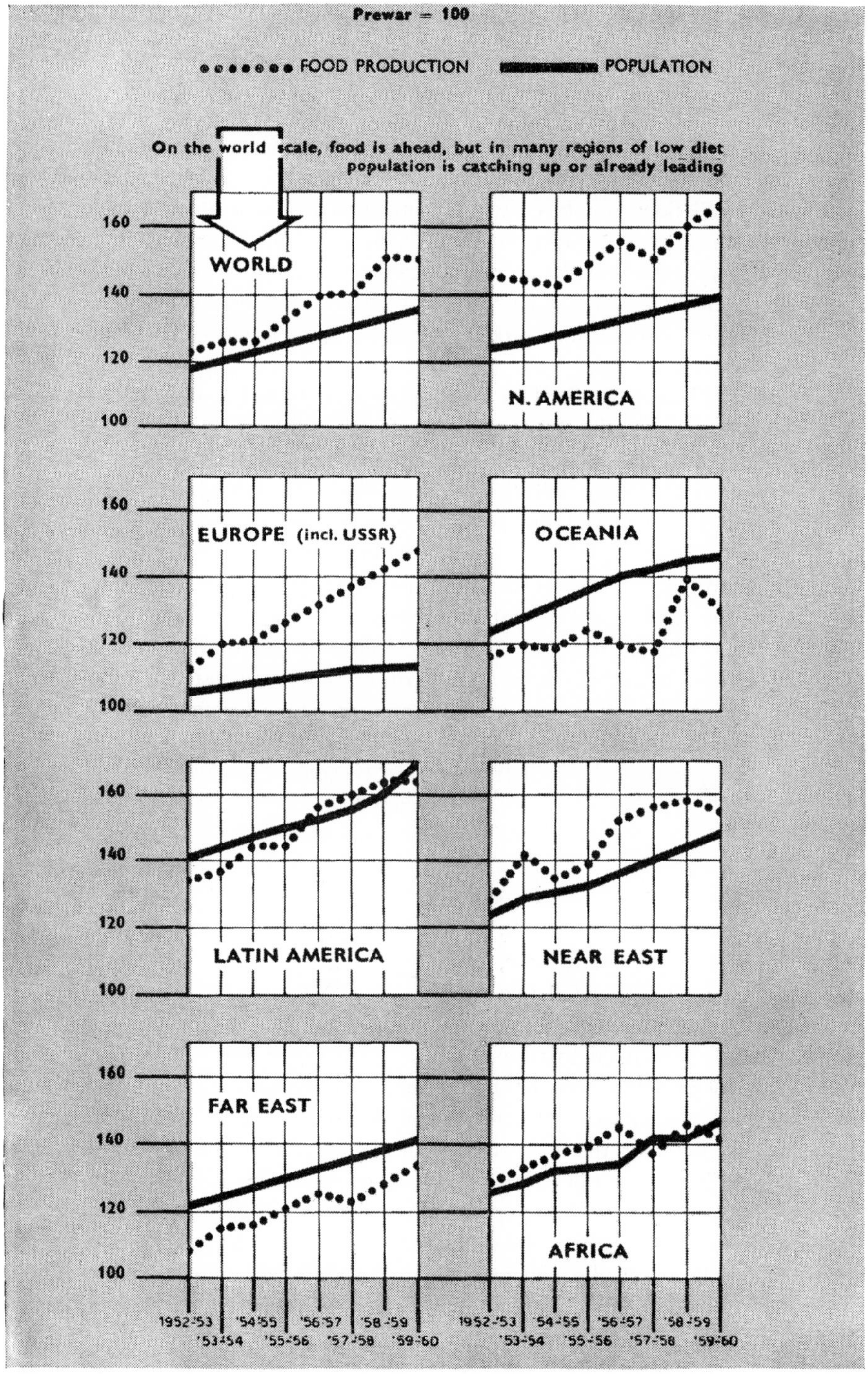

Fig. 11.2 The race between food and population. (Courtesy Food and Agriculture Organization.)

the world as a whole (top left), provide an unrealistic and overly optimistic picture of the problem as it actually exists in certain critical areas.

In the United States at the present time, food production is proceeding at a faster rate than population growth. Between 1939 and 1957, the aggregate farm output in this country increased about 40 percent, and the population increased 30 percent. Studies indicate that agricultural production is likely to outrun or keep pace with population into 1975 or beyond. The uncertainty of predicting for the future appears to lie in the population to be expected—in how many mouths there will be to feed—rather than in food production possibilities [2].

As these perennial and basic questions continue to occupy nutritional scientists, there will be other and entirely new ones to demand attention. Many of them will result from scientific discoveries in other fields. An example is the problem of adequate nutrition for persons who will travel in outer space.

Space Nutrition

With the space age already here, nutritionists are concerned with what one can eat and how one can be well nourished in outer space. Much research on this topic is under way. A great deal has been reported in current scientific literature. The need for information is real, but there are difficulties in obtaining it. The matter of weightlessness in outer space, for example, poses the elemental problem of getting food to the mouth. One solution is the collapsible "squeeze" tube that serves in place of forks. Semisolid foods and liquids in tubes can be conveyed directly into the mouth by applying pressure to the tube (Fig. 11.3). Ready-to-eat foods that can be grasped in the hand are also possibilities.

Such procedures are practical for short trips. The space traveller who is to be away from earth for months or even years may find himself dependent on a more primitive nutritional plan. He could carry neither the amount of food nor water necessary for conventional subsistence. Procedures are yet to be found. Scientists have proposed that green algae, produced en route, may offer possibilities as a single food item in a complete diet. Growing algae in the sealed space cabin would provide oxygen for him; carbon dioxide exhaled by the traveller would sustain the plants; the plants would be eaten by the traveller, and his waste products of metabolism would be used as nourishment for the plants to grow additional crops of the algae. This brief oversimplification of the intricacies of space nutrition merely suggests the involved and unfamiliar character of coming nutritional problems in the world and the ingenuity and breadth of knowledge required to solve them [7].

» PROGRAMS TO DEAL WITH NUTRITION PROBLEMS

As major nutrition problems are identified throughout the world, efforts are being made to deal with them. Some problems are being attacked on an international scale; others are approached at regional, national, and local levels. The tasks are being undertaken by agencies and organizations serving under many different auspices. Their purposes and scopes differ widely, but all are concerned in some measure with the betterment of human nutrition. It is important for citizens to know of such movements and to understand their objectives. An informed public, convinced of the importance of improved nutrition to human welfare, is the single most important factor in approaching the solution of nutrition problems. An acquaintance with activities within one's own country should be the starting point [8].

In the United States: Governmental Agencies

Among the agencies in this country concerned with nutrition are the long-established departments of the federal Government. These include the U.S. Department of Health, Education, and Welfare, with its Children's Bureau, its Office of Education, and its Public Health Service, and the U.S. Department of Agriculture, with its Nutrition and Consumer-use Research, its Experiment Stations, and its Extension Service. The research, the publications, and the program services of these departments as they relate to nutrition, have been cited repeatedly in preceding chapters. The Department of Agriculture, for example, provided you with certain of the tools you have used throughout the text, such as data on the nutritive values of common foods and information on the eating patterns of people in different regions of this country. These and other such aids are essential instruments in developing action programs for improved nutrition.

Nongovernmental agencies such as the Food and Nutrition Board of the Academy of Sciences—National Research Council, and the Council on Foods and Nutrition of the American Medical Association are composed of leaders in nutrition from medicine and other related fields. Their programs are largely concerned with national nutrition policy and the development of specialized nutrition materials. You have learned to know and to apply the recommended dietary allowances that originate with the Food and Nutrition Board.

Professional societies of nutritionists strengthen national and international programs through their official support and participation. Universities and colleges prepare nutritionists for teaching and other fields and carry on nutrition research through their departments of nutrition, biochemistry, medicine, and home economics. Foundations for research and education support nutrition research and make findings available to action groups. Food industry associations and individual food companies sponsor nutrition research and publicize the results. Finally, state, county, and local organizations and agencies, such as health departments, schools at all levels, extension services, visiting nurse associations, infant welfare societies, and official nutrition committees, are occupied to some degree with nutrition education.

This brief overview obviously cannot fully convey the breadth of effort represented by the vast array of organizations and agencies in the United States giving more or less emphasis to nutrition. Despite its magnitude, much is left to be done to strengthen individual programs and to unite them in creating a greater impact on their joint objective—better nutrition for the people of this country.

But efforts in behalf of good nutrition go beyond our own borders. Many agencies and organizations of the United States have been established to contribute specifically to the nutritional welfare of peoples in developing nations of the world. The official programs largely function under departments of the federal government that are concerned with international development [9]. The scope of such programs is broad and the types of aid are varied. As applied to nutritional needs of these peoples, they in-

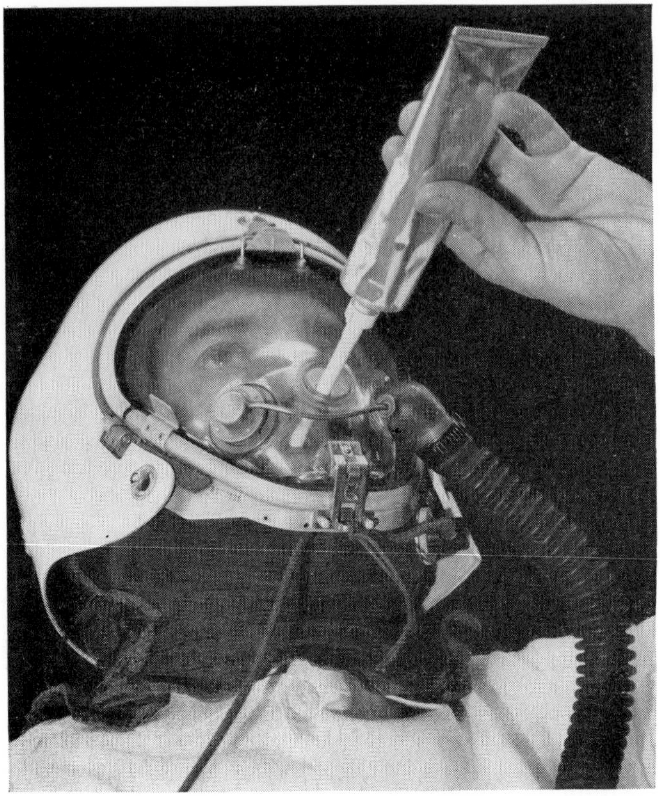

Fig. 11.3 Eating in outer space. New methods are continuously being tested. (Courtesy American Can Company.)

clude concrete assistance such as loans of money for the purchase of food, acceptance of payment for food in local currencies, and, when the need is indicated, gifts of food.

A less direct type of aid is that which offers developing countries technical assistance in meeting long-range food problems. This may take the form of providing trained personnel to a country requesting aid, or it may mean bringing representatives from that country to the United States for special training. In either case, it is part of a broad plan to help the country assess its nutrition problems, to develop plans for meeting them, and to adopt the procedures for doing so. Technicians, machinery, seeds, and fertilizer may all be elements in the assistance program. As pointed out earlier, in many countries a major need is to know how to increase the production and utilization of local food supplies. Along with help in production problems goes aid in educational programs to encourage use of the foods. These community programs often extend to the school lunch, to family meals, and to child feeding. Experience has shown that more food does not guarantee better diets. There must be continuing nutrition education to assure that food habits are influenced for the better as food supplies become more plentiful.

International Agencies and Programs

The vast problems of malnutrition cannot be met by any one country, or even by a small group of countries. It requires the combined efforts of many nations. Joint concern for the nutritional welfare of the peoples of the world stems from World War I, when the League of Nations was formed, and a nutrition division was added to its small health section. This agency sought to find in nutrition the solution to a situation that created food surpluses in one part of the world and hunger in others. World War II temporarily halted this effort.

By the onset of World War II, the newer knowledge of nutrition was being applied. There was an awareness of the prevalence of inadequate diets in the world and. of the consequences that follow. The war gave the opportunity to study the nutrition of adults and children under stress conditions. and to observe the outcomes. The findings brought renewed realization of the need for nations to work together for good nutrition. The obvious solution was the establishment of international organizations that could deal competently with the food situation on a world-wide basis. This was accomplished by setting up agencies for that purpose within the organization of the United Nations, which was just then becoming a reality. The United States has taken an active role in these agencies from their beginnings.

Agencies of the United Nations

The *Food and Agriculture Organization* (FAO) (Fig. 11.4) was the first of the UN subgroups to come into existence (1945)[10]. One of its 5 technical divisions is devoted exclusively to nutrition. In general, FAO programs deal with nutrition in relation to the production, distribution, and consumption of food in all areas of the free world. On this broad base, FAO works with the health, nutrition, and agricultural authorities in the countries being served to bring to each the specific help it needs most to achieve higher nutritional status for its

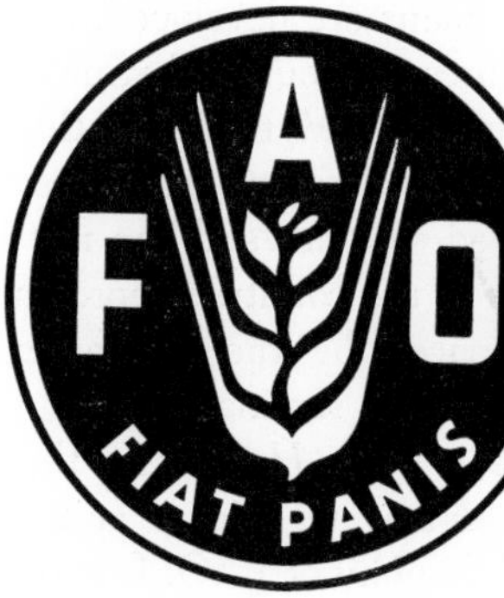

Fig. 11.4 Seal of the Food and Agriculture Organization of the United Nations.

people. Much of the effort made to raise food production levels in needy countries may be attributed to the programs of FAO.

The nutrition activities of FAO are too numerous and varied to consider here in detail. Technical assistance has received an important share of its attention and has been integrated with the other activities of the organization. Technical assistance has consisted of working with local governments to analyze their problems and to set up projects, of providing experts to help with the projects and making fellowships available for more advanced training of leaders. In the past decade FAO has sent upwards of 3000 technicians into the field in more than 60 countries to help them develop their own resources.

A distinctive and far-reaching type of FAO assistance is that given through seminars, workshops, and institutes with local and regional nutrition leaders in different sections of the world. Such conferences are often sponsored jointly with other international agencies and/or regional organizations. They may consider a wide variety of nutritional problems common in the area [11,12]. Or they may concentrate on a topic such as school feeding [13]. Representatives from countries in the region present data on their local conditions. Ideas are exchanged, plans are developed, and desirable procedures are outlined. Such sessions serve to refresh and to guide the participants. Trade policies and programs, as they relate to food supplies and the nutrition of populations in the countries represented, are often influenced by the recommendations formulated at such seminars.

Freedom From Hunger for the nations of the world may be said to epitomize the working philosophy of FAO. It is under this arresting slogan that FAO is seeking to dramatize the need for redoubling efforts on an international scale to improve the world food situation [14]. The campaign calls for cooperation among agencies of the United Nations and with all other governmental and private groups everywhere to tackle, with renewed seriousness and dedication, the unsolved problems of providing adequate diets for the peoples of the world.

Other UN organizations with certain specific concerns for nutrition came into existence soon after the formation of FAO: in 1946, the United Nations Children's Fund (UNICEF); in 1946, also, the United Nations Educational, Scientific and Cultural Organization (UNESCO); and in 1948, the World Health Organization (WHO). Booklets outlining the purpose, scope, and working plans of each of these organizations are included in the reference list [15]. Briefly, the particular province of WHO is that of nutrition in relation to the maintenance of health and prevention of disease. UNICEF is concerned in part with providing needed foods or the equipment required to make foods edible and safe, such as milling and pasteurization machinery. UNESCO concentrates on raising the educational and cultural level of peoples to help them acquire an understanding of the world's foods and ways in which they can help to make it available to all. Each of these agencies of the United Nations has its specific program area; all cooperate to strengthen the over-all effort. FAO and WHO, for example, conduct research jointly on critical nutrition problems. A typical problem, that of protein deficiency, has received vigorous investigation and follow-up as a result of the concentrated effort.

Thus, we have in the world a network of official agencies, organizations, programs, and activities, all of which seek to deal with phases of nutrition and nutrition education. In addition many international programs—too many even to enumerate—are carried on by nongovernmental groups of many types. One notable example is the International Congress on Nutrition, which meets every 3 years under the auspices of the International Union of Nutrition Sciences [3].

The International Congress on Nutrition This group is composed of hundreds of nutritionists representing nearly every country of the world. Exchange fellowships, sponsored by the Congress, and regular meetings of the body, have proved to be powerful devices for establishing scientist-to-scientist contacts. Rapport and communication among members tend to uphold high standards of nutrition research and to stimulate productive investigations that benefit the peoples in the countries represented.

» FOOD—A COMMON DENOMINATOR AMONG NATIONS

International nutrition agencies have set in motion many activities designed to improve the food habits of the peoples of the world. None is of more practical importance than the establishment of suitable dietary allowances toward which nations

Fig. 11.5 There are many ways to obtain an adequate diet: A sampling of daily food patterns from 5 continents—Africa, South America, North America, Asia, and Europe.

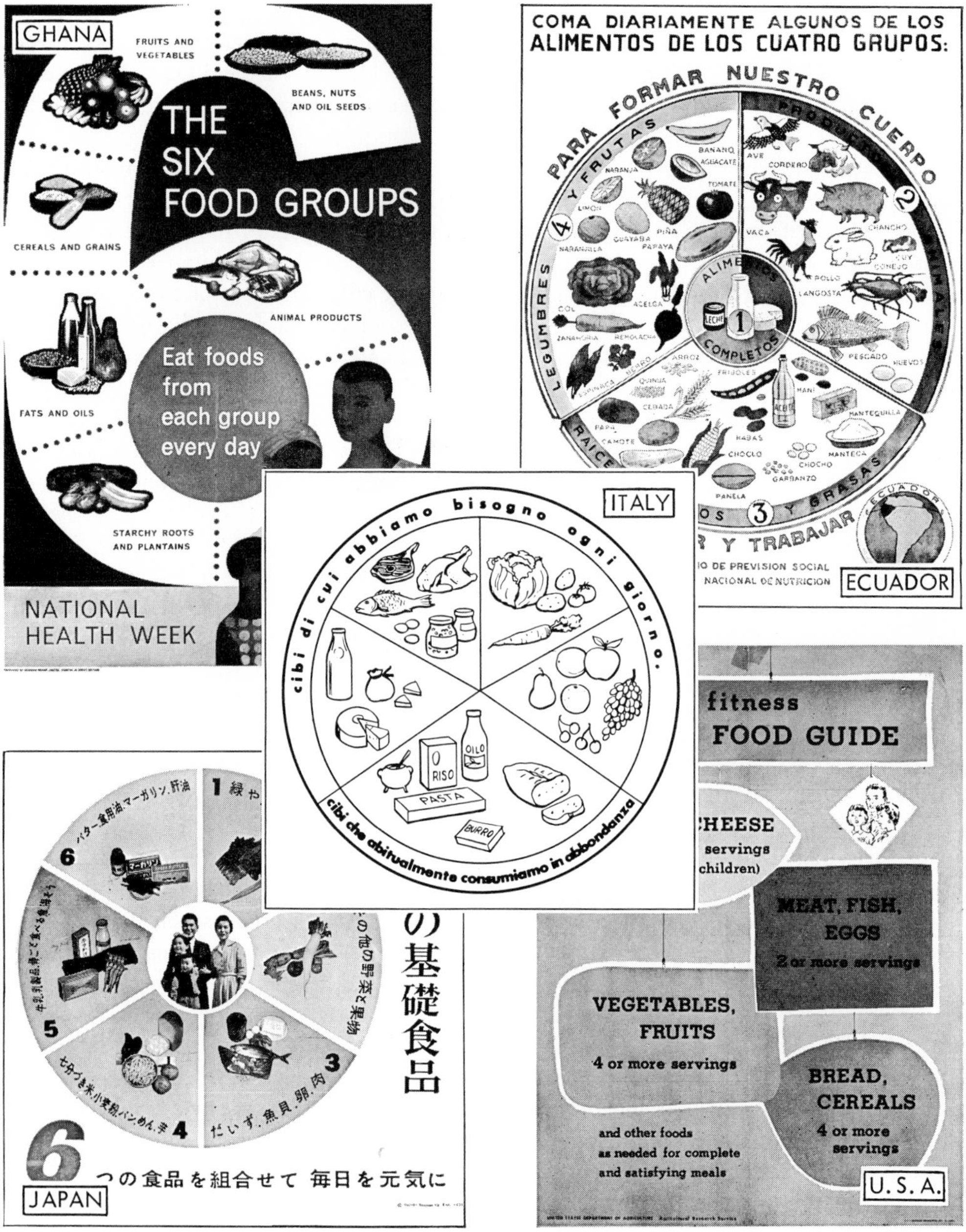

(Courtesy U.S. Department of Agriculture, Agricultural Research Service; Newman Neame, Ltd., Great Britain; Ministerio de Prevision Social, Instituto Nacional de Nutricion; Daiichi Shuppan Co., Ltd.; La Scuola Editrice.) (Only upper part of Japanese poster reproduced.)

can set their sights. Scientists in a number of individual countries have translated these goals into the foods familiar to their own people, thus establishing guide lines to desirable eating practices.

Figure 11.5 shows a group of these daily food patterns issued by official agencies in countries of representative regions of the world. Each pattern, properly interpreted and applied, would guide a person to the selection of a satisfactory diet in his own country. This display illustrates better than words the fact, stressed throughout this text, that there are many ways to obtain an adequate diet and that no one way is the "right" way. Developed locally, these patterns take into consideration the food supplies available to the respective countries and the preferences and meal habits of the peoples. At the same time, the patterns establish reasonable goals for nutritional improvement in terms of locally obtainable foods. Application of this principle to one item—vegetables—is demonstrated in the Daily Food Guide of the United States. This guide recommends a dark green or deep yellow vegetable at least every other day [16]. People in this country are eating less than that amount, despite the fact that such vegetables are plentiful and relatively inexpensive. Increasing the quantity of these vegetables to amounts recommended in the Daily Food Guide would raise the level of vitamin A intake and tend to wipe out the existing deficit of vitamin A in many diets.

A study of Figure 11.5 reveals similarities and differences in the daily food patterns of the various continents. The similarities lie in the broad groupings of foods known to be important for nourishing the body in certain respects. The chief differences lie in the number of divisions on the patterns and in the kinds of foods within the groupings. It will be noted, for example, that certain groupings are common to all of the patterns, i.e., milk, meat, vegetables, fruits, and cereals. But foods within these groups vary not only in kind but also in the emphasis given them. A comparison of the daily food pattern of Japan with that of the United States illustrates some of these similarities and differences (Table 11-1).

For convenience let us examine Table 11-1 under the 4 food groupings suggested in the United States food pattern listed at the left. The center column consists of the kinds of common foods of this country that are recommended for daily use [16]. The right hand column lists the corresponding groupings of foods from the Japanese food pattern (Fig. 11.5). Group numbers are indicated as a guide to the numerals on the Japanese chart. Similarities and differences in the two lists are evident immediately. The lists are similar, for example, in that each of the corresponding groupings has some of the same foods. They are different in 2 important respects: the Japanese groupings include several foods that do not appear on the other list, and there is a different emphasis in the use of some of the foods common to both countries. The Japanese foods that are entirely foreign to American diets are easily identified: seaweeds, soybean curd, soybean paste, and lotus root. Seaweeds are used in Japanese diets as a source of minerals, and soybeans occupy an important place as a source of protein.

The difference in emphasis in use of foods in the 2 countries is also evident from the listings. Milk, which supplies the major portion of the calcium in the United States food supply, plays a secondary role in Japan because of the relatively small amount available. Native foods are substituted, notably the bones of fish, which are obtainable from small fish, eaten whole, or from whole dry fish taken in powdered form (Group 5). This is not a wholly satisfactory solution

TABLE 11-1

A CLOSER LOOK AT DAILY FOOD PATTERNS OF THE UNITED STATES AND JAPAN

FOUR FOOD GROUPS	UNITED STATES Foods Recommended	JAPAN* Foods Recommended	Group Numbers on Japanese Pattern (Fig. 11.5)
MILK GROUP (calcium)	Milk Cheese Ice cream	Small fish (with bones for calcium) Powdered dry fish Seaweeds Milk for children	Group 5
MEAT GROUP	Lean meats beef, pork, lamb, veal Poultry Fish Eggs Legumes (dry)	Soybean curd Soybean paste Fish and shellfish Meat Eggs	Group 3
VEGETABLE-FRUIT GROUP	Green and Yellow (vitamin A) "greens" carrots apricots	Green and Yellow (vitamin A) pumpkin spinach carrots green pepper	Group 1
	Citrus and others for ascorbic acid: oranges, grapefruit, tomatoes Others: potatoes, beets, peas, apples, bananas	Citrus and others for ascorbic acid: tangerines, oranges, tomatoes Others: white radishes, lotus roots, green onions, sweet potatoes, white potatoes	Groups 2 and 4
BREAD-CEREAL GROUP	Breads Breakfast foods Cereal foods (noodles)	Rice Noodles Bread	Group 4

* Group 6 on the Japanese pattern contains butter, margarine, vegetable oils, and liver to signify liver oils. High fat consumption in the United States makes it unnecessary to include such a grouping.

from the standpoint of the amount of calcium available, but it is more feasible in Japan than it would be in this country. In Japan, fish and shellfish are eaten in far greater amounts than here. The annual per capita consumption of fish in Japan is well over 40 lbs, that of the United States about 10 lbs. In the world's catch of fish, the Japanese take twice that of the United States, which is next in line among the nations [17]. Efforts are being made to increase consumption of milk in Japan, especially among the children.

Rice is another food used with different emphasis in the 2 countries. In Japan it is the basic carbohydrate food that takes the place of our cereal grains, such as wheat and corn. Still other differences will be noted in Figure 11.5. For example, in Japan, large white radishes, cooked or raw, play a more prominent part in the diet than do our own small radishes, used chiefly as a relish.

Table 11-2 shows how these same recommended foods, in both daily food patterns may be grouped into family meals. Similarities and differences again are apparent. In both cases, the foods associated in each meal represent combinations of flavors and textures that are pleasing to the peoples in the 2 countries. Table 11-2 lists the foods, so far as possible, in a way that indicates comparable choices in the 2 sets of meals. It shows, for example, that rice in Japanese meals corresponds with our toast, bread, and rolls; that their tea takes the place of our coffee, and that the general construction of the 2 sets of meals is similar. The most striking difference lies in the content of the breakfasts. However, if the nutritive values of the 2 meals were calculated, they might prove to be surprisingly similar.

An attempt has been made to present here 2 sets of meals that are fairly representative for the 2 countries [18]. Foods are never "typical" in any country for all seasons and all situations. The recommended daily food pattern for Japan has been drawn upon for the Japanese meals. (Fig. 11.5). The pattern takes into account home-produced foods that are available in different parts of the country at different times of the year and form the basis of the traditional Japanese diet. As in all other countries, Japanese homes today are influenced by international contacts, which have their effect on eating practices as well as on other living habits.

Although daily food patterns of different nations basically have much in common, they represent completely different habits of eating. The comparison of the United States-Japanese daily food patterns could be repeated for almost any other 2 countries with similar results. The forms of the foods, the ways they are prepared, their groupings in meals, and even the manner in which they are eaten epitomize the eating customs that are unique to a country. It is these characteristics which, taken together, make the native food habits of one country distinctive from those of another country.

Food Speaks a Universal Language

Familiar foods have deep significance for entire populations as well as for individuals (Chap. 1). Adhering to long-established eating customs tends to create a feeling of permanence and solidarity among peoples of a country. It often symbolizes security in the face of other basic changes. And the very importance that individual countries attach to their own native foods and eating customs enhances a common, world-wide interest and concern for food.

As rapid transportation and communication have made neighbors of all peoples,

TABLE 11-2

SAMPLE MEALS THAT MIGHT BE SELECTED FROM THE FOOD PATTERNS OF THE UNITED STATES AND JAPAN

	UNITED STATES*	JAPAN [18]
BREAKFAST	Fruit	Seaweed with soy sauce
	Egg	Soybean soup with bean curd
	Toast	Rice ball
	Milk	Pickled plums
	Coffee	Green tea
LUNCH	Ham sandwich with lettuce	Fish, raw, fried or broiled
	Celery	Vegetables: bamboo shoots, bean sprouts, tomatoes, cucumbers, or dried mushrooms
	Baked apple	Pickles (cucumber or radish)
	Cookie	Rice ball
	Milk	Green tea
SNACK	Banana	
DINNER	Pot roast	Soup: fish, chicken or vegetable
		Beef, pork, chicken or fish
	Peas, carrots	Vegetables: white radish, lotus root, onion, green beans or potatoes
	Lettuce salad	
	Rolls	Rice ball
	Ice cream	Seasonal fresh fruit: orange, apple, pear, grapes or banana.
	Coffee	Green tea

* Menu for Diet B, young adult, Chap. 8.

the average citizen better understands the way families eat and live in far-off places. Many persons are making these discoveries for themselves as a result of world travel, service in the armed forces overseas, and through the myriad of cultural exchange programs under which people live, study, and work in countries other than their own. Such first-hand experiences have helped to demonstrate that basic nutrition needs are similar everywhere and that essentially the same kinds of foods nourish all peoples, even though the foods themselves may look and taste unlike those served at home.

Eating together is a symbol of good will in every culture. This simple rite tends to remove barriers to friendship that are often resistant to more ambitious efforts. Urging appreciation of the foods of other cultures is not to suggest that national food customs should be abandoned, and that, eventually all people should learn to like and eat the same foods. Quite the contrary! It *does* suggest the importance of increased acceptance and respect for the distinctive features of the diets of nations other than one's own. Such understanding is an essential element in recognizing world nutrition problems, and a long step toward solving them.

» THE SCENT OF VICTORY

What is being accomplished by all of these national and international efforts in behalf of improved nutrition? What, if any, are the signs of improvement? Progress may be measured in many different ways. One authority has said that mere recognition of the nature and distribution of main nutritional disorders in the world and the organized national and international efforts to do something about them constitute a major advance [19]. Another world figure has cited as evidence of progress the fact that we are the first generation that has dared to think in terms of food enough for all, and that we have progressed even to the point of considering *quality* as well as quantity of food for the world's peoples [3]. These are only "straws in the wind," but the fact that we already possess the technical "know how" to increase the food supplies of the world gives added encouragement. This knowledge has scarcely been tapped as yet. With all agencies working in their respective fields and cooperating on problems of joint concern, it should be possible soon to "catch the scent of victory."

REFERENCES

1. Stiebeling, H. K., "Food in Our Lives," *Food—The Yearbook of Agriculture.* Washington, D.C.: U.S. Department of Agriculture, 1959. p. 1.
2. Wells, O. V., "The Years Ahead," *Food—The Yearbook of Agriculture.* Washington, D.C.: U.S. Department of Agriculture, 1959. p. 701.
3. *Proceedings of the Fifth International Congress on Nutrition.* Federation Proceedings, American Societies for Experimental Biology. Vol. 20, No. 1, Part III, Suppl. 7, March 1961.
4. Judd, J. E., "Century-old Dietary Taboos in 20th Century Japan," *J. Am. Dietet. Assoc.,* 33 (May 1957) pp. 489–91.
5. *Control of Malnutrition in Man.* New York: American Public Health Association, 1960.
6. *Food for The Future through Research.* Agriculture Information Bull. 220. Washington, D.C.: U.S. Department of Agriculture, 1960.
7. Finkelstein, B., "Progress in Space Feeding Research," *J. Am. Dietet. Assoc.,* 40 (June 1962) pp. 528–31.
8. Adelson, S. F., and Wilson, C. S., *Nutrition Committee News (Some Organized Efforts in Nutrition).* Washington, D.C.: U.S. Department of Agriculture, Nov. 1958–April 1959.
9. *An Act for International Development, 1962.* Washington, D.C.: U.S. Department of State.
10. Akroyd, W. R., "FAO," *Nutrition Abstracts and Reviews,* 23 (April 1953) pp. 229–43.
11. *Report of FAO/WHO Seminar on Problems of Food and Nutrition in Africa South of the Sahara.* Rome, Italy: Food and Agriculture Organization, 1961.*
12. *Report of Technical Meeting on Nutrition in Food Policy and Planning in Asia and The Far East.* Rome, Italy: Food and Agriculture Organization, 1961.*
13. *Report on Regional Seminar on School Feeding in South America.* Rome, Italy: Food and Agriculture Organization, 1959.*

14. *Freedom From Hunger Campaign—A Statement of Philosophy and Plan.* Rome, Italy: Food and Agriculture Organization, 1961.*
15. *FAO—What It Is, What It Does, How It Works.* Washington, D.C.: Food and Agriculture Organization, Regional Office, North America.
WHO—What It Is, What It Does, How It Works. Washington, D.C.: Food and Agriculture Organization, Regional Office, North America.
UNICEF—What It Is, What It Does, How It Works. New York: U.S. Commission for UNICEF, United Nations.
UNESCO—What It Is, What It Does, How It Works. New York: United Nations Educational Scientific and Cultural Organization.
16. *Food For Fitness—A Daily Food Guide.* Leaflet No. 424, Washington, D.C.: U.S. Department of Agriculture, 1958.
17. Anderson, A. W., "Fishing and the Fishing Industry," *Food—The Yearbook of Agriculture.* Washington, D.C.: U.S. Department of Agriculture, 1959. p. 353.
18. All material on Japanese foods in meals was prepared in consultation with Miss Chieko Goh of Gakushuin Junior College, Tokyo, Japan, and with Miss Mieko Nasu, Chicago.
19. Scrimshaw, N. S., "Progress in Solving World Nutrition Problems," *J. Am. Dietet. Assoc.,* 35 (May 1959) pp. 441–47.

READINGS†

The Food We Eat. Miscell. Pub. 870. Washington, D.C.: U.S. Department of Agriculture, 1961.

Finkelstein, B., "Nutrition Research for the Space Traveller," *J. Am. Dietet. Assoc.,* 36 (April 1960) pp. 313–17.

Foreign Agricultural Service, *The World Food Deficit—A First Approximation.* Washington, D.C.: U.S. Department of Agriculture, March 1961.

Harris, R. S., "Nutrients in Breads from Fourteen Countries," *J. Am. Dietet. Assoc.,* 38 (Jan. 1961) pp. 27–31.

Hungry Angels. (16 mm film; color, 20 min.) UNICEF Information Service, Suite 220, 20 E Street, N.W., Washington, D.C.

Man and Hunger. World Food Problems No. 2. Rome, Italy: Food and Agriculture Organization, 1961.*

Nuestra Huerta Escolar, Manual De Nutrición Y Horticultura. Rome, Italy: Food and Agriculture Organization, 1960. (A manual developed and tested for 3 years in Guatemala in training courses for rural school teachers working in the FAO/WHO/UNICEF-assisted program being carried out there. Printed in Spanish.)

"Nutrition for Man In Space," *Nutrition Reviews,* 18 (April 1960) pp. 100–101.

White, R. B. "Turkish and American Women Study Feeding the Family," (An experiment in teaching nutrition in Ankara.) *J. Home Economics,* 54 (May 1962) pp. 390–93.

---

* FAO publications may be obtained in the United States from the Regional Office of North America in Washington, D.C.

† See also "Suggestions for further readings" on the following page. Many of the references on that list contribute to the topic of global nutrition discussed in Chapter 11.

Suggestions for further readings

Now that you have been introduced to nutrition you will want to continue and broaden your interest in it. Everyday, new books and pamphlets are published which show the basic relationship of foods and nutrition to the well-being of people and the affairs of the world. You will find in the following listing exciting reading that will take you beyond your present concept of nutrition.

Calder, R., *Common Sense about a Starving World.* New York: The Macmillan Company, 1962.

———, *Men against the Desert.* London: George Allen & Unwin Ltd., 1951.

———, *Men against the Jungle.* New York: The Macmillan Company, 1954. These three fascinating books were written by the widely-read Ritchie Calder, science editor for a London newspaper. He has described his experiences with peoples in all parts of the world, recounting how they live, what they eat, how they survive their environments, ways they may be helped.

Desrosier, N. W., *Attack on Starvation.* Westport, Conn.: The AVI Publishing Co., Inc., 1961.
This book was written by a specialist in the field of food technology. He is explicit on ways to approach the problem. It is not sufficient, says the author, to hope that starvation will eliminate itself: we must be willing to do something about the situation.

Food and Nutrition Board, *The Role of Nutrition in International Programs.* Washington, D.C.: National Academy of Sciences–National Research Council, 1961. This is a booklet developed by the Committee on International Nutrition Programs of the Food and Nutrition Board. It outlines basic principles that could serve as a guide to the proper emphasis on nutrition in international programs.

Gerard, R. W., *Food For Life.* Chicago: University of Chicago Press, 1952.
Several well-known physicians and other scientists contributed to the content of this book. It covers in rather popular style basic information about food and its significance in the nutrition of people.

Hemming, J. *Mankind Against the Killers.* New York: Longmans, Green & Co., Inc., 1956.
As the title suggests, this book deals more with bacteriology than with nutrition. However, emphasis is placed on the need for control of the "killers" in behalf of good health, not on the details of control methods. The style of writing invites reading.

McCollum, E. V., *The History of Nutrition.* Boston: Houghton Mifflin Company, 1957.
A scholarly, well-documented treatise on the history of nutrition. It traces in considerable detail nutrition research in several major areas.

Mead, M. (Ed.), *Cultural Patterns and Technical Change.* Paris: UNESCO, 1953. Studies of cultures in various parts of the world are reported. Principles involved in developing mental health during technical change are given special emphasis.

Riedman, S. R., *Food For People.* New York: Abelard-Schuman Ltd., 1961.

Lord John Boyd Orr, who has written the introduction to this unusual book, says: "Food is a common daily need of all mankind, and in this now small world the task of increasing the food supply to meet the needs of all the people in all countries should be a common task of all governments."

Roberts, L. J., and Stefani, R. L., *Patterns of Living in Puerto Rican Families.* Rio Piedras: The University of Puerto Rico, 1949.

A picture of the living conditions in Puerto Rico in the late 1940's is presented. It is based on an island-wide study of a representative sample of families. The report describes in detail the food and living habits of the people at that time.

Sen, B. R., *The Basic Freedom—Freedom From Hunger.* Rome, Italy: Food and Agriculture Organization, 1960. (Obtainable from North American Regional Office, 1325 C St., S.W., Washington, D.C.

This booklet is composed of selections from speeches made by Dr. Sen, Director General of FAO. It stresses particularly the *Freedom from Hunger* campaign and the critical need for achieving this goal for all the world.

Simoons, F. J., *Eat Not This Flesh.* Madison: University of Wisconsin Press, 1961.

The author outlines 2 objectives: to consider the use and avoidance of certain foods of animal origin in the old world and to explain their occurrence in historical terms; and to demonstrate that foodways behave like other culture traits. The book contains an amazing collection of food customs and taboos. It will stimulate you to use its extensive reference list to read still more on the subject.

Stefansson, V., *The Fat of the Land.* New York: The Macmillan Company, 1956.

The author lived for many years in the Arctic and ate the native diet, consisting chiefly of meat. He has written extensively of his experiences. The present book includes some of his earlier material.

Stewart, M. S., *That No Man Shall Hunger.* New York: Public Affairs Pamphlet No. 304, 1960.

What *should* be done and what is *being* done by FAO and other organizations to free the world of hunger is outlined in this booklet.

Todhunter, E. N., "The Story of Nutrition," *Food–The Yearbook of Agriculture.* Washington, D.C.: U.S. Department of Agriculture, 1959. p. 7.

An account of men and women throughout the world who have contributed to the development of the science of nutrition. What they have contributed and how each step in progress has depended on the one before it makes a fascinating story.

———, *Human Nutrition—Past and Present.* Reprinted from Centennial Symposium, "Nutrition of Plants, Animals, Man," sponsored by the College of Agriculture, Michigan State University (Lansing), February 14–16, 1955.

This report summarizes present nutrition knowledge in a group of concepts; traces briefly the development of scientific thought leading to the emergence of nutrition as a science; describes some of the tools of nutrition research; and indicates some of the classical studies, past and present, in human nutrition.

Ward, B., *The Rich Nations and the Poor Nations.* New York: W. W. Norton & Company, Inc., 1962.

A British woman economist is concerned with the gap between the rich nations and the poor nations. She analyzes the reasons for the gap and suggests ways to narrow it.

Williams, R. J., *The Human Frontier*. New York: Harcourt, Brace & World, Inc., 1946.

A well-known scientist discusses some of the areas in nutrition and chemistry about which we know little and need to know more. His comments on his own informal explorations of some of these problems make this an interesting book.

Williams, R. R., *Williams-Waterman Fund For the Combat of Dietary Diseases*. New York: Research Corporation, 1956.

The engrossing story of the fight against dietary deficiency diseases around the world. It is particularly concerned with thiamine, the results of a deficiency of this vitamin, and cereal enrichment as a way of combating this deficiency.

Appendixes

APPENDIX A

Sample form for three-day meal record: instructions

FIRST DAY (sample day's meals, Chap. 3)			SECOND DAY			THIRD DAY	
Meals	Amount of Food	Additional Information	Meals	Amount of Food	Additional Information	Meals	Amount of Food
Breakfast			**Breakfast**			**Breakfast**	
Pineapple juice	1 glass	½ standard cup	Prunes				
Cornflakes	1⅓ cup	fortified	Egg				
sugar	2 tsp	white					
milk	¼ cup	whole					
Toast	2 sl	white, enrich.	Muffin				
butter*	2 tsp		butter*				
jelly	1 tbsp	fruit jelly					
Coffee	if desired		Cocoa				
Morning Snack			**Morning Snack**				
None			Apple				
Lunch			**Lunch**				
Baked beans	¾ cup	with pork	Ham sandwich				
Celery	1 stalk	raw	bun				
Applesauce	½ cup	sweetened	ham				
Gingerbread	1 piece	2x2x2 in.	butter* relish				
Milk	1 glass	8 oz whole	Orange				
			Milk shake				
Afternoon Snack			**Afternoon Snack**				
Kola-type drink	6 oz	¾ cup	Cookies				
Dinner			**Dinner**				
Hamburger	1–3 oz	3 in. diam. ¾ in. thick	Pork chop				
Potato	1 med	white, boiled	Potato				
butter*	1 tsp		butter*				
Green beans	½ cup		Carrots				
butter*	1 tsp		butter*				
Cole slaw	½ cup	raw cabbage	Green salad				
Roll	1 (yeast)	white, enriched	Bread				
butter*	1 tsp		butter*				
Lemon meringue pie	1/7 pie	9 in. pie	Rice pudding				
Evening Snack			**Evening Snack**				
Cupcake	1 cake, iced	2¾ in. dia	Orange				

Suggestions for Recording Meals
(use form shown on this page)

1. List all the foods you eat for a period of 3 days.
   Record everything you put into your mouth and swallow.
   List foods as soon after eating as possible, preferably at the table. Do not trust your memory.
   Provide "additional information" for each food (see form). This is needed to identify foods properly for calculation.
   Include all "extras": snacks, butter for bread, butter or sauce for vegetables, dressings for salads, jelly, jam, nuts, etc. Include vitamin pills or other concentrates.
   List separately the different foods that compose one diet item, such as the "makings" of a ham sandwich (see sample second day), or cereal with milk and sugar (see sample first day). Indent accompanying foods for ease in interpreting the menu.
2. Measure or estimate quantities of foods.
   Measure foods in standard measuring cups or spoons. Learn to visualize quantities.
   Examine measures of foods in Appendix G to assist you in recognizing denominations of foods to be used in calculating their nutritive content. For equivalents in weights and measures and for abbreviations, see Appendix F.
3. *Select one day's meals* from the 3 recorded to be used as a basis for calculating calorie and nutrient values.
   Choose the day most representative of your regular eating habits. Weekend meals are often atypical.
   Avoid, so far as feasible, a day with several complicated food mixtures. They introduce errors because of the difficulty in estimating quantities of ingredients.
   Set up your chosen day's meals on the form used for the specimen diet in Appendix B. Use a large piece of paper to avoid crowding. Crossbar paper is useful.

* Or margarine fortified with vitamin A.

APPENDIX B

Calculation of specimen diet

Diet based on sample day's meals, chapter 3

MEALS	Amounts of Foods	Cal.	Pro-tein g	Cal-cium mg	Iron mg	Vita-min A IU	Thia-min mg	Ribo-flavin mg	Ascorbic acid mg
BREAKFAST									
Pineapple juice	½ cup	60	1	19	0.6	100	0.07	0.02	11
Cornflakes	1⅓ cups	110	2	3	0.5		0.12	0.03	
sugar	2 tsp	35							
milk, whole	¼ cup	41	2	71		98	0.02	0.11	
Toast (enriched)	2 sl.	120	4	38	1.2		0.10	0.10	
butter*	2 tsp	70				307			
jelly	1 tbsp	50		2	0.1				1
Coffee	if desired								
Breakfast Totals		486	9	133	2.4	505	0.31	0.26	12
LUNCH									
Baked beans	¾ cup	250	12	129	3.3	105	0.10	0.08	4
Celery	1 stalk	5	1	20	0.2		0.02	0.02	3
Applesauce	½ cup	90		5	0.5	40	0.03	0.02	2
Gingerbread	1 piece	180	2	63	1.4	50	0.02	0.05	
Milk (whole)	1 cup	165	9	285	0.1	390	0.08	0.42	2
Lunch Totals		690	24	502	5.5	585	0.25	0.59	11
DINNER									
Hamburger	1, 3 in.	245	21	9	2.7	30	0.07	0.02	
Potato	1 med.	90	3	9	0.7		0.10	0.04	20
Green beans	½ cup	15	1	23	0.5	415	0.05	0.06	9
Cole slaw	½ cup	50	1	24	0.3	40	0.03	0.03	25
Roll, soft	1	115	3	28	0.7		0.11	0.07	
Butter* for roll, beans, potato	1 tbsp	100				460			
Lemon meringue pie (9 in.)	1/7	300	4	24	0.6	210	0.04	0.10	1
Dinner Totals		915	33	117	5.5	1155	0.40	0.32	55
SNACKS (all other intake)									
Kola-type drink	6-oz glass	80							
Cupcake, iced	1, 2¾ in.	160	3	58	0.2	50	0.01	0.04	
Snack Totals		240	3	58	0.2	50	0.01	0.04	
Grand Totals for day		2331	69	810	13.6	2295	0.97	1.21	78
Recommended Daily Allowances for Young Adult Woman		2300	58	800	12.0	5000	1.20	1.50	70
Estimated Daily Calorie Need (Personal activity, Chap. 4)—2246.									

* Or margarine fortified with vitamin A.

APPENDIX C

*Recommended daily dietary allowances,** REVISED 1958

Food and Nutrition Board, National Research Council

(Allowances are intended for persons normally active in a temperate climate)

	Age Years	Weight kg (lb)	Height cm (in.)	Calories	Protein g	Calcium mg	Iron mg	Vitamin A IU	Thiam. mg	Ribo. mg	Niacin† mg equiv.	Asc. Acid mg	Vitamin D IU
Men	25	70 (154)	175 (69)	3200‡	70	800	10	5000	1.6	1.8	21	75	
	45	70 (154)	175 (69)	3000	70	800	10	5000	1.5	1.8	20	75	
	65	70 (154)	175 (69)	2550	70	800	10	5000	1.3	1.8	18	75	
Women	25	58 (128)	163 (64)	2300	58	800	12	5000	1.2	1.5	17	70	
	45	58 (128)	163 (64)	2200	58	800	12	5000	1.1	1.5	17	70	
	65	58 (128)	163 (64)	1800	58	800	12	5000	1.0	1.5	17	70	
	Pregnant (second half)			+300	+20	1500	15	6000	1.3	2.0	+3	100	400
	Lactating (850 ml daily)			+1000	+40	2000	15	8000	1.7	2.5	+2	150	400
Infants	0–1/12§				See								
	2/12–6/12	6 (13)	60 (24)	kg × 120	Footnote	600	5	1500	0.4	0.5	6	30	400
	7/12–12/12	9 (20)	70 (28)	kg × 100	§	800	7	1500	0.5	0.8	7	30	400
Children	1– 3	12 (27)	87 (34)	1300	40	1000	7	2000	0.7	1.0	8	35	400
	4– 6	18 (40)	109 (43)	1700	50	1000	8	2500	0.9	1.3	11	50	400
	7– 9	27 (60)	129 (51)	2100	60	1000	10	3500	1.1	1.5	14	60	400
	10–12	36 (79)	144 (57)	2500	70	1200	12	4500	1.3	1.8	17	75	400
Boys	13–15	49 (108)	163 (64)	3100	85	1400	15	5000	1.6	2.1	21	90	400
	16–19	63 (139)	175 (69)	3600	100	1400	15	5000	1.8	2.5	25	100	400
Girls	13–15	49 (108)	160 (63)	2600	80	1300	15	5000	1.3	2.0	17	80	400
	16–19	54 (120)	162 (64)	2400	75	1300	15	5000	1.2	1.9	16	80	400

* The allowance levels are intended to cover individual variations among most normal persons as they live in the United States under usual environmental stresses. The recommended allowances can be attained with a variety of common foods, providing other nutrients for which human requirements have been less well defined.

† Niacin equivalents include dietary sources of the preformed vitamin and the precursor, tryptophan. Sixty mg tryptophan equals 1 mg niacin.

‡ Calorie allowances apply to individuals usually engaged in moderate physical activity. For office workers or others of sedentary occupations they are excessive. Adjustments must be made for variations in body size, age, physical activity, and environmental temperature.

§ The Board recognizes that human milk is the natural food for infants and feels that breast feeding is the best and desired procedure for meeting nutrient requirements in the first months of life. No allowances are stated for the first month of life. Breast feeding is particularly indicated during the first month when infants show handicaps in homeostasis due to different rates of maturation of digestive, excretory, and endocrine functions. Recommendations as listed pertain to nutrient intake as afforded by cow's milk formulas and supplementary foods given the infant when breast feeding is terminated. Allowances are not given for protein during infancy.

APPENDIX D

Desirable weights for men and women

Weight in Pounds According to Frame (in indoor clothing)

	HEIGHT (with shoes on) 1-in. heels Feet	Inches	SMALL FRAME	MEDIUM FRAME	LARGE FRAME
	5	2	112–120	118–129	126–141
	5	3	115–123	121–133	129–144
	5	4	118–126	124–136	132–148
DESIRABLE	5	5	121–129	127–139	135–152
	5	6	124–133	130–143	138–156
WEIGHTS	5	7	128–137	134–147	142–161
	5	8	132–141	138–152	147–166
FOR MEN	5	9	136–145	142–156	151–170
	5	10	140–150	146–160	155–174
of ages 25	5	11	144–154	150–165	159–179
	6	0	148–158	154–170	164–184
and over	6	1	152–162	158–175	168–189
	6	2	156–167	162–180	173–194
	6	3	160–171	167–185	178–199
	6	4	164–175	172–190	182–204

	HEIGHT (with shoes on) 2-in. heels Feet	Inches	SMALL FRAME	MEDIUM FRAME	LARGE FRAME
	4	10	92– 98	96–107	104–119
	4	11	94–101	98–110	106–122
	5	0	96–104	101–113	109–125
DESIRABLE	5	1	99–107	104–116	112–128
	5	2	102–110	107–119	115–131
WEIGHTS	5	3	105–113	110–122	118–134
	5	4	108–116	113–126	121–138
FOR WOMEN	5	5	111–119	116–130	125–142
	5	6	114–123	120–135	129–146
of ages 25	5	7	118–127	124–139	133–150
	5	8	122–131	128–143	137–154
and over	5	9	126–135	132–147	141–158
	5	10	130–140	136–151	145–163
	5	11	134–144	140–155	149–168
	6	0	138–148	144–159	153–173

For girls 18–25, subtract 1 lb for each year under 25.

METROPOLITAN LIFE INSURANCE COMPANY

APPENDIX E

Specimen weight chart

Young woman: medium frame, 5 ft 4 in. tall
Desirable weight zone: 113–126 lbs

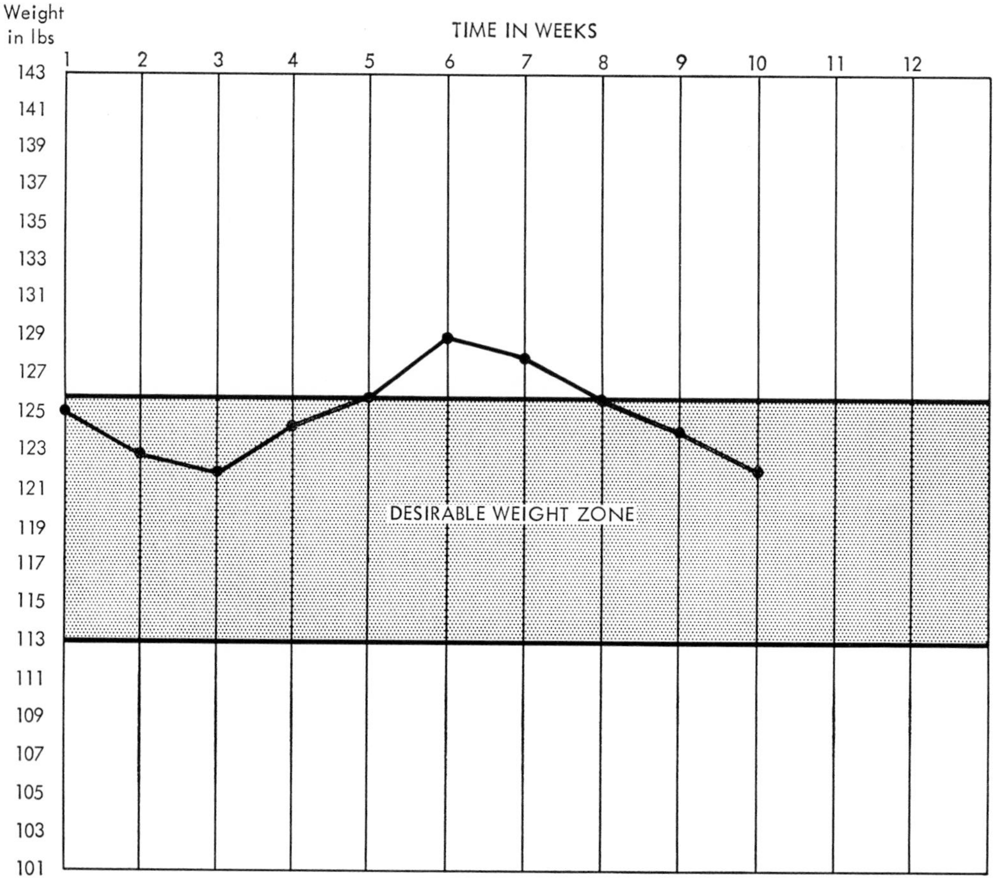

Weekly weights in lbs:	125	129
	123	128
	122	126
	124	124
	126	122

APPENDIX F

Equivalents in weights and measures; abbreviations

1. Equivalents of Commonly Used Weights and Measures

1 tablespoon	3 teaspoons
1 cup	16 tablespoons (or ½ pt, or ¼ qt)
1 pint, liquid	2 cups
1 quart, liquid	2 pints (or 4 cups)
1 liter	1.06 quarts (or 1000 milliliters)
1 ounce	28.4 grams
1 pound	453.6 grams (or 16 oz)
1 kilogram	2.2 pounds
1 gram	1,000 milligrams
1 milligram	1,000 micrograms
1 microgram	1/1,000,000 gram

2. Abbreviations Used in Text and Tables

Units of Measurement

cal	calorie
g	gram
in.	inch
kg	kilogram
l	liter
lb	pound
μg	microgram
mg	milligram
ml	milliliter
oz	ounce
pt	pint
qt	quart
tbsp	tablespoon
tsp	teaspoon

Miscellaneous

bk'd	baked
can'd	canned
dia	diameter
enrch'd	enriched
hd	head
indiv.	individual
med.	medium
pl.	plain
serv.	serving
sl.	slice
tr	trace
vit.	vitamin

APPENDIX G

Nutritive values of foods in household units

Foods largely in forms ready to eat

Dots appearing on the Table in place of numerical values indicate there may be a measurable amount of a constituent present, but no evidence is available to verify its presence. For abbreviations and equivalents in weights and measures, see Appendix F.

Sources of Data Used in Development of Appendix G

Nutritive Value of Foods. Home and Garden Bulletin No. 72. Washington, D.C.: U.S. Department of Agriculture, 1960.

Composition of Foods (Raw, Processed, Prepared). Agriculture Handbook No. 8, Washington, D.C.: U.S. Department of Agriculture, 1950.

Composition of Puerto Rican foods: Dr. Lydia J. Roberts, University of Puerto Rico. Personal communication, 1962.

Food Composition Table for use in Latin America: The Institute of Nutrition of Central America and Panama, and The Interdepartmental Committee on Nutrition for National Defense. Bethesda, Maryland: National Institutes of Health, 1961.

The calorie and nutritive values of several dishes (combination of foods): calculated by the author using recipes from M. Heseltine and U. M. Dow, *The New Basic Cook Book,* Boston: Houghton Mifflin Company, 1957. Dishes were prepared and weights and measures recorded.

Food	Weight oz	Approximate Measure and Description	Calories	Protein g	Fat g	Carbohydrate g	Calcium mg	Iron mg	Vit. A Value IU	Thiamine mg	Riboflavin mg	Asc. acid mg
Almonds, shelled	0.5	12 nuts or 2 tbsp	90	3	8	3	35	0.7	0	0.04	0.14	tr
Apple, baked	4.6	1 med. apple, 2½ in. dia	120	tr	tr	30	8	0.4	50	0.04	0.02	3
Apple, raw	5.3	1 med. apple, 2½ in. dia	70	tr	tr	18	8	0.4	50	0.04	0.02	3
Apple, brown Betty	4.0	½ cup	175	2	4	35	21	0.7	135	0.07	0.05	tr
Apple pie (see Pies)												
Applejuice (sweet cider)	4.4	½ cup, fresh or can'd	60	tr	0	17	8	0.6	45	0.03	0.04	1
Applesauce	4.4	½ cup, sweetened, can'd	90	tr	tr	25	5	0.5	40	0.03	0.02	2
Apricots, canned	4.3	½ cup or 4 med. halves, 2 tbsp juice, sirup pack	105	1	tr	27	13	0.4	2130	0.02	0.03	5
Apricots, raw	1.3	1 med apricot	20	tr	tr	5	6	0.2	963	0.01	0.01	3
Apricots, dried, cooked	3.8	½ cup (scant) or 8 halves, 2 tbsp juice, sweetened	135	2	tr	34	26	1.5	2287	tr	0.04	3
Apricot whip	3.3	½ cup made with whipped nonfat dry milk	130	4	tr	30	64	1.2	2342	0.02	0.12	4
Asparagus, green, cooked	3.1	½ cup or 9 green stalks 4½ in. long	20	2	tr	3	17	0.9	910	0.12	0.15	20
Avocado, raw	3.8	½ avocado, 3⅓ x 4¼ in. peeled and pitted	185	2	18	6	11	0.6	310	0.12	0.21	15
Bacon, broiled or fried	0.6	2 sl., cooked crisp	95	5	8	1	2	0.5	0	0.08	0.05	...
Bacon, Canadian, cooked	1.5	3 sl., cooked crisp	100	18	12	tr	13	2.2	0	0.62	0.12	0
Banana, raw	5.3	1 med banana, 6 x 1½ in.	85	1	tr	23	8	0.7	190	0.05	0.06	10
Bavarian cream	3.5	½ cup (orange)	210	2	10	30	27	0.1	627	0.10	0.05	54
Bean sprouts, raw	1.6	½ cup, Mung sprouts	10	2	tr	2	13	0.4	5	0.03	0.04	7
Beans, white, dry, can'd	6.9	¾ cup, with pork and tomato or molasses	250	12	5	41	129	3.3	105	0.10	0.08	4
Beans, white, dry, can'd	6.9	¾ cup, without pork and with tomato or molasses	240	12	1	45	137	3.9	105	0.10	0.08	4
Beans, Lima, dry, cooked	5.0	¾ cup	195	12	1	36	42	4.2	tr	0.20	0.09	tr
Beans, Lima, green, cooked	2.8	½ cup	75	4	1	15	23	1.4	230	0.11	0.07	12
Beans, pinto, dry, raw	3.5	½ cup (Mexican red beans)	350	23	1	64	160	6.9	0	0.65	0.24	2

Beans, red, dry, can'd	6.7	¾ cup	175	11	1	32	56	3.5	0	0.10	0.10	tr
Beans, snap, green, cooked	2.2	½ cup	15	1	tr	3	23	0.5	415	0.05	0.06	9
Beef, corned, can'd	3.0	3 sl., 3 x 2 x ¼ in.	180	22	10	0	17	3.7	20	0.01	0.20	. . .
Beef, corned, hash, can'd	4.5	¾ cup	180	18	8	9	33	1.7	15	0.03	0.17	. . .
Beef, dried or chipped	2.0	4 thin sl., 4 x 5 in.	115	19	4	0	11	2.9	. . .	0.04	0.18	. . .
Beef, hamburger, cooked	3.0	1 patty, 3 in. dia (market ground)	245	21	17	0	9	2.7	30	0.07	0.02	. . .
Beef, heart, braised	3.0	2 round sl., 2½ in. dia, ½ in. thick	160	26	5	1	14	5.9	30	0.23	1.05	3
Beef, liver (see Liver)												
Beef, loaf (see Meat loaf)												
Beef, pot roast, cooked	3.0	1 piece, 4 x 3¾ x ½ in.	245	23	16	0	10	2.9	30	0.04	0.18	. . .
Beef, potpie, bkd.	7.9	1 indiv. pie, 4¼ in. dia	460	18	28	32	20	2.5	2830	0.07	0.14	tr
Beef, roast, oven cooked	3.0	2 sl., 6 x 3¼ x ⅛ in.	255	22	18	0	9	2.8	30	0.06	0.16	0
Beef steak, broiled	3.0	1 piece, 3½ x 2 x ¾ in., no bone	375	19	32	0	9	2.6	60	0.06	0.16	0
Beef Stroganoff, cooked	4.6	½ cup	250	17	18	6	41	2.6	395	0.12	0.29	2
Beef tongue, boiled	3.0	7 sl., 2¼ x 2¼ x ⅛ in.	205	18	14	tr	7	2.5	. . .	0.04	0.26	. . .
Beets, cooked	2.9	½ cup, diced	35	1	tr	8	18	0.6	15	0.02	0.04	6
Beverages												
Beer	8.4	1 glass, 4 percent alcohol*	115	1	tr	11	10	tr	0	tr	0.06	0
Eggnog	4.0	½ cup (holiday type)*	225	3	11	12	56	0.4	536	0.03	0.12	. . .
Ginger ale	7.0	⅞ cup, carbonated soft drink	70	. . .	. . .	18	. . .	. . .	. . .	. . .	. . .	. . .
Kola-type	6.0	¾ cup, carbonated soft drink	80	. . .	. . .	21	. . .	. . .	. . .	. . .	. . .	. . .
Biscuits, baking powder	1.3	1 biscuit, 2½ in. dia, (enrch'd flour)	130	3	4	18	61	0.7	tr	0.09	0.09	tr
Blackberries, raw	2.5	½ cup	40	1	1	10	23	0.7	145	0.03	0.03	15
Blueberries, raw	2.5	½ cup	45	1	1	11	11	0.7	70	0.02	0.04	10
Bluefish, cooked	3.0	1 piece, 3½ x 2 x ½ in.	135	22	4	0	25	0.6	40	0.09	0.08	. . .
Bologna (see Sausage)												
Bouillon cubes	0.14	1 cube, ⅝ in.	2	tr	tr	0	. . .	. . .	. . .	. . .	0.07	0
Branflakes	1.0	¾ cup (40% bran), added thiamine)	85	3	1	22	17	1.1	0	0.13	0.07	0

Food	Weight oz	Approximate Measure and Description	Calories	Protein g	Fat g	Carbohydrate g	Calcium mg	Iron mg	Vit. A Value IU	Thiamine mg	Riboflavin mg	Asc. acid mg
Bread, Boston brown	1.7	1 sl., 3 in. dia, ½ in. thick, (degermed cornmeal)	100	3	1	22	43	0.9	0	0.05	0.03	0
Bread, cracked wheat	0.8	1 sl., 3¾ x 3¾ x ⅓ in.	60	2	1	12	20	0.3	tr	0.03	0.02	tr
Bread, French or Vienna	0.7	1 sl., 3¼ x 2 x 1 in. (enrch'd flour)	60	2	1	11	9	0.4	tr	0.06	0.04	tr
Bread, Italian	0.7	1 sl., 3¼ x 2 x 1 in. (enrch'd flour)	55	2	tr	11	3	0.4	0	0.06	0.04	0
Bread, pumpernickel	1.2	1 sl., 4¾ x 3½ x ⅜ in. (dark rye flour)	85	3	0	19	30	0.8	0	0.08	0.05	0
Bread, raisin	0.8	1 sl., 3¾ x 3¾ x ⅓ in.	60	2	1	12	16	0.3	tr	0.01	0.02	tr
Bread, rye, light	0.8	1 sl., 2¾ x 2¼ x ½ in. (American type: ⅓ rye, ⅔ wheat)	55	2	tr	12	17	0.4	0	0.04	0.02	0
Bread, white	0.8	1 sl., 3¾ x 3¾ x ⅓ in. (enrch'd flour, 3–4% nonfat dry milk)	60	2	1	12	19	0.6	tr	0.06	0.05	tr
Bread, white	0.8	1 sl., 3¾ x 3¾ x ⅓ in. (unenrch'd flour, 3–4% nonfat dry milk)	60	2	1	12	19	0.2	tr	0.02	0.02	tr
Bread, white, toasted	0.7	1 sl., 3¾ x 3¾ x ⅓ in. (enrch'd flour, 3–4% nonfat dry milk)	60	2	1	12	19	0.6	tr	0.05	0.05	tr
Bread, whole-wheat	0.8	1 sl., 3¾ x 3¾ x ⅓ in. (graham or entire wheat bread	55	2	1	11	23	0.5	tr	0.06	0.05	tr
Bread crumbs	0.8	¼ cup, dry	85	3	1	16	27	0.8	tr	0.05	0.07	tr
Broccoli, cooked	2.6	½ cup	20	3	tr	4	98	1.0	2550	0.05	0.11	56
Brussels sprouts, cooked	2.3	½ cup or 5 med sprouts	30	3	1	6	22	0.9	260	0.03	0.08	30
Bun (see Rolls)												
Butter	0.5	1 tbsp or 1 pat, ½ in. thick	100	tr	11	tr	3	tr	460	. . .	. . .	0

Buttermilk, cultured from skim milk (see Milk, skim)												
Cabbage, cooked	3.0	½ cup, cooked briefly, little water	20	1	tr	5	39	0.4	75	0.04	0.04	27
Cabbage, raw	1.8	½ cup, finely shredded	10	1	tr	3	23	0.3	40	0.03	0.03	25
Cabbage, Chinese, raw	1.8	½ cup, 1 in. pieces	8	1	tr	1	22	0.5	130	0.02	0.02	16
Cake, angel food	1.4	2 in. sector or 1/12 of cake 8 in. dia without icing	110	3	tr	23	2	0.1	0	tr	0.05	tr
Cake, chocolate, layer	4.2	2 in. sector or 1/16 of cake 10 in. dia, fudge icing	420	5	14	70	118	0.5	140†	0.03	0.10	tr
Cake, fruit, dark	1.1	1 piece, 2 x 2 x ½ in.	105	2	4	17	29	0.8	50†	0.04	0.04	tr
Cake, pl., cupcake	1.4	1 cupcake, 2¾ in. dia without icing	130	3	3	23	62	0.2	50†	0.01	0.03	tr
Cake, pl., cupcake	1.8	1 cupcake, 2¾ in. dia with icing	160	3	3	31	58	0.2	50†	0.01	0.04	tr
Cake, pl., layer	3.5	2 in. sector or 1/16 of cake 10 in. dia with icing	320	5	6	62	117	0.4	90†	0.02	0.07	tr
Cake, pl., loaf	1.9	1 piece, 3 x 2 x 1½ in. without icing	180	4	5	31	85	0.2	70†	0.02	0.05	tr
Cake, pound	1.1	1 sl., 2¾ x 3 x ⅝ in.	130	2	7	15	16	0.5	100†	0.04	0.05	tr
Cake, sponge	1.4	2 in. sector or 1/12 of cake, 8 in. dia	115	3	2	22	11	0.6	210†	0.02	0.06	tr
Candy, caramels	1.0	4 small	120	1	3	22	36	0.7	50	0.01	0.04	tr
Candy, chocolate bar, pl. milk chocolate, sweet	1.0	1 bar, 3¾ x 1½ x ¼ in.	145	2	9	16	61	0.3	40	0.03	0.11	0
Candy, chocolate bar, almond	1.75	1 bar, 5⅓ x 1⅞ x ⅓ in.	265	4	19	25	102	1.4	70	0.07	0.25	0
Candy, chocolate creams	1.0	2 pieces, 1¼ in. dia (base) ⅝ in. thick	110	1	4	20	. . .	. . .	. . .	. . .	. . .	0
Candy, chocolate fudge	1.0	1 piece, 1¼ x 1¼ x 1 in.	115	tr	3	23	14	0.1	60	tr	0.02	tr
Candy, hard	1.0	6 pieces, 1 in. dia ¼ in. thick	110	0	0	28	0	0	0	0	0	0
Candy, peanut brittle	1.0	1 piece, 3¼ x 2½ x ¼ in.	125	2	4	21	11	0.6	10	0.03	0.01	0
Cantaloup, raw	13.5	½ melon, 5 in. dia	40	1	tr	9	33	0.8	6950 (orange flesh)	0.09	0.07	63

Food	Weight oz	Approximate Measure and Description	Calories	Protein g	Fat g	Carbohydrate g	Calcium mg	Iron mg	Vit. A Value IU	Thiamine mg	Riboflavin mg	Asc. acid mg
Carrots, cooked	2.6	½ cup, diced	20	1	1	5	19	0.5	9065	0.04	0.04	3
Carrots, raw	1.9	½ cup, grated	20	1	tr	5	22	0.5	6600	0.03	0.03	4
Carrots, raw	1.8	1 carrot, 5½ in. long or 25 thin strips	20	1	tr	5	20	0.4	6000	0.03	0.03	3
Catsup, tomato (see Tomato)												
Cauliflower, cooked	2.1	½ cup, flower buds	15	2	tr	3	13	0.7	55	0.04	0.05	17
Celery, raw	1.8	½ cup, diced	10	1	tr	2	25	0.3	0	0.03	0.02	4
Celery, raw	1.4	1 stalk, large outer, 8 in. long	5	1	tr	1	20	0.2	0	0.02	0.02	3
Cheese, blue mold	1.0	¾ in. sector or 3 tbsp (Roquefort type)	105	6	9	tr	122	0.2	350	0.01	0.17	0
Cheese, cheddar (American)	1.0	1 cube, 1⅛ in.	115	7	9	1	221	0.3	380	0.01	0.15	0
Cheese, cheddar (American)	0.25	1 tbsp, grated	30	2	2	tr	55	0.1	90	0.02	0.03	0
Cheese food, cheddar	1.0	2 round sl., 1⅝ in. dia, ¼ in. thick or 2 tbsp	95	6	7	2	163	0.2	300	0.01	0.17	0
Cheese, cottage	2.0	¼ cup creamed cottage cheese (made from skim milk)	60	8	2	2	50	0.2	100	0.02	0.16	0
Cheese, cottage	1.0	2 tbsp uncreamed cottage cheese (made from skim milk)	25	5	tr	1	26	0.1	tr	0.01	0.08	0
Cheese, cream	0.5	1 tbsp	55	1	6	tr	9	tr	230	tr	0.04	0
Cheese, Swiss	1.0	1 sl., 7 x 4 x ⅛ in.	105	7	8	1	271	0.3	320	0.01	0.06	0
Cheese sauce	2.1	¼ cup	110	5	9	4	156	0.1	337	0.02	0.14	1
Cheese souffle	2.8	¾ cup	200	10	16	7	210	1.0	826	0.08	0.23	1
Cheesecake	5.7	1/10 of cake, 9 in. dia	400	15	23	35	128	0.8	958	0.08	0.33	1
Cherries, domestic, raw	4.0	1 cup, sour, sweet, hybrid	65	1	1	15	19	0.4	650	0.05	0.06	9
Cherries, West Indian, raw	0.4	2 med cherries (Ascerola)	3	...	...	1	1	...	...	...	0.01	100
Chick peas, dry, raw	3.7	½ cup (*garbanzos*)	380	22	5	64	97	7.5	tr	0.58	0.19	2
Chicken, broiled	3.0	¼ small broiler, flesh and skin	185	23	9	0	10	1.4	260	0.04	0.15	...

Chicken, can'd	3.0	⅓ cup, boned meat	170	25	7	0	12	1.5	160	0.03	0.14	. . .
Chicken, creamed‡	3.5	½ cup	222	20	12	6	84	1.1	445	0.04	0.20	1
Chicken, fried	3.3	½ breast, with bone	215	24	12	. . .	10	1.1	60	0.03	0.06	. . .
Chicken, fried	4.3	1 leg (thigh and drumstick)	245	27	15	. . .	13	1.8	220	0.05	0.18	. . .
Chicken pie (see Poultry potpie)												
Chile con carne, can'd	6.6	¾ cup, made with beans	250	14	11	23	74	3.2	113	0.06	0.15	. . .
Chile con carne, can'd	6.7	¾ cup, made without beans	385	20	29	11	73	2.7	285	0.04	0.23	. . .
Chili powder	0.5	1 tbsp (hot red peppers, ground)	50	2	1	9	20	1.2	11520	0.03	0.20	2
Chili sauce	0.6	1 tbsp (mainly tomatoes)	15	tr	tr	4	2	0.1	320	0.02	0.01	2
Chocolate, bitter	1.0	1 square baking chocolate	145	2	15	8	28	1.2	20	0.01	0.06	0
Chocolate candy (see Candy)												
Chocolate-flavored milk	8.8	1 cup chocolate milk drink	190	8	6	27	270	0.4	210	0.09	0.41	2
Chocolate morsels	0.5	30 morsels or 1½ tbsp	80	1	4	10	5	0.3	tr	tr	tr	0
Chocolate sirup	1.4	2 tbsp	80	tr	tr	22	6	0.6	. . .	. . .	. . .	. . .
Chop suey, cooked	4.3	¾ cup	325	19	20	16	43	2.9	85	0.11	0.13	17
Clams, can'd	3.0	½ scant cup or 3 med clams	45	7	1	2	74	5.4	70	0.04	0.08	. . .
Cocoa, beverage	6.4	¾ cup, made with milk	175	7	8	20	215	0.7	293	0.07	0.34	2
Cocoa, dry	0.25	1 tbsp, powder	21	1	1	3	9	0.8	tr	0.01	0.03	0
Coconut, dried	0.6	¼ cup, shredded, sweetened	86	1	6	8	3	0.4	0	0.01	0.01	0
Coconut, fresh	0.8	¼ cup, shredded	83	1	8	3	4	0.4	. . .	0.02	0.01	1
Codfish, dried	1.8	½ cup	190	41	2	0	25	1.8	0	0.04	0.23	0
Coffee cake	2.8	1 piece, frosted, 3 x 3 x 1¼ in.	260	4	11	37	25	1.0	477	0.12	0.13	0
Cole slaw	2.1	½ cup	50	1	4	5	24	0.3	40	0.03	0.03	25
Collards (see Greens)												
Cookies												
Brownies	0.9	1 piece, 1⅞ x 1⅞ x ⅝ in.	145	2	9	17	12	0.5	231	0.03	0.04	. . .
Chocolate chip	0.4	1 cookie, 2¼ in. dia	60	1	3	7	4	0.2	81	0.01	0.01	. . .
Coconut bar chews	0.4	1 cookie, 3 x ⅞ x ⅓ in.	55	tr	2	9	7	0.3	76	0.01	0.01	0
Oatmeal cookies	0.4	1 cookie, 2⅛ in. dia (raisins and nuts)	65	1	4	6	5	0.3	18	0.04	0.02	tr

Food	Weight oz	Approximate Measure and Description	Calories	Protein g	Fat g	Carbohydrate g	Calcium mg	Iron mg	Vit. A Value IU	Thiamine mg	Riboflavin mg	Asc. acid mg
Plain and assorted	0.9	1 cookie, 3 in. dia	110	2	3	19	6	0.2	0	0.01	0.01	0
Sugar cookies	0.3	1 cookie, 2½ in. dia	40	1	2	6	2	0.1	64	0.02	0.01	0
Corn, ears, cooked	4.9	1 ear sweetcorn, 5 in. long	65	2	1	16	4	0.5	300 (yellow corn)	0.09	0.08	6
Corn, sweet, can'd	4.5	½ cup, solids and liquid	85	3	1	21	5	0.7	260 (yellow corn)	0.04	0.07	7
Corned beef (see Beef)												
Corned beef hash (see Beef)												
Corn bread or muffin	1.7	1 muffin, 2¾ in. dia (enrch'd, degermed cornmeal)	155	4	5	22	79	0.9	240 (yellow corn)	0.10	0.15	tr
Cornflakes	1.0	1⅓ cup (added thiamine, niacin, and iron)	110	2	tr	24	3	0.5	0	0.12	0.03	0
Corn grits, cooked	5.6	⅔ cup, white (enrch'd degermed)	80	2	tr	18	1	0.5	tr	0.07	0.05	0
Corn meal, dry	5.0	1 cup, white or yellow (enrch'd, degermed)	525	11	2	114	9	4.2	430 (yellow corn)	0.64	0.38	0
Cow peas (see Peas)												
Crabmeat, cooked	3.0	½ cup flakes	90	14	2	1	38	0.8	...	0.04	0.05	...
Crackers, graham	0.3	1 cracker, 2½ in. square	30	1	1	5	2	0.2	0	0.02	0.01	...
Crackers, saltines	0.3	2 saltines, 2 in. square	35	1	1	6	2	0.1	0	tr	tr	0
Crackers, soda	0.2	1 cracker, 2½ in. square	25	1	1	4	1	tr	0	tr	tr	0
Cracker meal	0.4	1 tbsp	45	1	1	7	2	0.1	0	0.01	tr	0
Cranberry sauce, cooked	2.4	¼ cup, sweetened	140	tr	tr	36	6	0.2	20	0.02	0.02	1
Cream, half and half	0.5	1 tbsp (milk and cream)	20	tr	2	1	16	0	70	0	0.02	tr
Cream, heavy, whipping	0.5	1 tbsp unwhipped	55	tr	6	tr	10	0	240	0	0.02	tr
Cream, light coffee	0.5	1 tbsp	35	tr	3	1	15	0	130	0	0.02	tr
Cucumbers, raw	1.8	6 sl., pared, ⅛ in. thick	5	tr	tr	1	5	0.2	0	0.02	0.02	4
Custard, bkd.	4.3	½ cup	140	7	7	14	140	0.5	435	0.05	0.24	1
Dates, fresh or dried	1.6	¼ cup or 8 pitted dates	125	1	tr	34	26	1.4	25	0.04	0.04	0
Dessert topping, whipped	0.4	2 tbsp (low calorie, with nonfat dry milk)	17	1	...	3	29	...	1	0.01	0.04	1

Doughnuts	1.1	1 doughnut, cake type	135	2	7	17	23	0.4	40	0.05	0.04	0
Egg, raw, boiled, poached	1.8	1 whole egg	80	6	6	tr	27	1.1	590	0.05	0.15	0
Egg white, raw	1.2	1 egg white	15	4	tr	tr	3	tr	0	tr	0.09	0
Egg yolk, raw	0.6	1 egg yolk	60	3	5	tr	24	0.9	580	0.04	0.07	0
Egg, creamed	4.0	½ cup (1 egg in ¼ cup white sauce)	190	9	14	7	103	1.2	928	0.07	0.25	tr
Egg, fried	1.9	1 egg, cooked in 1 tsp fat	115	6	10	tr	28	1.1	590	0.05	0.15	0
Egg, scrambled	2.2	1 egg, with milk and fat	110	7	8	1	51	1.1	690	0.05	0.18	0
Escarole, raw	2.0	3 leaves	10	1	tr	2	45	1.0	1700	0.04	0.07	6
Farina, cooked	5.6	⅔ cup (enrch'd with iron, thiamine, riboflavin, niacin, calcium)	70	2	tr	15	21	0.5	0	0.07	0.05	0
Fats, cooking, vegetable	0.4	1 tbsp solid fat	110	0	12	0	0	0	0	0	0	0
Figs, dried	0.7	1 large fig, 2 x 1 in.	60	1	tr	15	40	0.7	20	0.02	0.02	0
Fish (see various kinds of fish)												
Fish, creamed‡	4.8	½ cup (tuna, salmon, other)	220	20	13	8	81	0.9	385	0.05	0.18	tr
Fishsticks, breaded, cooked	4.0	5 sticks, 3¾ x 1 x ½ in.	200	19	10	8	13	0.5	. . .	0.05	0.08	. . .
Frankfurter, cooked	1.8	1 frankfurter (hot dog)	155	6	14	1	3	0.8	. . .	0.08	0.10	. . .
French toast, fried	2.8	1 sl. (enrch'd bread)	180	6	12	14	78	1.0	568	0.09	0.17	tr
Fruit balls, raw	0.4	1 ball, 1 in. dia (dried apricots, dates, nuts)	45	1	1	8	10	0.4	285	0.02	0.02	tr
Fruit cocktail, can'd	4.5	½ cup, solids and liquid	100	1	1	25	12	0.5	180	0.02	0.02	3
Gelatin, dry pl.	0.4	1 tbsp	35	9	tr	0	0	0	0	0	0	0
Gelatin dessert, pl.	4.2	½ cup, ready to eat	80	2	tr	18	0	0	0	0	0	0
Gelatin dessert, with fruit	4.2	½ cup, ready to eat	85	2	tr	21	7	0.4	135	0.04	0.03	4
Gingerbread	1.9	1 piece, 2 x 2 x 2 in.	180	2	7	28	63	1.4	50	0.02	0.05	tr
Grapefruit, can'd	4.4	½ cup or 4 sections with 4 tbsp juice, sirup pack	80	1	tr	22	16	0.4	10	0.04	0.02	38
Grapefruit, white, raw	10.0	½ med, 4¼ in. dia	50	1	tr	14	21	0.5	10	0.05	0.02	50
Grapefruit juice, can'd	4.3	½ cup, unsweetened	50	1	tr	12	10	0.5	10	0.04	0.02	42
Grapes, American type, raw	5.4	1 cup or 1 med bunch (slip skin)	70	1	1	16	13	0.4	100	0.05	0.03	4

Food	Weight oz	Approximate Measure and Description	Calories	Protein g	Fat g	Carbohydrate g	Calcium mg	Iron mg	Vit. A Value IU	Thiamine mg	Riboflavin mg	Asc. acid mg
Grapes, European type, raw	5.6	1 cup or 40 grapes	100	1	tr	26	18	0.6	150	0.08	0.04	7
Grapejuice, can'd	4.4	½ cup, sweetened	80	1	tr	21	14	0.4	. . .	0.05	0.03	tr
Greens, collards, cooked	3.3	½ cup	40	4	1	7	237	1.5	7250	0.08	0.23	42
Greens, dandelion, cooked	3.2	½ cup	40	3	1	8	169	2.8	13655	0.12	0.11	15
Greens, kale, cooked	1.9	½ cup	20	2	1	4	124	1.2	4610	0.04	0.13	28
Greens, mustard, cooked	2.5	½ cup	15	2	tr	3	154	2.1	5025	0.04	0.13	32
Greens, spinach, cooked	3.2	½ cup	20	3	1	3	112 (not usable)	1.8	10600	0.07	0.18	27
Greens, turnip, cooked	2.6	½ cup	20	2	1	4	188	1.8	7685	0.05	0.30	44
Guavas, raw	2.8	1 guava	50	1	tr	12	21	0.5	180	0.05	0.03	212
Haddock, fried	3.0	1 fillet, 4 x 2½ x ½ in.	135	16	5	6	15	0.5	50	0.03	0.08	. . .
Ham, smoked, cooked	3.0	2 sl., 5½ x 3¾ x ⅛ in.	290	18	24	1	8	2.2	0	0.39	0.15	. . .
Ham, luncheon meat, can'd	2.0	4 tbsp (spiced or unspiced)	165	8	14	1	5	1.2	0	0.18	0.12	. . .
Ham, luncheon meat, cooked	2.0	1 sl., 6¼ x 3¾ x ⅛ in.	170	13	13	0	5	1.5	0	0.57	0.15	. . .
Hamburger (see Beef)												
Honey, strained	0.7	1 tbsp	60	tr	0	17	1	0.2	0	tr	0.01	1
Ice, orange	4.7	½ cup	140	0	0	35	5	0.1	45	0.04	0.01	20
Ice cream, pl.	2.2	1 container, 3½ fluid oz, factory packed	130	2	8	13	76	0.1	320	0.03	0.12	1
Ice cream, pl., brick	2.5	1 sl., or cut (⅛ brick), factory packed	145	3	9	15	87	0.1	370	0.03	0.13	1
Ice cream, vanilla	3.5	1/6 qt scoop	200	4	12	21	117	0.12	720	0.04	0.34	0
Ice cream soda, chocolate	9.0	1 fountain-size serv.	255	3	8	46	75	0.7	297	0.03	0.13	1
Ice milk	3.3	½ cup	140	5	5	21	146	0.1	195	0.05	0.21	1
Jams, marmalades, preserves	0.7	1 tbsp	55	tr	tr	14	2	0.1	tr	tr	tr	1
Jellies	0.7	1 tbsp	50	0	0	13	2	0.1	tr	tr	tr	1

Kale (see Greens)													
Lamb chop, broiled	4.8	1 shoulder chop, 5 x 3½ x ½ in., fat trimmed with bone	405	25	33	0	10	3.1	. . .	0.14	0.25	. . .
Lamb, leg, roasted	3.0	2 sl., 3 x 3¼ x ⅛ in. lean and fat, no bone	235	22	16	0	9	2.8	. . .	0.13	0.23	. . .
Lard	0.5	1 tbsp	135	0	14	0	0	0	0	0	0	0
Lemon juice, fresh	0.5	1 tbsp	5	tr	tr	1	1	tr	tr	tr	tr	7
Lemonade	8.7	1 cup, ready to serve, (from concentrate, frozen, sweetened)	110	tr	tr	28	2	0.1	10	0.01	0.01	17
Lentils, dry, cooked	3.5	½ cup	120	9	tr	22	12	2.5	200	0.20	0.09	0
Lettuce, headed, raw	16.0	1 hd., compact, 4¾ in. dia	70	5	1	13	100	2.3	2470	0.20	0.38	35
Lettuce, headed, raw	1.8	2 large leaves or 4 small	5	1	tr	1	11	0.2	270	0.02	0.04	4
Liver, beef, fried	2.0	1 sl., 3½ x 3 x ½ in.	120	13	4	6	5	4.4	30330	0.15	2.25	18
Liver, calf, fried	2.6	1 sl., 5 x 2 x ⅓ in. (dredged in flour)	230	15	15	4	5	9.0	19130	0.18	2.65	30
Liver, chicken, fried	3.0	3 med. livers (dredged in flour)	235	20	15	5	15	6.4	27370	0.19	2.11	17
Liver, pork, fried	2.5	1 sl., 3¾ x 1¾ x ½ in. (dredged in flour)	225	17	15	3	8	15.3	12070	0.34	2.53	19
Macaroni, cooked	3.7	¾ cup (enrch'd)	115	4	1	24	8	1.0	0	0.14	0.08	0
Macaroni and cheese, bk'd	5.8	¾ cup (macaroni enrch'd)	350	14	19	33	296	1.5	728	0.17	0.35	tr
Mackerel, can'd	3.0	3/5 cup, solids and liquid	155	18	9	0	221	1.9	20	0.02	0.28	. . .
Mangoes, raw	7.0	1 med. mango	90	1	. . .	23	12	0.3	8380	0.08	0.07	55
Margarine	0.5	1 tbsp or 1 pat ½ in. thick (fortified with vit. A)	100	tr	11	tr	3	tr	460	. . .	. . .	0
Marshmallows	0.3	marshmallow, 1¼ in. dia	25	tr	0	6	0	0	0	0	0	0
Meat and bean stew, cooked	8.6	1 cup (Mexican dish)	345	17	16	34	90	4.6	1177	0.37	0.22	59
Meatloaf, beef, bak'd	2.7	1 sl., 3¾ x 2¼ x ¾ in.	240	19	17	3	34	2.9	138	0.10	0.21	. . .
Milk, dry skim (nonfat)	0.7	¼ cup powder	73	7	tr	11	260	0.1	5	0.07	0.36	2
Milk, evaporated, can'd	4.4	½ cup, undiluted, unsweetened	170	9	10	12	318	0.2	410	0.05	0.42	2

Food	Weight oz	Approximate Measure and Description	Calories	Protein g	Fat g	Carbohydrate g	Calcium mg	Iron mg	Vit. A Value IU	Thiamine mg	Riboflavin mg	Asc. acid mg
Milk, fluid, skim	8.6	1 cup (same as buttermilk)	90	9	tr	13	298	0.1	10	0.10	0.44	2
Milk, fluid, whole	8.5	1 cup	165	9	10	12	285	0.1	390	0.08	0.42	2
Milk, goat's, fluid, whole	8.5	1 cup	165	8	10	11	3.5	0.2	390	0.10	0.27	2
Milk, malted, pl., beverage	11.8	1 fountain-size glass	350	16	15	40	455	1.0	838	0.21	0.70	3
Milk, malted, pl., dry	0.4	1 tbsp (8 tablets)	40	1	1	6	28	0.2	92	0.03	0.05	0
Milkshake, chocolate	12.0	1 fountain-size glass	420	11	18	58	363	0.9	687	0.12	0.55	4
Molasses, cane, blackstrap	0.7	1 tbsp third extraction	45	...	...	11	116	2.3	...	0.02	0.04	...
Molasses, cane, light	0.7	1 tbsp first extraction	50	...	...	13	33	0.9	...	0.01	0.01	...
Muffins, pl.	1.7	1 muffin 2¾ in. dia (enrch'd white flour)	135	4	5	19	74	0.7	60	0.08	0.11	tr
Mushrooms, can'd	4.3	½ cup, solids and liquid	15	2	tr	5	9	1.0	0	0.02	0.30	...
Noodles, egg, cooked	4.2	¾ cup, enrch'd	150	5	2	28	12	1.1	45	0.17	0.11	0
Nuts, cashew, roasted	1.2	¼ cup	195	6	16	9	13	1.3	...	0.12	0.12	...
Nuts, peanuts, roasted	0.5	20 kernels, or about 2 tbsp	90	4	7	3	11	0.3	0	0.05	0.02	0
Nuts, pecan halves	0.5	10 med. halves	100	1	11	2	11	0.4	20	0.13	0.02	tr
Nuts, walnut halves	0.5	8 med. halves	100	2	10	2	15	0.5	5	0.05	0.02	tr
Oatmeal or rolled oats, cooked	5.5	⅔ cup, regular or quick cooking	100	3	2	17	14	1.1	0	0.15	0.03	0
Oils, salad or cooking	0.5	1 tbsp	125	0	14	0	0	0	...	0	0	0
Okra, cooked	1.5	4 pods, 3 x ⅝ in.	15	1	tr	3	35	0.3	315	0.03	0.03	9
Olives, green, pickled	0.8	4 extra large	22	tr	2	tr	16	0.3	57	tr	...	...
Olives, ripe	0.8	4 extra large	30	tr	3	1	15	0.3	13	tr	tr	...
Onions, cooked	3.7	½ cup or 5 onions 1¼ in. dia	40	1	tr	9	34	0.5	55	0.02	0.03	7
Onions, raw	3.9	1 onion, 2½ in. dia	50	2	tr	11	35	0.6	60	0.04	0.04	10
Onions, raw	0.4	1 tbsp chopped	5	tr	0	1	3	0	tr	tr	tr	1
Orange, raw	7.4	1 orange, 3 in. dia, med.	70	1	tr	18	63	0.3	290	0.12	0.03	66
Orange juice, can'd	4.4	½ cup or 1 small glass (unsweetened)	60	1	tr	14	13	0.5	250	0.09	0.03	50

Orange juice, fresh	4.3	½ cup or 1 small glass	60	1	tr	13	13	0.3	250	0.11	0.03	46
Orange juice, frozen	4.3	½ cup or 1 small glass (diluted ready to serve)	55	1	tr	14	11	0.1	250	0.11	0.02	56
Oyster stew	8.1	1 cup with 3–4 oysters	200	11	12	11	269	3.3	640	0.12	0.40	. . .
Oysters, raw	4.2	½ cup or 6–10 oysters	80	10	2	4	113	6.6	370	0.15	0.20	. . .
Pancakes, wheat	0.9	1 griddlecake, 4 in. dia (enrch'd flour)	60	2	2	8	34	0.3	30	0.05	0.06	tr
Papayas, raw	3.2	½ cup, in ½ in. cubes	35	1	tr	9	18	0.3	1595	0.04	0.04	51
Parsley, raw	0.12	1 tbsp chopped	1	tr	tr	tr	7	0.2	290	tr	0.01	7
Parsnips, cooked	2.7	½ cup	50	1	1	11	44	0.6	0	0.05	0.08	10
Peaches, can'd	4.1	2 med. halves with 2 tbsp juice, sirup pack	90	tr	tr	24	5	0.4	500	0.01	0.03	3
Peaches, raw	2.9	½ cup sl.	30	1	tr	8	8	0.4	1115 (yellow flesh)	0.02	0.04	6
Peaches, raw	4.0	1 med. 2½ in. dia	35	1	tr	10	9	0.5	1320 (yellow flesh)	0.02	0.05	7
Peanut butter	0.6	1 tbsp	90	4	8	3	12	0.4	0	0.02	0.02	0
Peanuts (see Nuts)												
Pears, can'd	4.1	2 med. halves with 2 tbsp juice, sirup pack	90	tr	tr	23	6	0.2	tr	0.01	0.02	2
Pears, raw	6.4	1 pear, 3 x 2½ in. dia	100	1	1	25	13	0.5	30	0.04	0.07	7
Peas, chick (see Chick peas, *garbanzos*)												
Peas, cowpeas, dry, cooked	4.3	½ cup (blackeye peas or frijoles)	95	7	1	17	21	1.6	10	0.21	0.06	tr
Peas, green, cooked	2.8	½ cup	55	4	1	10	18	1.5	575	0.20	0.11	12
Peas, pigeon, dry, raw	3.5	6 tbsp (gandules)	310	22	2	50	140	4.0	169	0.45	0.34	0
Peas, split, dry, cooked	4.4	½ cup	145	10	1	26	14	2.1	60	0.18	0.11	tr
Peppers, green, sweet, raw	0.7	¼ cup, diced	5	tr	tr	1	2	0.1	87	0.02	0.02	26
Peppers, green, stuffed, cooked	4.0	1 med. pepper (meat stuffing)	200	12	14	12	31	1.9	637	0.09	0.14	64
Peppers, red, sweet, raw	2.1	1 med. pod	20	1	tr	4	8	0.4	2670	0.05	0.05	122
Perch, ocean, fried	3.0	4 x 3 x ½ in.	195	16	11	6	14	1.3	50	0.09	0.10	. . .
Persimmon, raw	4.4	1 persimmon, 2½ in. dia (Japanese)	75	1	tr	20	6	0.4	2740	0.03	0.02	11

Food	Weight oz	Approximate Measure and Description	Calories	Protein g	Fat g	Carbohydrate g	Calcium mg	Iron mg	Vit. A Value IU	Thiamine mg	Riboflavin mg	Asc. acid mg
Pickle relish	0.4	1 tbsp	15	tr	tr	3	2	0.2	10	0	tr	1
Pickles, cucumber, bread and butter	1.5	6 sl., ¼ x 1½ in. dia	30	tr	tr	7	13	0.8	80	0.01	0.02	4
Pickles, cucumber, dill	4.7	1 large pickle, 4 x 1¾ in. dia	15	1	tr	3	34	1.6	420	tr	0.09	8
Pickles, cucumber, sweet	0.7	1 pickle, 2¾ x ¾ in. dia	20	tr	tr	5	3	0.3	20	0	tr	1
Pie, apple	4.7	4-in. sector or 1/7 of pie 9 in. in dia	330	3	13	53	9	0.5	220	0.04	0.02	1
Pie, cherry	4.7	4-in. sector or 1/7 of pie 9 in. in dia	340	3	13	55	14	0.5	520	0.04	0.02	2
Pie, custard	4.6	4-in. sector or 1/7 of pie 9 in. in dia	265	7	11	34	162	1.6	290	0.07	0.21	0
Pie, lemon meringue	4.2	4-in. sector or 1/7 of pie 9 in. in dia	300	4	12	45	24	0.6	210	0.04	0.10	1
Pie, mince	4.7	4-in. sector or 1/7 of pie 9 in. in dia	340	3	9	62	22	3.0	10	0.09	0.05	1
Pie, pumpkin	4.6	4-in. sector or 1/7 of pie 9 in. in dia	265	5	12	34	70	1.0	2480	0.04	0.15	0
Pimientos, can'd	1.3	1 med. pod (sweet pepper)	10	tr	tr	2	3	0.6	870	0.01	0.02	36
Pineapple, can'd	4.3	1 large or 2 small sl., 2 tbsp juice, sirup pack	95	tr	tr	26	35	0.7	100	0.09	0.02	11
Pineapple, raw	2.5	½ cup, diced, unsweetened	35	1	tr	10	11	0.2	90	0.06	0.02	17
Pineapple juice, can'd	4.4	½ cup or 1 small glass	60	1	tr	16	19	0.6	100	0.07	0.02	11
Pizza pie (cheese)	2.6	5½ in. sector or ⅛ of pie 14 in. in dia	180	8	6	23	157	0.7	570	0.03	0.09	8
Plantain, green, raw	3.5	1 baking banana, 6 in. long	135	1	...	32	8	.08	380	0.07	0.04	28
Plums, can'd	4.3	½ cup or 3 plums with 2 tbsp juice, sirup pack	90	tr	tr	25	10	1.3	280	0.03	0.03	1
Plums, raw	2.1	1 plum, 2 in. dia	30	tr	tr	7	10	0.3	200	0.04	0.02	3
Popcorn, popped, buttered	0.5	1 cup	90	2	5	11	2	0.4	153	0.05	0.02	0

Pork, chop, cooked	3.4	1 chop, with bone	260	16	21	0	8	2.2	0	0.63	0.18	. . .
Pork, roast, cooked	3.0	2 sl., 5 x 4 x ⅛ in.	310	21	24	0	9	2.7	0	0.78	0.22	. . .
Potato, white, bk'd	3.4	1 med. 2½ in. dia	90	3	tr	21	9	0.7	tr	0.10	0.04	20
Potatoes, French fried	2.0	10 pieces, 3 x ½ x ¼ in.	155	2	7	20	9	0.7	tr	0.06	0.04	8
Potatoes, mashed	3.4	½ cup (milk added)	70	2	1	15	24	0.5	25	0.09	0.06	9
Potatoes, mashed	3.4	½ cup (milk and butter added)	115	2	6	14	23	0.5	235	0.08	0.05	8
Potato chips	0.7	10 med. chips, 2 in. dia	110	1	7	10	6	0.4	tr	0.04	0.02	2
Poultry potpie	7.9	1 individual pie, 4¼ in. dia (chicken or turkey)	485	17	28	39	41	1.6	1860	0.07	0.14	tr
Pretzels	0.2	5 small sticks	20	tr	tr	4	1	0	0	tr	tr	0
Prune juice, can'd	4.2	½ cup or small glass	85	1	tr	23	17	4.9	. . .	tr	0.02	2
Prunes, dried, cooked	3.7	5 med. prunes with 2 tbsp juice sweetened	160	1	tr	42	21	1.5	733	0.03	0.06	1
Pudding, chocolate	4.6	½ cup (chocolate blanc-mange)	190	6	8	26	158	0.9	211	0.06	0.27	1
Pudding, cornstarch	4.3	½ cup (plain blancmange)	140	5	5	20	145	0.1	195	0.04	0.20	1
Pudding, rice with raisins	4.8	½ cup (old-fashioned)	300	8	8	52	243	0.8	313	0.10	0.35	3
Pudding, tapioca	2.6	½ cup	140	5	5	12	104	0.4	327	0.04	0.19	1
Radishes, raw	1.4	4 small, without tops	10	tr	tr	2	15	0.4	10	0.01	0.01	10
Raisins, dried	0.4	1 tbsp	30	tr	tr	8	6	0.4	2	0.01	0.01	tr
Raspberries, red, raw	2.2	½ cup	35	1	1	9	14	0.6	80	0.02	0.05	16
Rhubarb, cooked	4.8	½ cup (sugar added)	190	1	tr	49	56 (not usable)	0.6	35	0.01	. . .	9
Rice, parboiled, cooked	4.6	¾ cup	150	3	tr	34	11	0.4	0	0.08	0.02	0
Rice, puffed	0.5	1 cup (added thiamine, niacin, and iron)	55	1	tr	12	2	0.3	. . .	0.06	0.01	0
Rice flakes	1.1	1 cup (added thiamine, niacin, and iron)	115	2	tr	26	9	0.5	. . .	0.11	0.01	0
Roll, barbecue bun	1.3	1 bun, 3½ in. dia (enrch'd)	115	3	2	20	28	0.7	tr	0.11	0.07	tr
Roll, hard, white	1.8	1 round roll	160	5	2	31	24	0.4	tr	0.03	0.05	tr
Roll, soft, white	1.3	1 roll (enrch'd)	115	3	2	20	28	0.7	tr	0.11	0.07	tr
Roll, sweet, pan	1.5	1 roll	135	4	4	21	37	0.3	30	0.03	0.06	0
Rutabagas, cooked	2.7	½ cup	25	1	tr	6	43	0.3	270	0.04	0.06	18

Food	Weight oz	Approximate Measure and Description	Calories	Protein g	Fat g	Carbohydrate g	Calcium mg	Iron mg	Vit. A Value IU	Thiamine mg	Riboflavin mg	Asc. acid mg
Salads§												
Salad, chicken	4.4	½ cup, with mayonnaise	280	25	19	1	20	1.7	200	0.04	0.15	1
Salad, egg	4.5	½ cup, with mayonnaise	190	6	18	1	35	1.3	630	0.06	0.16	1
Salad, fresh fruit	4.4	½ cup with French dressing (orange, apple, banana, grapes)	130	...	6	21	25	0.6	154	0.06	0.05	22
Salad, jellied, vegetable	4.3	½ cup, no dressing	70	3	...	16	14	0.2	25	0.03	0.02	20
Salad, lettuce	4.6	¼ solid hd., with French dressing	80	1	6	5	28	0.7	618	0.05	0.10	9
Salad, potato	4.9	½ cup with mayonnaise	185	2	12	17	21	0.8	40	0.11	0.05	17
Salad, tomato aspic	4.2	½ cup, no dressing	45	5	0	7	12	0.5	1441	0.07	0.05	22
Salad, tuna fish	3.6	½ cup, with mayonnaise	250	21	18	1	14	1.2	98	0.04	0.09	1
Salad dressing, blue cheese	0.6	1 tbsp	90	1	10	1	11	tr	30	tr	0.02	tr
Salad dressing, boiled	0.6	1 tbsp (homemade)	30	1	2	3	15	0.1	80	0.01	0.03	tr
Salad dressing, commercial	0.5	1 tbsp (plain, mayonnaise type)	60	tr	6	2	2	tr	30	tr	tr	0
Salad dressing, cottage cheese	0.9	2 tbsp (low calorie, no oil, nonfat dry milk)	17	2	0	2	31	0	18	0.01	0.06	1
Salad dressing, French	0.5	1 tbsp	60	tr	6	2	3	0.1	0	0	0	0
Salad dressing, mayonnaise	0.5	1 tbsp	110	tr	12	tr	2	0.1	40	tr	tr	0
Salad dressing, Thousand Island	0.5	1 tbsp	75	tr	8	1	2	0.1	60	tr	tr	2
Salmon, boiled or bk'd	4.2	1 steak, 4 x 3 x ½ in.	200	34	7	tr	...	1.4	...	0.12	0.33	...
Salmon, can'd	3.0	½ cup, pink salmon	120	17	5	0	159 (includes bones)	0.7	60 (pink)	0.03	0.16	...
Salmon loaf	4.0	½ cup or 1 sl., 4 x 1¼ x 1¼ in.	235	29	10	5	43	1.8	332	0.08	0.20	2
Sandwiches‖												
Sardines, can'd	2.0	5 pieces, 3 x 1 x ¼ in. (can'd in oil)	120	15	6	1	245	1.7	127	0.01	0.12	...
Sauce, chocolate	1.4	2 tbsp	75	1	4	9	32	0.2	87	0.01	0.05	...

Sauce, custard	1.1	2 tbsp (low calorie, with nonfat dry milk)	45	2	1	7	56	0.17	89	0.02	0.09	...
Sauce, hard	0.6	1 tbsp	90	...	6	11	1	0	231	0	0	0
Sauce, hollandaise (mock)	0.9	2 tbsp	75	2	7	3	36	0.2	353	0.02	0.06	1
Sauce, lemon	1.0	2 tbsp	40	0	1	8	...	...	34	...	...	2
Sauerkraut, can'd	2.6	½ cup, drained solids	15	1	tr	4	27	0.4	30	0.03	0.05	12
Sausage, bologna	2.0	3 sl., 3¼ in. dia 1/10 in. thick	170	7	16	1	4	1.0	...	0.09	0.12	...
Sausage, frankfurters (see Frankfurters)												
Sausage, liverwurst	2.0	3 sl., 2½ in. dia, ¼ in. thick	150	10	12	1	5	3.1	3260	0.10	0.63	0
Sausage, pork, bulk, can'd	2.0	3 small patties, 2 in. dia, ¼ in. thick	170	9	15	0	5	1.3	0	0.12	0.14	...
Sausage, salami	1.1	1 sl., 4½ in. dia, ⅛ in. thick	135	7	11	0	5	1.1	0	0.16	0.15	0
Sausage, Vienna, can'd	2.0	3 sausages, 2 in. long, ¾ in. dia	125	9	9	0	5	1.4	0	0.06	0.07	0
Shad, bk'd	3.0	1 piece, 4 x 3 x ½ in.	170	20	10	0	20	0.5	20	0.11	0.22	...
Sherbet	3.4	½ cup, factory packed	120	2	tr	29	48	0.05	0	0.02	0.08	0
Shrimp, can'd	3.0	½ cup, meat only	110	23	1	...	98	2.6	50	0.01	0.03	...
Sirup	0.7	1 tbsp, table blends	55	0	0	15	9	0.8	0	0	tr	0
Soup, bean, can'd	8.8	1 cup, ready-to-serve	190	8	5	30	95	2.8	...	0.10	0.10	...
Soup, chicken noodle, can'd	6.7	4/5 cup or ⅓ can, ready-to-serve	70	2	4	6	16	0.2	...	...	...	...
Soup, clam chowder, can'd	8.9	1 cup, ready-to-serve	85	5	2	12	36	3.6	...	...	...	...
Soup, consomme, broth, can'd	8.4	1 cup, ready-to-serve	10	2	...	0	2	1.0	0	0	0.05	0
Soup, cream, vegetable, can'd	8.9	1 cup, ready-to-serve (asparagus, celery, or mushroom)	200	7	12	18	217	0.5	200	0.05	0.20	0
Soup, minestrone	8.5	1 cup (homemade)	130	6	5	16	59	2.5	5177	0.13	0.15	31
Soup, tomato, can'd	8.6	1 cup, ready-to-serve	90	2	2	18	24	1.0	1230	0.02	0.10	10
Soup, vegetable, can'd	8.8	1 cup, ready-to-serve	80	4	2	14	32	0.8	...	0.05	0.08	8
Spaghetti, cooked	3.7	¾ cup, enrch'd	115	4	1	24	8	1.0	0	0.14	0.08	0
Spaghetti with meat sauce	6.6	¾ cup	215	10	8	26	19	1.5	518	0.05	0.08	10

Food	Weight oz	Approximate Measure and Description	Calories	Protein g	Fat g	Carbohydrate g	Calcium mg	Iron mg	Vit. A Value IU	Thiamine mg	Riboflavin mg	Asc. acid mg
Spaghetti with tomato sauce	6.6	¾ cup (with cheese)	160	5	4	27	34	0.8	623	0.05	0.06	11
Spinach (see Greens)												
Squash, summer, cooked	3.7	½ cup, diced	20	1	tr	4	16	0.4	275	0.04	0.08	12
Squash, winter, bk'd	3.6	½ cup, mashed	50	2	1	12	25	0.8	6345	0.05	0.16	7
Stew, beef and vegetable	6.2	¾ cup	140	11	8	11	23	2.1	1898	0.10	0.14	11
Strawberries, raw	2.6	½ cup, capped	30	1	1	7	16	0.8	45	0.02	0.05	44
Sugar, brown	0.5	1 tbsp (dark brown, firmly packed)	50	0	0	13	10	0.4	0	0	0	0
Sugar, granulated	0.4	1 tbsp (beet or cane)	50	0	0	12	...	...	0	0	0	0
Sugar, powdered	0.3	1 tbsp	30	0	0	8	...	...	0	0	0	0
Sugar, loaf	0.3	1 loaf (domino) 1⅛ x ¾ x ⅜ in.	25	0	0	7	...	...	0	0	0	0
Sweet potatoes, bk'd	3.9	1 med. potato, 5 x 2 in., peeled	155	2	1	36	44	1.0	8970	0.10	0.07	24
Sweet potatoes, candied	3.1	½ potato, 3½ x 2¼ in.	150	1	3	30	33	0.8	5515	0.05	0.04	9
Tangerine, raw	4.0	1 med., 2½ in. dia	40	1	tr	10	34	0.3	360	0.05	0.01	26
Toast, melba	0.2	1 sl., 3¾ x 1¾ in.	20	1	tr	3.9	5	0.1	0	0.01	0.01	0
Tomato, raw	5.3	1 med., 2 x 2½ in. dia	30	2	tr	6	16	0.9	1640	0.08	0.06	35
Tomatoes, can'd	4.2	½ cup	25	1	tr	5	14	0.8	1270	0.07	0.04	20
Tomato catsup	0.6	1 tbsp	15	tr	tr	4	2	0.1	320	0.02	0.01	2
Tomato juice, can'd	4.2	½ cup or 1 small glass	25	1	tr	5	9	0.5	1270	0.06	0.04	19
Tongue (see Beef)												
Tortillas	0.7	1 tortilla, 5 in. dia	50	1	1	10	22	0.4	40 (yellow corn)	0.04	0.01	...
Tuna, can'd	3.0	½ cup, drained solids	170	25	7	0	7	1.2	70	0.04	0.10	...
Tuna salad (see Salad)												
Turnip greens (see Greens)												
Turnips, cooked	2.7	½ cup	20	1	tr	5	31	0.4	tr	0.03	0.05	14
Veal, roast, cooked	3.0	2 sl., 3 x 2½ x ¼ in. (medium fat)	305	23	14	0	10	2.9	...	0.11	0.26	...

Veal cutlet, broiled	3.0	1 med. cutlet, 3¾ x 3 x ½ in. (without bone)	185	23	9	0	9	2.7	. . .	0.06	0.21	. . .
Veal cutlet, (breaded), cooked	4.8	2 sl., 2½ x 2½ x ¾ in. (wiener schnitzel)	315	26	21	5	37	4.2	295	0.22	0.41	. . .
Vinegar	0.5	1 tbsp	2	0	. . .	1	1	1.0	. . .	. . .	. . .	. . .
Waffles	2.6	1 waffle, 4½ x 5½ x ½ in. with enrch'd flour	240	8	9	30	124	1.4	310	0.14	0.21	tr
Watermelon, raw	32.4	1 wedge, 4 x 8 in. (with rind)	120	2	1	29	30	0.9	2530	0.20	0.22	26
Welsh rarebit	4.4	½ cup	330	19	26	6	534	0.7	1118	0.04	0.40	. . .
Wheat flakes	1.0	1 cup	100	3	tr	23	13	1.2	0	0.16	0.05	0
Wheat flour, white	3.9	1 cup, enrch'd flour	400	12	1	84	18	3.2	0	0.48	0.29	0
Wheat flour, white	3.9	1 cup, unenrch'd flour	400	12	1	84	18	0.9	0	0.07	0.05	0
Wheat flour, whole-wheat	4.2	1 cup	400	16	2	85	49	4.0	0	0.66	0.14	0
Wheat germ	0.3	2 tbsp	30	2	1	4	7	0.7	0	0.17	0.07	0
Wheat, rolled, cooked	5.5	⅔ cup	120	3	1	27	13	1.1	0	0.11	0.04	0
Wheat, shredded	1.0	1 large biscuit, 4 x 2¼ in.	100	3	1	23	13	1.0	0	0.06	0.03	0
White sauce (medium)	2.3	¼ cup	110	3	8	6	76	0.1	338	0.02	0.11	tr
Yeast, brewer's, dry	0.3	1 tbsp	25	3	tr	3	17	1.4	tr	1.25	0.34	tr
Yoghurt	8.6	1 cup, from partially skimmed milk	120	8	4	13	295	0.1	170	0.09	0.43	2

* See page 286 for calorie values of additional alcohol beverages.

† Vitamin A value varies with the kind of fat used in making cakes. Butter or fortified margarine used in cakes listed in this Appendix.

‡ One-half cup of a creamed dish calls for ¼ cup white sauce and about ⅓ cup of any one of a wide variety of meats, vegetables, or other foods which may be combined. (See Egg, creamed and Fish, creamed.)

§ Only a few common types of salad are listed here. The calorie and nutritive values of any combination of foods in a salad are easily estimated. The ½ cup servings of salad in this table, using mayonnaise, were made with ⅓ cup of the main ingredient, such as chicken, plus 2 tbsp of a crisp vegetable, such as celery, plus 1 tbsp of mayonnaise. One tbsp of French dressing was used in the fruit and lettuce salads. The total calorie yield of a salad may vary greatly, depending on the kind and the amount of salad dressing added.

‖ Sandwiches, as such, are not included in this list, but the "makings" are available for any type desired. For example, a simple sandwich might consist of 2 slices of enriched bread, 2 tsp butter, 1 slice salami sausage, 1 tsp mayonnaise, plus 2 leaves of lettuce. The sum of the calories and of the nutrients gives the total contribution of the sandwich. For salad sandwiches, the procedure is essentially the same. Chicken, egg, or tuna salads, in the measures given in Appendix G, provide the amount of filling needed for a sandwich made with a large bun or 2 slices of bread.

ALCOHOLIC BEVERAGES

Beverage	Amount	Number of Calories
Beer (4 percent alcohol)	8-oz glass	115
Eggnog (holiday variety made with whiskey and rum)	½ cup	225
Whiskey, Gin, Rum		
100 proof	1 jigger (1½ oz)	125
90 proof	1 jigger (1½ oz)	110
86 proof	1 jigger (1½ oz)	105
80 proof	1 jigger (1½ oz)	100
70 proof	1 jigger (1½ oz)	85
Wines		
Table wines (such as Chablis, claret, Rhine wine and sauterne)	1 wine glass, about 3 oz	70–90
Sweet or dessert wines (such as muscatel, port, sherry or Tokay)	1 wine glass, about 3 oz	120–160

All values, except for Eggnog, from *Food and Your Weight*. Home and Garden Bulletin, No. 74. Washington, D.C. U.S. Department of Agriculture, 1960.

INDEX

INDEX[1]

[1] For practical considerations, the names of individual foods have, for the most part, been omitted from the Index. Some of these foods appear repeatedly in text and tables throughout the book. A complete, alphabetical list of such foods, with their nutritive values, appears in Appendix G, pp. 267-286.